METHODS IN MOLECULAR BIOLOGY™

Series Editor
**John M. Walker
School of Life Sciences
University of Hertfordshire
Hatfield, Hertfordshire, AL10 9AB, UK**

For further volumes:
http://www.springer.com/series/7651

Kinase Inhibitors

Methods and Protocols

Edited by

Bernhard Kuster

*LS für Proteomik und Bioanalytik, Technische Universität München,
Freising, Germany*

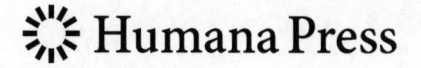

💥 Humana Press

Editor
Bernhard Kuster
LS für Proteomik und Bioanalytik
Technische Universität München
Emil Erlenmeyer Forum 5
85354 Freising
Germany
kuster@tum.de

ISSN 1064-3745   e-ISSN 1940-6029
ISBN 978-1-61779-336-3   e-ISBN 978-1-61779-337-0
DOI 10.1007/978-1-61779-337-0
Springer New York Dordrecht Heidelberg London

Library of Congress Control Number: 2011936748

© Springer Science+Business Media, LLC 2012
All rights reserved. This work may not be translated or copied in whole or in part without the written permission of the publisher (Humana Press, c/o Springer Science+Business Media, LLC, 233 Spring Street, New York, NY 10013, USA), except for brief excerpts in connection with reviews or scholarly analysis. Use in connection with any form of information storage and retrieval, electronic adaptation, computer software, or by similar or dissimilar methodology now known or hereafter developed is forbidden.
The use in this publication of trade names, trademarks, service marks, and similar terms, even if they are not identified as such, is not to be taken as an expression of opinion as to whether or not they are subject to proprietary rights.

Printed on acid-free paper

Humana Press is part of Springer Science+Business Media (www.springer.com)

Preface

Protein and lipid kinases are often the master regulators of cell signaling in eukaryotic systems. The human genome codes for more than 500 of these enzymes and their misregulation has been shown to be involved in the onset and progression of many diseases including cancer and inflammation. Therefore, small molecule kinase inhibitors have become important research tools for the elucidation of many biological roles of kinases and their mechanisms of action. In addition, kinase inhibitors are now successful drugs in a number of liquid and solid tumors. In fact, about one dozen molecules are currently approved for clinical use and 200 more molecules are in different stages of clinical evaluation. Kinase inhibitors thus contribute significantly to the drug pipelines of pharmaceutical and biotechnology industries and to the growing need for the treatment of cancer and inflammation.

There are many challenges in the discovery and development of kinase inhibitors both for research and clinical use and thus, many methods are being devised and applied to understand the often complex functional relationships between kinases and the respective inhibitors. In this book, experts in kinase biology, drug discovery, and clinical research present a series of exemplary methods that can be used to address these challenges.

To set the scene, two introductory reviews discuss how kinase inhibitors can be used to target cancer and inflammation. The themes covered span a wide range of topics from the structural basis of kinase inhibition, to mechanistic aspects, resistance formation, and animal models. The following three chapters present biochemical kinase activity assays for protein and lipid kinases. These include the classical recombinant enzyme assays which today still are workhorses in the evaluation of kinase inhibitor potency and selectivity. However, the discovery of novel kinase inhibitors increasingly attempts to target protein domains that are distinct from the kinase domain and its ATP pocket. The rational for these approaches is to provide better selectivity of the inhibitors because they might better reflect the actual mechanisms of action of kinase activation and deactivation.

Two major and often related issues in the development of kinase inhibitors as drugs or research tools are their selectivity and toxicity which is why six chapters of this book are devoted to these topics. Apart from issues such as hepatotoxicity, which is a major problem in all areas of drug development, the structural conservation of kinase domains in general and ATP binding sites in particular pose a number of extra challenges as many small molecules have the propensity to inhibit many kinases. In cancer therapy, this may sometimes be advantageous because many cancers represent a molecularly heterogeneous group of diseases. However, multikinase inhibition may also lead to toxicity which may prevent the use of these agents particularly in chronic applications. Classically, selectivity profiling is performed using large panels of recombinant kinase assays. More recently, proteomic approaches are being followed as they provide a means to study inhibitor selectivity in cells or tissues, which is thought to represent a more realistic biological assay context than individual kinases tested in the absence of other cellular components.

Kinase inhibitors may impact a biological system very specifically or rather broadly. The full appreciation of the potential of a kinase inhibitor should therefore include an evaluation of its impact at the level of individual signaling pathways, cellular model systems, or the entire biological system. As examples, the last five chapters in this book describe methods that identify individual kinase–substrate relationships, measure the phosphorylation status of proteins in response to kinase inhibitor treatment, and identify resistance mechanisms by which many tumors eventually escape therapeutic intervention.

It is obviously beyond the scope of this book to cover the field of kinase inhibitors in its entirety. However, the individual chapters aim to provide modern and relevant exemplary methods that scientists may implement in their laboratories to accelerate or strengthen their research and drug discovery programs.

Freising, Germany   *Bernhard Kuster*

Contents

Preface... *v*
Contributors... *ix*

1. Targeting Cancer with Small-Molecular-Weight Kinase Inhibitors... 1
   Doriano Fabbro, Sandra W. Cowan-Jacob, Henrik Möbitz, and Georg Martiny-Baron

2. Small-Molecule Protein and Lipid Kinase Inhibitors in Inflammation and Specific Models for Their Evaluation... 35
   Matthias Gaestel and Alexey Kotlyarov

3. Measuring the Activity of Leucine-Rich Repeat Kinase 2: A Kinase Involved in Parkinson's Disease... 45
   Byoung Dae Lee, Xiaojie Li, Ted M. Dawson, and Valina L. Dawson

4. Measuring PI3K Lipid Kinase Activity... 55
   Elisa Ciraolo, Alessia Perino, and Emilio Hirsch

5. A Fluorescence Polarization Assay for the Discovery of Inhibitors of the Polo-Box Domain of Polo-Like Kinase 1... 69
   Wolfgang Reindl, Klaus Strebhardt, and Thorsten Berg

6. Assessment of Hepatotoxicity Potential of Drug Candidate Molecules Including Kinase Inhibitors by Hepatocyte Imaging Assay Technology and Bile Flux Imaging Assay Technology... 83
   Jinghai J. Xu, Margaret C. Dunn, Arthur R. Smith, and Eric S. Tien

7. Kinase Inhibitor Selectivity Profiling Using Differential Scanning Fluorimetry... 109
   Oleg Fedorov, Frank H. Niesen, and Stefan Knapp

8. Chemoproteomic Characterization of Protein Kinase Inhibitors Using Immobilized ATP... 119
   James S. Duncan, Timothy A.J. Haystead, and David W. Litchfield

9. Proteome-Wide Identification of Staurosporine-Binding Kinases Using Capture Compound Mass Spectrometry... 135
   Jenny J. Fischer, Olivia Y. Graebner (neé Baessler), and Mathias Dreger

10. Affinity Purification of Proteins Binding to Kinase Inhibitors Immobilized on Self-Assembling Monolayers... 149
    Marcus Bantscheff, Scott Hobson, and Bernhard Kuster

11. Kinase Inhibitor Profiling Using Chemoproteomics... 161
    Markus Schirle, Eugene C. Petrella, Scott M. Brittain, David Schwalb, Edmund Harrington, Ivan Cornella-Taracido, and John A. Tallarico

12. Covalent Cross-Linking of Kinases with Their Corresponding Peptide Substrates... 179
    Alexander V. Statsuk and Kevan M. Shokat

13 Receptor Tyrosine Kinase Inhibitor Profiling Using Bead-Based
    Multiplex Sandwich Immunoassays.. 191
    *Oliver Pötz, Nicole Schneiderhan-Marra, Tanja Henzler,
    Thomas Herget, and Thomas O. Joos*

14 Monitoring Phosphoproteomic Response to Targeted Kinase Inhibitors
    Using Reverse-Phase Protein Microarrays... 203
    Gabriela Lavezzari and Mark R. Lackner

15 Measuring Phosphorylation-Specific Changes in Response to Kinase Inhibitors
    in Mammalian Cells Using Quantitative Proteomics................................. 217
    Nurhan Özlü, Marc Kirchner, and Judith Jebanathirajah Steen

16 Investigation of Acquired Resistance to EGFR-Targeted Therapies
    in Lung Cancer Using cDNA Microarrays... 233
    Kian Kani, Rafaella Sordella, and Parag Mallick

Index.. 255

Contributors

Marcus Bantscheff • *Cellzome AG, Heidelberg, Germany*
Thorsten Berg • *University of Leipzig, Institute for Organic Chemistry, Leipzig, Germany*
Scott M. Brittain • *Novartis Institutes for Biomedical Research, Cambridge, MA, USA*
Elisa Ciraolo • *Department of Genetics, Biology and Biochemistry, Molecular Biotechnology Center, University of Torino, Torino, Italy*
Ivan Cornella-Taracido • *Novartis Institutes for Biomedical Research, Cambridge, MA, USA*
Sandra W. Cowan-Jacob • *Novartis Institutes for Biomedical Research, Structural Biology Platform, Basel, Switzerland*
Ted M. Dawson • *Department of Neurology, Neuroregeneration and Stem Cell Program, Institute for Cell Engineering, Johns Hopkins University School of Medicine, Baltimore, MA, USA; Solomon H. Snyder Department of Neuroscience, Neuroregeneration and Stem Cell Program, Institute for Cell Engineering, Johns Hopkins University School of Medicine, Baltimore, MA, USA*
Valina L. Dawson • *Department of Neurology, Neuroregeneration and Stem Cell Program, Institute for Cell Engineering, Baltimore, MA, USA; Solomon H. Snyder Department of Neuroscience, Neuroregeneration and Stem Cell Program, Institute for Cell Engineering, Baltimore, MA, USA; Department of Physiology, Johns Hopkins University School of Medicine, Baltimore, MA, USA*
Mathias Dreger • *caprotec bioanalytics GmbH, Berlin, Germany*
James S. Duncan • *Department of Biochemistry, Schulich School of Medicine & Dentistry, University of Western Ontario, London, ON, Canada; Department of Pharmacology, University of North Carolina, School of Medicine, Chapel Hill, NC, USA*
Margaret C. Dunn • *Pfizer Research Technology Center, Cambridge, MA, USA*
Doriano Fabbro • *Novartis Institutes for Biomedical Research, Expertise Platform Kinases, Basel, Switzerland*
Oleg Fedorov • *Structural Genomics Consortium, Oxford University, Oxford, UK*
Jenny J. Fischer • *caprotec bioanalytics GmbH, Berlin, Germany*
Matthias Gaestel • *Hannover Medical School, Institute of Biochemistry, Hannover, Germany*
Olivia Y. Graebner (neé Baessler) • *caprotec bioanalytics GmbH, Berlin, Germany*
Edmund Harrington • *Novartis Institutes for Biomedical Research, Cambridge, MA, USA*
Timothy A.J. Haystead • *Department of Pharmacology & Cancer Biology, Duke University Medical Centre, Durham, NC, USA*

TANJA HENZLER • *Merck KGaA, Darmstadt, Germany*
THOMAS HERGET • *Merck KGaA, Darmstadt, Germany*
EMILIO HIRSCH • *Molecular Biotechnology Center, University of Torino, Torino, Italy*
SCOTT HOBSON • *Cellzome AG, Heidelberg, Germany; Department for CNS Research, Boehringer Ingelheim GmbH & Co KG, Biberach an der Riß, Germany*
THOMAS O. JOOS • *NMI Natural and Medical Sciences Institute at the University of Tuebingen, Reutlingen, Germany*
KIAN KANI • *University of Southern California, Los Angeles, CA, USA*
MARC KIRCHNER • *Department of Pathology, Children's Hospital Boston, John F. Enders Research Laboratories, Boston, MA, USA*
STEFAN KNAPP • *Structural Genomics Consortium, Oxford University, Oxford, UK*
ALEXEY KOTLYAROV • *Hannover Medical School, Institute of Biochemistry, Hannover, Germany*
BERNHARD KUSTER • *TU München LS für Proteomik, Freising, Germany*
MARK R. LACKNER • *Department of Development Oncology Diagnostics, Genentech Inc., South San Francisco, CA, USA*
GABRIELA LAVEZZARI • *Theranostics Health, Rockville, MA, USA*
BYOUNG DAE LEE • *Neuroregeneration and Stem Cell Programs, Institute for Cell Engineering, Johns Hopkins University School of Medicine, Baltimore, MD, USA*
XIAOJIE LI • *Cell and Molecular Medicine Graduate Training Program, Johns Hopkins University School of Medicine, Baltimore, MA, USA*
DAVID W. LITCHFIELD • *Department of Biochemistry, Schulich School of Medicine & Dentistry, University of Western Ontario, London, ON, Canada*
PARAG MALLICK • *University of Southern California, Los Angeles, CA, USA; Stanford University, Stanford, CA, USA*
GEORG MARTINY-BARON • *Novartis Institutes for Biomedical Research, Expertise Platform Kinases, Basel, Switzerland*
HENRIK MÖBITZ • *Novartis Institutes for Biomedical Research, Global Discovery Chermistry, Basel, Switzerland*
FRANK H. NIESEN • *Structural Genomics Consortium, Oxford University, Oxford, UK*
NURHAN ÖZLÜ • *Center for Life Science, F.M. Kirby Center for Neurobiology, Children's Hospital Boston, Istanbul, Turkey*
ALESSIA PERINO • *Department of Genetics, Biology and Biochemistry, Molecular Biotechnology Center, University of Torino, Torino, Italy*
EUGENE C. PETRELLA • *Novartis Institutes for Biomedical Research, Cambridge, MA, USA*
OLIVER PÖTZ • *NMI Natural and Medical Sciences Institute at the University of Tuebingen, Reutlingen, Germany*
WOLFGANG REINDL • *Department of Molecular Biology, and Center for Integrated Protein Science Munich (CIPSM), Max Planck Institute of Biochemistry, Martinsried, Germany*
MARKUS SCHIRLE • *Novartis Institutes for Biomedical Research, Cambridge, MA, USA*
NICOLE SCHNEIDERHAN-MARRA • *NMI Natural and Medical Sciences Institute at the University of Tuebingen, Reutlingen, Germany*

DAVID SCHWALB • *Novartis Institutes for Biomedical Research, Cambridge, MA, USA*
KEVAN M. SHOKAT • *Department of Cellular and Molecular Pharmacology, University of California San Francisco, San Francisco, CA, USA*
ARTHUR R. SMITH • *Pfizer Research Technology Center, Cambridge, MA, USA*
RAFAELLA SORDELLA • *Cold Spring Harbor Laboratory, Cold Spring Harbor, NY, USA*
ALEXANDER V. STATSUK • *Department of Chemistry, Northwestern University, Evanston, IL, USA*
JUDITH JEBANATHIRAJAH STEEN • *Center for Life Science, F.M. Kirby Center for Neurobiology, Children's Hospital Boston, Boston, MA, USA*
KLAUS STREBHARDT • *Department of Gynecology and Obstetrics, Johann Wolfgang Goethe-University, Medical School, Frankfurt, Germany*
JOHN A. TALLARICO • *Novartis Institutes for Biomedical Research, Cambridge, MA, USA*
ERIC S. TIEN • *Pfizer Research Technology Center, Cambridge, MA, USA*
JINGHAI J. XU • *Knowledge Discovery & Knowledge Management, Merck & Co., Inc., RY86-235, Rahway, NJ, USA*

Chapter 1

Targeting Cancer with Small-Molecular-Weight Kinase Inhibitors

Doriano Fabbro, Sandra W. Cowan-Jacob, Henrik Möbitz, and Georg Martiny-Baron

Abstract

Protein and lipid kinases fulfill essential roles in many signaling pathways that regulate normal cell functions. Deregulation of these kinase activities lead to a variety of pathologies ranging from cancer to inflammatory diseases, diabetes, infectious diseases, cardiovascular disorders, cell growth and survival. 518 protein kinases and about 20 lipid-modifying kinases are encoded by the human genome, and a much larger proportion of additional kinases are present in parasite, bacterial, fungal, and viral genomes that are susceptible to exploitation as drug targets. Since many human diseases result from overactivation of protein and lipid kinases due to mutations and/or overexpression, this enzyme class represents an important target for the pharmaceutical industry. Approximately one third of all protein targets under investigation in the pharmaceutical industry are protein or lipid kinases.

The kinase inhibitors that have been launched, thus far, are mainly in oncology indications and are directed against a handful of protein and lipid kinases. With one exception, all of these registered kinase inhibitors are directed toward the ATP-site and display different selectivities, potencies, and pharmacokinetic properties. At present, about 150 kinase-targeted drugs are in clinical development and many more in various stages of preclinical development. Kinase inhibitor drugs that are in clinical trials target all stages of signal transduction from the receptor protein tyrosine kinases that initiate intracellular signaling, through second-messenger-dependent lipid and protein kinases, and protein kinases that regulate the cell cycle. This review provides an insight into protein and lipid kinase drug discovery with respect to achievements, binding modes of inhibitors, and novel avenues for the generation of second-generation kinase inhibitors to treat cancers.

Key words: Kinase inhibitors, Cancer, CML, Oncogene, Small-molecular-weight compounds, Kinase inhibitor binding mode

Abbreviations

AML   Acute myeloid leukemia
B-ALL B-cell acute lymphoblastic leukemia
CEL   Chronic eosinophilic leukemia

CML	Chronic myeloid leukemia
CMML	Chronic myelomonocytic leukemia
RCC	Renal cell cancer
NSCLC	Non-small-cell lung cancer
GIST	Gastrointestinal stromal cancer
CSF1R	colony-stimulating factor 1 receptor
EGFR	Epidermal growth factor receptor
FLT3	FMS-related tyrosine kinase 3
GIST	Gastrointestinal stromal tumor
NSCLC	Non-small-cell lung cancer
PDGFR	Platelet-derived growth factor receptor
RCC	Renal cell carcinoma
Ph+	Philadelphia chromosome positive
VEGFR	Vascular endothelial growth factor receptor

1. Introduction

Protein and lipid kinases represent, after GPCRs and proteases, one of the most important target classes for treating human disorders. In fact, one third of the protein targets under investigation by pharmaceutical companies are protein or lipid kinases. Deregulation of the reversible phosphorylation that governs cellular processes leads to the development of a number of malignant pathological disorders (1–7). Many human malignancies are associated with activated protein or lipid kinases or inactivated phosphatases due to mutations, chromosomal rearrangements, and/or gene amplification (1, 8–11). Approximately 50 of the 100 known genes that have been directly linked to the induction and maintenance of cancer encode protein kinases (8, 12–15).

Given the role played by various protein and lipid kinases in cancer, it is not surprising that the majority of kinase inhibitors are being developed in life-threatening oncology indications, a therapeutic area in which there is a greater tolerance for side effects. All protein and lipid kinases share a conserved catalytic kinase domain. The kinase domain is a bilobal structure where the N-terminal lobe consists mainly of β-sheets and the C-terminal domain contains alpha helices (8, 12–17). The two lobes are connected by the so-called hinge region, which lines the ATP-binding site that is targeted by the majority of small-molecular-weight kinase inhibitors (8, 12–17). In the past decade, 11 of these small-molecule kinase inhibitors have been approved for clinical use (Table 1). These registered kinase inhibitors target only a few members of the kinome, including the tyrosine receptor kinases EGFR, ERBB2, VEGFRs, Kit, PDGFRs, the nonreceptor tyrosine kinases ABL and SRC, and only one Ser/Thr-specific kinase, the atypical protein kinase mTOR (Table 1). The commercial success of imatinib has

Table 1
Registered kinase inhibitors

Compound	Kinase target	Cancer target	Company
Imatinib (Glivec, Gleevec, STI571)	ABL 1–2, PDGFR, KIT	CML, Ph+ B-ALL, MML, CEL, GIST	Novartis
Gefitinib (Iressa, ZD1839)	EGFR	NSCLC	AstraZeneca
Erlotinib (Tarceva, OSI-774)	EGFR	NSCLC, pancreatic cancer	OSI, Genentech Inc, Roche
Lapatinib (Tykerb, GW2016)	EGFR, ERBB2	Breast cancer	Glaxo SmithKline
Dasatinib (Sprycel, BM-354825)	ABL1–2, PDGFR, KIT, SRC	CML	Bristol Myers
Nilotinib (Tasigna, AMN107)	ABL1–2, PDGFR, KIT	CML	Novartis
Sunitinib (Sutent, SU11248)	VEGFR1–3, KIT, PDGFR, RET, CSF1R, FLT3	RCC, GIST	Pfizer
Sorafenib (Nexavar, Bay 43-9006)	VEGFR2, PDGFR, KIT, FLT3, BRAF	RCC	Onyx and Bayer Pharmaceuticals
Pazopanib (Votrient, GW-786034)	VEGFR1–3, PDGFR, KIT,	RCC	GlaxoSmithKline
Everolimus (Afinitor, Rad001)	mTOR	RCC	Novartis
Temsirolimus (Torisel, CCI-779)	mTOR	RCC	Wyeth

attracted considerable interest and has triggered many efforts leading to the identification of broad-spectrum inhibitors of BCR-ABL1 and its imatinib-resistant mutants, while targets such as phosphoinositide-3 kinases (PI3Ks), mTOR, AKT, and cell-cycle regulating kinases are getting increasing attention (18–22).

The major challenge that kinase drug discovery for the treatment of cancer is currently facing is related to the molecular mechanisms underlying the various forms of cancer, and research is mainly geared to identify the following: the "addiction of tumors" to the target kinase (4, 5), the emerging resistance to kinase inhibition (23–25), the patients most likely to respond to a given kinase inhibitor treatment as well as the identification and validation of novel kinase targets for the treatment of cancer. Genome-wide screening for kinase mutations has revealed how the mutational status of the inherited variants of the various kinome members may be associated with increasing risk of various cancer conditions (8–10). Additional investigation of deregulated kinase activities in cancer by phosphoproteomics, analysis of gene amplifications/mutations will not only lead to the identification of new kinase targets but also allow a better prediction of drug responses in patients (1, 12, 13, 25, 26). The finding that protein kinases with a gain of function mutation appear to be either more sensitive or resistant to inhibition by kinase inhibitors compared to the wild type variant has opened new avenues to kinase drug discovery approaches (1, 23, 25, 27, 28). In addition, multiple clinical studies have revealed that various protein kinases escape resistance by either mutating key residues in their catalytic domains or by developing compensatory mechanisms allowing to bypass the kinase target by overexpression of alternative kinases or other oncogenes (3, 29–34). All of these issues have prompted the pharmaceutical industry and small biotech companies to come up with strategies that may allow them to override these various types of resistances including compounds capable of circumventing the target related drug resistance (35–40).

Another important area of kinase drug discovery is focused on understanding the selectivity profile of kinase inhibitors as well as of targeting kinases by novel approaches (41, 42). Although there is a continuous debate on how selective a kinase inhibitor needs to be when used in cancer indications, the development of kinase inhibitors with outstanding selectivity is likely to be important not only for minimizing side effects and allowing chronic treatment of non-life-threatening diseases but also to better understand the on- and off-target pharmacology of kinase inhibitors.

2. Current Status of Protein and Lipid Kinase Drug Discovery

2.1. Approved Protein Kinase Inhibitors for the Treatment of Cancer

To date, 11 small-molecular-weight kinase inhibitors have been launched for cancer indications (Table 1). These include imatinib (Glivec®, STI571, Novartis AG) (43), gefitinib (Iressa™, ZD1839. AstraZeneca Inc.) (44), erlotinib (Tarceva™, OSI-774, Genentech Inc.) (45, 46), Lapatinib (Tykerb®, GW2016, GlaxoSmithKline) (47), sorafenib (Nexavar®, Bay 43–9006, Onyx and Bayer Pharmaceuticals) (48), sunitinib (Sutent®, SU11248; Pfizer, Inc.) (49), dasatinib (SPRYCEL®, BM-354825, Bristol-Myers Squibb) (39), nilotinib (Tasigna®, AMN107, Novartis) (36), pazopanib (Votrient™, GW-786034, GlaxoSmithKline) (50), torisel (Temsirolimus®, CCI-779, Wyeth Pharmaceuticals) (51), and everolimus (Afinitor®, RAD001, Novartis AG) (52). Everolimus, an orally active and potent immunosuppressive agent that inhibits T cell proliferation (53), has been already approved as Certican® for the prophylaxis of organ rejection of heart and kidney (54).

This rapalog is to date the only kinase inhibitor that has been registered for nononcology indications. All other approved kinase drugs are active against more than one type of cancer where the pivotal registration trials are ongoing (55).

Imatinib, a phenyl-amino-pyrimidine derivative targeting the inactive conformation of the ABL1 kinase, was the first kinase inhibitor used in clinical trials for the treatment of chronic myelogenous leukemia (CML) (23, 56). The ABL1 kinase is constitutively activated in more than 95% of CML due to a chromosomal translocation leading to the Philadelphia (Ph) chromosome (43, 56). The success of imatinib in CML patients may be considered unique among cancers, as CML is caused by a single molecular abnormality and during its chronic phase can be regarded as a myeloproliferative disorder rather than leukemia (23, 57). Owing to its multitargeted nature, imatinib, has since then been approved for various other cancer indications including Ph+ALL (targeting ABL1) (57), gastrointestinal stromal tumors (GIST) (targeting mutant forms of KIT and PDGFR) (27, 58–61), recurrent and/or metastatic dermatofibrosarcoma protuberans (targeting PDGFR) (62), myelodysplastic and/or myeloproliferative diseases (targeting PDGFR, KIT, and/or ABL1) (57, 63), and hypereosinophilic syndrome (targeting PDGFR) (57). Imatinib has also been used in nononcology indications (targeting PDGFR) for the treatment of pulmonary arterial hypertension, a severe, incurable blood vessel disorder (64). Imatinib and other kinase inhibitors are known to generate target dependent resistance, in particular in advanced stages of GIST, CML, or non-small-cell lung cancer (NSCLC) (23, 24, 61). More potent drugs, such as nilotinib, another phenyl-amino-pyrimidine with a selectivity profile similar to imatinib or drugs with a binding mode different from imatinib, such as the amino-thiazole dasatinib, a potent BCR-ABL1 inhibitor with a broad selectivity spectrum, have been approved for imatinib-resistant CML (65).

The indolinone-derivative sunitinib, a multikinase inhibitor, with a broad selectivity spectrum targeting the active conformation of VEGFR, PDGFR, FGFR, KIT, and FLT3, was approved for the treatment of renal cancer as well as second-line therapy in imatinib-resistant GIST (66–68). Although sorafenib is a multikinase inhibitor like sunitinib, its kinase specificity, chemical structure and mode of binding are quite distinct from sunitinib. Sorafenib is a urea derivative that was originally designed to target the RAF kinase was found later to bind to the inactive conformation of the VEGFR kinase (69). Owing its potent activity against VEGFR and PDGFR, sorafenib was first approved for the treatment of renal cell and hepato-cellular carcinoma (70). Similarly, pazopanib, a 2-amino pyrimidine targeting VEGFR, PDGFR, and KIT has been approved for the treatment of advanced renal cell carcinoma (50) (Table 1).

Another important cancer target is the EGFR family of RTPKs, which comprises four members with various ligands, with a complex signaling through their homo- or heterodimerization (71, 72). The 4-anilino-quinazolines gefitinib and erlotinib target the active conformation of the EGFR kinase, while lapatinib, a dual kinase inhibitor, binds to a particular inactive conformation of EGFR and ERBB2 (HER2/neu) (73–75). Both, gefitinib and erlotinib have been approved for the use in second- and third-line therapy for advanced NSCLC (73, 74). Interestingly, gefitinib demonstrated a much higher response rate and survival benefit in Asian than in American patients, due to specific activating mutations in the EGFR receptor in a small subset of the Asian patients conferring enhanced sensitivity to gefitinib (24). Recently, erlotinib in combination with gemcitabine has been approved for the treatment of patients with metastatic pancreatic cancer, while lapatinib has been approved for the treatment of a particular set of advanced or metastatic breast cancers overexpressing ERBB2 (74, 75). The clinical successes of these EGFR kinase inhibitors have been hampered by the fact that the late stage NSCLC displays many levels of cross talk along several pathways of signal transduction, allowing cancer cells to escape these types of targeted therapies in multiple ways.

The only Ser/Thr-specific kinase inhibitors approved to date are two immunosuppressant macrolide rapamycin derivatives (rapalogs) temsirolimus and everolimus, which without binding to the ATP-site block specifically the raptor function of mTOR (*m*ammalian *Target of* *R*apamycin), an atypical protein kinase that is the major downstream mediator of the PI3K/AKT pathway (21, 53). These two rapalogs are the most selective kinase inhibitors on the market as they target a particular allosteric site of the mTOR kinase that results in the abrogation of only one aspect of the many mTOR functions. The orally administered everolimus has been registered as an immunosuppressant for the treatment of transplant rejection in 2001 as Certican® (54). Temsirolimus as Torisel® was approved in 2007 for the treatment of renal cell carcinoma (76), while everolimus as Afinitor® has been registered for advanced metastatic renal cancer in 2008 (52, 77). Both rapalogs are currently being tested in multiple clinical Phase II/III studies in various cancer indications as single agents and in combination with other drugs (52, 77) (Table 1).

With the exception of the rapamycin derivatives, these first-generation kinase drugs bind to the hinge region of the target kinase and can be, therefore, considered broadly as ATP mimetics. Except for the two rapalogs and lapatinib, which display outstanding selectivity profiles, all of the other registered kinase drugs also have many other kinase targets as demonstrated by recently published comprehensive biochemical profiling (78, 79). Although these profiling data should be taken with a grain of salt, as not all of the biochemically identified protein kinases have been shown to be inhibited in cell based assays (80), they represent the most comprehensive selectivity profile with the broadest kinome coverage.

Table 2
Kinase inhibitors in phase III clinical trials

Code name	Name	Target	Indication	Company
CGP-41251; PKC-412	Midostaurin	PKC, FLT3, KIT	AML, Systemic Mastocytosis	Novartis
317615; LY-317615	Enzastaurin	PKC-beta	Multiple cancers	Lilly
BPI-2009H	Icotinib	EGFR	NSCLC	Beta Pharma
BIBW-2992		EGFR, ERBB2	NSCLC, Head and Neck, Prostate and Breast Cancers	Boehringer Ingelheim
HKI-272; WAY-179272	Neratinib	EGFR, ERBB2	NSCLC; Solid Tumors Therapy; Breast Cancer Therapy	Wyeth
PTK/ZK; PTK-787; ZK-222584	Vatalanib	VEGFR1-3, KIT, PDGFR	Multiple cancer, angiogenesis	Novartis
NSC-732208; AZD-2171	Cediranib	VEGFR1-3	Multiple cancers	AstraZeneca
AMG-706	Motesanib	VEGFR1-3, KIT	Multiple cancers	Amgen
BIBG-1120		VEGFR1-3, FGFR, PDGFR	Multiple cancers	Boehringer Ingelheim
ZD-6474; CH-331; AZD-6474	Vandetanib	RET, VEGFR1-2, FGFR, EGFR	Multiple cancers, angiogenesis	AstraZeneca
XL-184; BMS-907351		RET, KIT, MET, VEGFR, FLT3, TIE2, PDGFR	NSCLC; Endocrine Cancer; Glioblastoma	Exelexis/ Bristol Myers
BMS-582664	Brivanib	FGFR1, VEGFR2	Multiple cancer	Bristol Myers
AB-1010	Masitinib	KIT, FGFR-3	Multiple cancer	AB Science
SKI-606	Bosutinib	SRC, ABL1-2	NSCLC, Colorectal, Breast, and Pancreatic Cancers; AML	Wyeth
AG-013736; AG-13736	Axitinib	PDGFR	Multiple cancers	Pfizer
PF-02341066; PF-2341066		MET	NSCLC; Solid Tumors; Lymphoma	Pfizer
OSI-906		IGF1R	Ovarian, Endocrine, and Breast Cancers	OSI Pharma
AP-23573; MK-8669 (Ridaforolimus)	Deforolimus	mTOR	Multiple cancers	Ariad/Merck & Co
INCB-18424; INCB-018424		JAK1, JAK2, TYK2	Hematological Cancers, Myeloma	Incyte

This type of profiling also revealed that the lipid and protein kinase inhibitors, which either are currently used as clinical drugs or are still under development, display a broader selectivity then originally intended (78–80). Together, these results clearly indicate that, with a few exceptions, it appears rather difficult to obtain a protein kinase inhibitor with a high degree of selectivity by targeting the ATP binding site. On the other hand, targeting multiple kinases in cancer indications may not necessarily be a disadvantage as many more clinical trials are ongoing with these registered kinase drugs seeking for line extensions.

2.2. Protein Kinase Inhibitors in Development for the Treatment of Cancer

More than 130 kinase inhibitors are reported to be in Phase I–III clinical development (14, 55). In addition to ongoing Phase III clinical studies (Table 2), many more are in clinical Phase I–II and preclinical stages (55). It is beyond the scope of this review to discuss all the protein kinase inhibitors that are in preclinical development and/or clinical Phase I–II. Protein kinase inhibitors not listed in Table 2 that are in advanced stages of clinical trials include the Flt3/JAK2 inhibitor lestaurtinib (Cephalon) for the treatment of acute myeloid leukemia, apatinib (YN968D1) yet another VEGFR inhibitor for renal cell cancer, and the cyclin-dependent kinase inhibitor alvocidib (flavopiridol, HMR-1275, Sanofi-Aventis) for the treatment of chronic lymphocytic leukemia and a variety of solid tumors (81, 82). Also not listed in Table 2 is the VEGF-R2 inhibitor vatalinib (PTK787, Novartis), which failed in a pivotal clinical trial in colon cancer (83, 84). Additional protein and lipid kinase inhibitors in Phase II include those targeting MEK, PI3K, and the cell cycle kinases, while many other protein kinase inhibitors that are in Phase I–II target ABL1, EGFR, VEGFR, MET, and IGF-R1 (81, 82). It should be noted that of the ongoing Phase II clinical studies, a large proportion accounts for inhibitors of the p38, which are used for treatment of nononcology indications such as rheumatoid arthritis. The large numbers of kinase inhibitors in clinical development which are for the vast majority targeting oncology indications reflect not only the more acute nature of the disease but also the greater tolerability with respect to potential side effects.

3. Kinase Structure, Selectivity Determinants, and Binding Modes

3.1. The ATP Binding Site

Protein and lipid kinases have evolved to have many different regulatory mechanisms and domain structures (1, 11, 12, 15, 17, 85). Although we have a good knowledge of the structural determinants for kinase inhibition by small molecules binding to the ATP-binding site (1, 11, 12, 15, 17, 85), the selectivity and the limited set of chemotypes targeting the ATP-binding site, a highly crowded area, have become major issues in kinase drug discovery. The molecular and structural understanding of the regulation of kinase activity, both at the level of the kinase domain as well as at the level of the full length protein kinase has improved significantly in the past 10 years. Protein and lipid kinases bind ATP in a cleft between the N- and C-terminal lobe of the kinase domain where the adenine group of ATP is surrounded by two hydrophobic surfaces and makes contact via hydrogen bonds to the connector of the two lobes, which is also referred to as the hinge (1, 11, 12, 15, 17, 85). The ATP cleft is lined by structural elements responsible for the catalytic activity of the kinase. These include the flexible activation loop (A-loop), which comes either in an open – the hallmark for the active ATP bound state of the kinase – or various closed conformations, where the substrate sites are either occluded and/or other elements of the kinase domain are displaced locking the protein kinase in the inactive state (Fig. 1) (1, 11, 12, 15, 17, 85). Additional important structures are the DFG motif at the start of the A-loop, helix-C and the P-loop which contributes to coordination of the phosphates of ATP (17, 86). The position of the A-loop, including the DFG motif at its N-terminal which can adopt different conformations from fully active to fully inactive, represents the hallmark for the active or inactive state of the protein kinase (Fig. 1) (11, 17, 86, 87). Owing to the spatial arrangement of residues important for catalysis, the structures of protein kinases in the active state are all very similar, despite the fact that they have

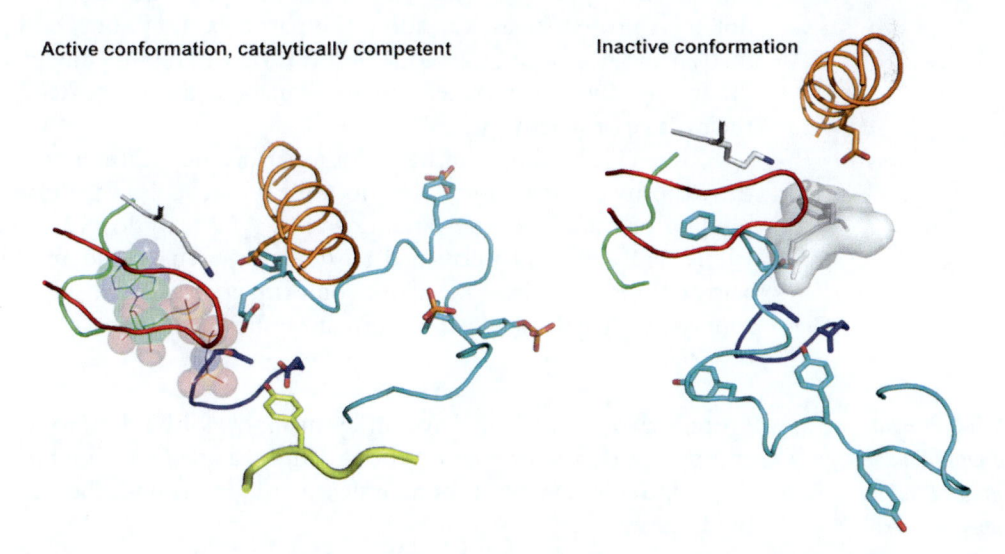

Fig. 1. Details of the binding of an ATP. The ATP analog (*transparent spheres*) and substrate peptide (*yellow*) in active IRK (PDB entry 1IR3, *left*) and the location of the same features in inactive IRK (PDB entry 1IRK, *right*) showing structural elements and residues important for the mechanism of action: helix-C (*orange*), P-loop (*red*), hinge region (*green*), catalytic loop (*blue*), activation loop (*cyan*), conserved lysine (*gray*). In the *right-hand panel*, the location of the DFG motif of the active conformation is shown by a transparent surface (*gray*).

different substrate specificities and different regulatory mechanisms (Fig. 1) (17). In the active state, the Asp in the DFG motif coordinates one magnesium ion, positioning the phosphates of ATP for the transfer of the phosphoryl group, while the Phe in the DFG motif packs under helix-C positioning both helix-C and A-loop for catalysis – this is the so-called DFG-in conformation (17, 87, 88). The position of the catalytic Lys from the β3 strand, often stabilized by the formation of a salt bridge with the conserved Glu residue from helix-C is responsible for facilitating the phosphoryl group transfer (Fig. 1). The extended β-sheet conformation of the P-loop helps coordinating the phosphates of ATP, while the β6 strand forms part of the catalytic loop that facilitates the phosphor transfer to either tyrosine, serine or threonine of the substrate (17, 86) (Fig. 1). The catalytic loop is the only element that does not differ between the active and inactive states (Fig. 1). The short EF-helix at the end of the A-loop with the conserved Glu forms the substrate binding site. The A-loop in the active conformation can be stabilized by phosphorylation (Fig. 1) (17, 86). Once the protein kinase has transferred the phosphoryl group from ATP to a tyrosine, serine or threonine of the substrate protein the protein kinase can return to its inactive conformation. In many kinases this involves returning the A-loop to the inactive (closed) position where one or both substrate sites (ATP and protein) become occluded. This can also involve the movement of the A-loop from the DFG-in (active) to the DFG-out (inactive) conformation, thus exposing an additional hydrophobic binding site directly adjacent to the ATP-binding site (11, 17, 86, 87) (Fig. 1). It should be mentioned that not every protein kinase can adopt this particular DFG-out conformation and it is out of the scope of this review to discuss the many other ways by which protein kinases can be activated or kept in their active or inactive states.

The ATP-binding site has additional distinct features which the majority of kinase inhibitors do not exploit, such as the ribose binding or the phosphate binding site of ATP (17, 86, 89). The whole ATP site can be classified on the basis of shape and amino-acid composition where the active conformation shows the highest similarity, while the inactive conformation shows the highest degree of variation.

3.2. The Protein and Lipid Kinase Inhibitor Binding Modes

Protein kinase inhibitors have different modes of binding to lipid and protein kinases which can be broadly classified into inhibitors that bind covalently or noncovalently to or around the ATP-binding site.

3.2.1. Covalent Protein and Lipid Kinase Inhibitors

Inhibitors which bind covalently may have reversible or irreversible binding modes depending on whether they have a Michel-acceptor, an alkylating or an acylating group (Fig. 2 and Table 3) (1, 11, 12, 15, 17, 85). Many inhibitors, which bind covalently to the ATP site,

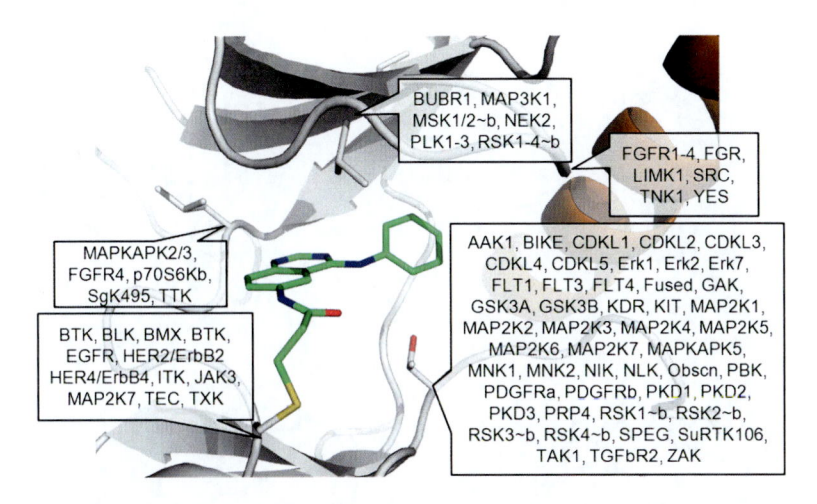

Fig. 2. Major cysteine sites in the ATP pocket. A close-up of the ATP pocket of EGFR bound covalently to a quinazoline inhibitor via its gk+7 Cys (pdb 2j5e). Frequently occurring Cys sites are shown as sticks and labeled with the kinases in which they occur. The sites are named by distance to the closest key residue (*clockwise from top*: Phi+3, Phi-1, DFG-1, gk+7, gk+2; Phi is the F/Y in the GXGXF/YG motif of the P-loop, gk = gatekeeper).

Table 3
Covalent kinase inhibitors

Kinase	Cys-site	Inhibitors	PDB code	References
JAK3	gk+7	CI-1033, PD168393		(155)
PI3Kγ	Catalytic lysine	Wortmannin (LY294002)	1e7u	(156)
EGFR	gk+7	CI-1033, PD168393	2j5e, 2j5f, 2jiv	(157, 155)
ERK2	DFG-1	Hypothemycin	3c9w, 2e14	(158)
PLK1	Catalytic lysine	Wortmannin (LY294002)	3d5x	(159)
BTK	gk+7	CI-1033, PD168393		(155)
HER4/ErbB4	gk+7	CI-1033, PD168393		(155)
HER2/ErbB2	gk+7	CI-1033, PD168393		(155)
BMX	gk+7	CI-1033, PD168393		(155)
RSK1/2	Phi+3	fluoroketone		(98)
SRC	DFG-1	quinazoline	2qq7, 2qlq, 2hwo, 2hwp	(160, 161)

The Cys sites are named based on the distance to the closest key residue (see Fig. 2). Kinases are named according to Manning.

usually form a bond to a Cys residue in or around the active site, preventing the binding of ATP to the protein kinase (Table 3) (90, 91). The Cys residue in the bottom part of the ATP binding site in EGFR and near the DFG-motif of ERK2 kinase (92) was successfully targeted with covalent inhibitors (Fig. 3). In the EGFR field these

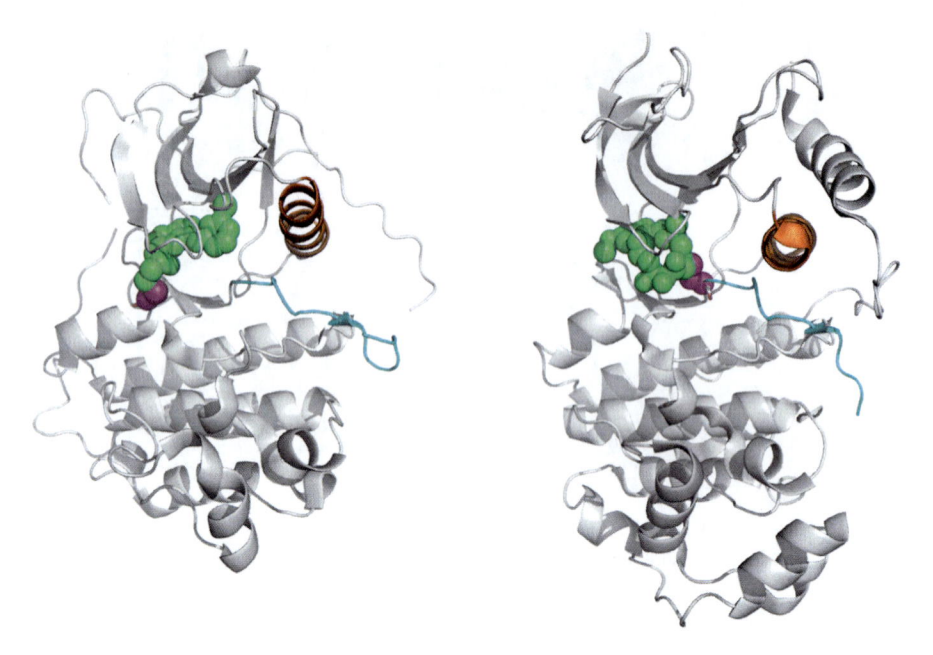

Fig. 3. Binding modes of covalent binders. Ribbon diagrams showing two examples of ATP site inhibitors covalently bound to the kinase. On the left a compound (*green*) is covalently linked to Cys797 (*magenta*) of EGFR at gk+7 (*the lower hinge*), while on the right hypothemycin (*green*) is linked to Cys164 (*magenta*) of ERK2. The sites are named by distance to the closest key residue. In both images the helix-C is colored *orange* and the activation loop is *cyan*.

covalent inhibitors have progressed to clinical stages where they are being evaluated in NSCLC (90, 93, 94). Various other covalent kinase inhibitors targeting a Cys have been designed for Fes (95), VEGF-R2 (96), BTK (97) and RSK2 (98) (Fig. 2 and Table 3). In addition, there are many more protein kinases that appear to have a Cys located in or around the ATP-binding pocket which could be potentially targeted (Table 3 and Fig. 2) (1, 11, 12, 15, 17, 85). Another type of covalent binder is exemplified by Wortmannin which binds to a the catalytic Lys in the ATP binding site of the PI3K (99).

The jury is still out as to whether these covalent kinase inhibitors are of clinical use. At least the covalent EGFR kinase inhibitors may become useful in targeting the most resistant form of the EGFR kinase that emerges upon treatment with the noncovalent EGFR inhibitors.

3.2.2. Noncovalent Protein and Lipid Kinase Inhibitors

The noncovalent kinase inhibitors can be classified into those which either bind (hinge binder) or do not bind (nonhinge binder) to the hinge region of the kinase (2, 89). A more refined classification for the noncovalent reversible kinase inhibitors is based on whether the kinase inhibitors work in an ATP- or non-ATP-competitive manner and whether the kinase inhibitors bind to an active or an inactive conformation of the kinase (2, 89). The ATP-site-directed hinge binders, which are competitive with respect to ATP, represent the vast majority of kinase inhibitors independent of whether they bind to the active or inactive form of the kinase domain (87).

Table 4
Structurally characterized allosteric kinase inhibitors

Kinase	PDB code apo/active	PDB code allosteric	Ligand	pIC50	Type	DFG
MEK1	3eqc	1s9j	CI-1040-like	9.0	Allosteric backpocket	In
CDK2	1fq1	3pxf	ANS	4.4	Allosteric backpocket	In
AKT1	3mv5	3o96	Cpd. 16h	7.2	Allosteric backpocket	Out
IGF1R	1m7n	3lw0	Cpd. 10	6.4	Allosteric backpocket	Out
CHK1	1ia8	3f9n	Cpd. 38	5.9	Substrate region	In
ABL	1iep	3k5v	GNF-2	8.0	Myristate pocket	Out
PDK1	1h1w	3hrf	Cpd. 2Z	5.0	PIF pocket	In

As a reference, the corresponding apo or active structure is given. Kinases are named according to Manning.

Another distinct, albeit heterogeneous, group of kinase inhibitors, which work in a non-ATP-competitive manner, is represented by those inhibitors targeting allosteric or remote sites on MEK, mTOR, CHK1, ABL, IKK, and AKT, just to name a few (38, 53, 100–105) (Table 4).

The hinge binding ATP-site-directed compounds targeting the active conformation which are often referred to as DFG-in or type I protein kinase inhibitors constitute the vast majority of the ATP-competitive inhibitors (11, 87). In this case, the A-loop adopts the active open conformation typical for the ATP-bound state of the kinase where the Asp in the DFG motif coordinates the phosphates of ATP and the Phe in the DFG motif stabilizes the position of helix-C and the A-loop for catalysis (Figs. 1 and 4b) (11, 17, 86, 87). The structures of protein kinases in the active ATP-bound state are all very similar, despite the fact that they have different substrate specificities and different regulations (Figs. 1 and 4b) (17). There is also a subset of type I kinase inhibitors that binds to inactive kinase conformations and depending on the features of these inhibitors, the structures of type-I inhibitor-kinase complexes can show remarkable differences (11, 17, 86, 87). For example, EGFR liganded to lapatinib adopts a DFG-in conformation typical of an active kinase, but helix-C is pushed out by lapatinib into an inactive state effectively disrupting the ion pairing between the catalytic Lys and the Glu from the helix-C (106) (Figs. 1 and 4a). This "DFG-in inactive" conformation has also been observed in other kinases and is often referred to as a SRC-like inactive conformation (107, 108).

There are now plenty of examples to create more selective inhibitors that take advantage of either a particular inactive conformation like lapatinib for EGFR (106) or other particular hallmarks in the kinase domain that can confer selectivity. For example, many

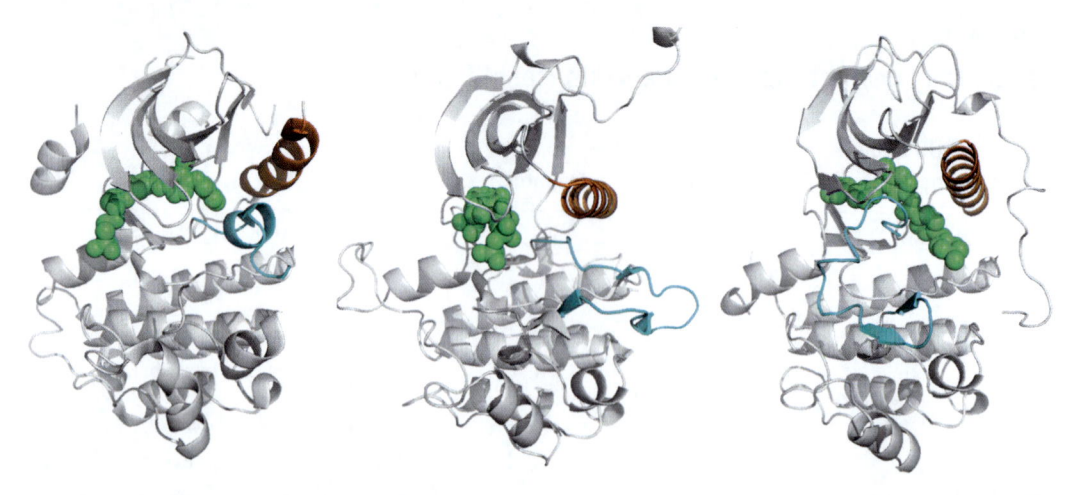

Fig. 4. Binding modes of ATP site inhibitors. Lapatinib (*green*) is bound to a confirmation of EGFR (*left*) in which the helix-C (*orange*) is pushed out and the activation loop (*cyan*) is folded inward compared to the conserved active conformation represented by IRK (*middle*) shown with ATP (*green*). Imatinib (*green*) is a type II inhibitor which binds to an inactive conformation of KIT (*right*) in which the DFG-motif at the start of the activation loop (*cyan*) is flipped out to make room for the inhibitor, but the helix-C (*orange*) is not significantly shifted.

of the type I kinase inhibitors that target the active conformation utilize the variation in the size, shape, and polarity of the gatekeeper residue at the back of the ATP site to gain selectivity, and knowledge about the various inactive conformations of different kinases allows one to combine these features (11).

The bias toward kinase inhibitors that target the active conformation of the kinase stems from the early days of kinase drug discovery where an ATP mimetic design together with the use of enzymatic assays displaying the highest level of activity were used. Classical examples for this type of kinase inhibitor class are gefitinib, erlotinib, dasatinib, sunitinib, and most notably staurosporine.

Kinase inhibitors that preferentially bind to the inactive conformation of the protein kinase and still have contacts to the hinge region are referred to as inhibitors binding to the DFG-out conformation or type II kinase inhibitors (11, 17, 86, 87) (Figs. 1 and 4c). These kinase inhibitors usually show ATP competitive behavior similar to those kinase inhibitors that target the active conformation. In this case, the movement of the A-loop from the DFG-in to the DFG-out conformation exposes an additional hydrophobic pocket adjacent to the ATP site that is used by these type II kinase inhibitors (11, 17, 86, 87) (Figs. 1 and 4c). In addition, these inhibitors share a similar pharmacophore where the Glu residue from the helix-C and the backbone amide of the Asp from the DGF motif are engaged in hydrogen bonds with the inhibitor (11, 17, 23). The energetic preference of a kinase to adopt this particular DFG-out conformation or not can be used to gain selectivity in

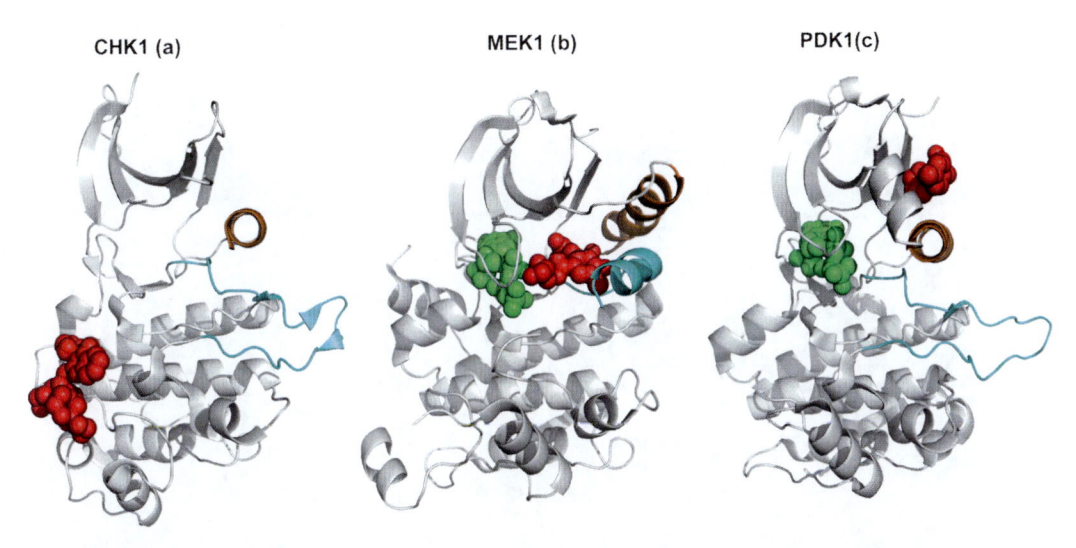

Fig. 5. Examples of non-ATP-competitive, non-ATP site binders. Ribbon diagrams showing non-ATP site binding modes (*red*) compared to the ATP site (*green*). A thioquinazoline binds to a surface-exposed site on CHK1 (**a**), which retains an active conformation and is, therefore, noncompetitive with ATP. By contrast, the uncompetitive MEK1 (**b**) inhibitor binds adjacent to ATP, causing large conformational changes in the helix-C (*orange*) and the A-loop (*cyan*). In PDK1 (**c**), compounds binding in the PIF-peptide pocket are found to be activators of the kinase.

the design of inhibitors, as done for TIE2 (109) or MET (110). The ground rules defining which of the protein kinases in the human kinome can adopt the DFG-out remain to be established. Kinase inhibitors binding to or stabilizing this inactive DFG-out conformation are, for example, imatinib, nilotinib, sorafenib, or vatalinib.

The non-ATP-competitive or allosteric kinase inhibitors that display no contact to the hinge – also referred to as type III inhibitors, show the highest degree of selectivity by exploiting binding sites and regulatory mechanisms that are unique to a particular kinase (11, 17, 86, 87) (Figs. 5 and 6). In addition to the DFG-in and DFG-out conformations mentioned above, analysis of multiple structures of protein kinases show that combinations of different conformational states of helix-C, the DFG motif, the A- and/or the P-loop can generate various inactive conformations of the kinase domain. Moreover, elements outside the kinase domain such as the juxta-membrane region or other N-terminal elements, the C-terminal tails as well as linkers, and/or other regulatory domains required for protein–protein interactions are all important elements in the regulation of the catalytic domain (17). Therefore, each individual kinase has a preferred inactive conformation, depending on its phosphorylation state and regulatory mechanisms involving structures outside the kinase domain. The unique combinations of all these structural elements create a structural diversity that can be used to design selective inhibitors. Inhibitors binding to the DFG-out and other inactive conformations

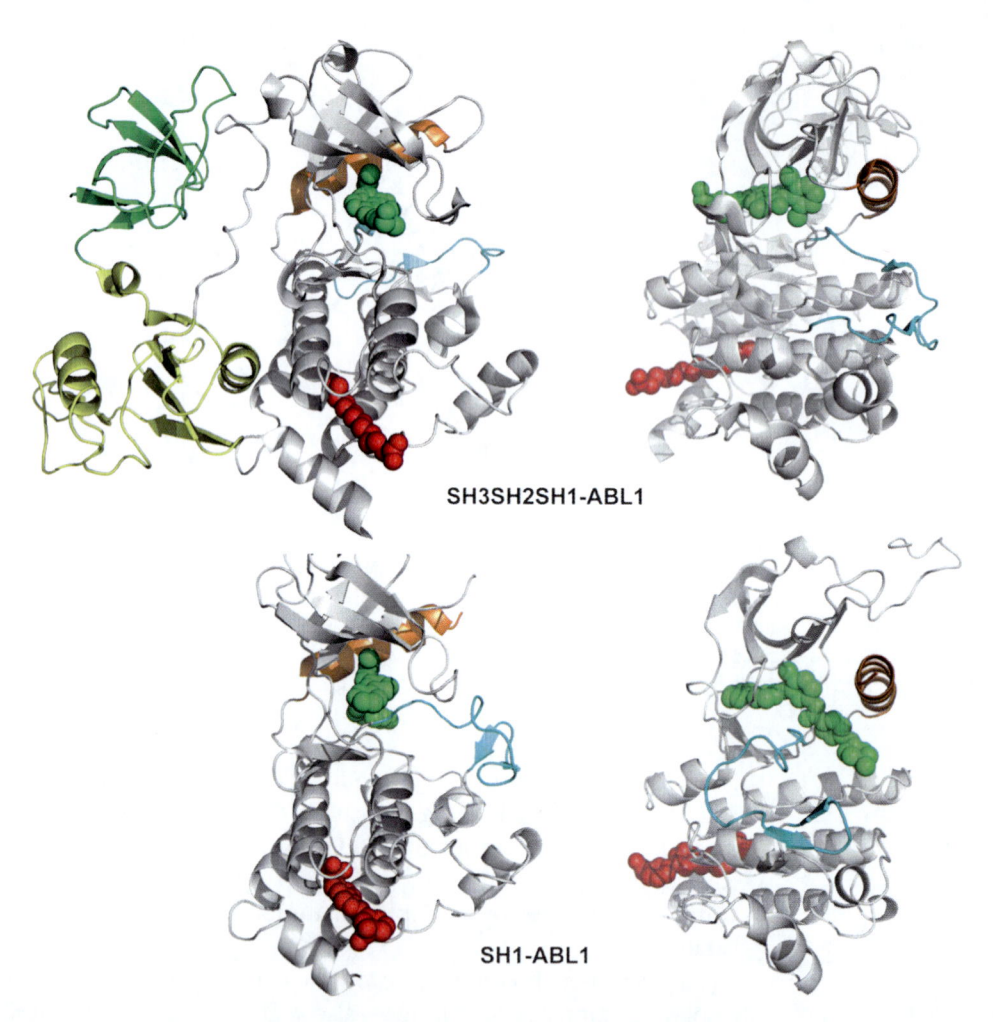

Fig. 6. Non-ATP site inhibitor (ABL1). *Top panel*: Ribbon diagrams showing two views about 90° apart of the assembled inactive state of Abl kinase induced on the binding of myristate (SH3 domain, *green*; SH2 domain, *yellow*; type I inhibitor, *green*; myristate, *red*; helix-C, *orange*; A-loop, *cyan*). *Bottom panel*: Similar views of the isolated kinase domain (SH1) in complex with a type II inhibitor (imatinib, *green*) and an ATP-competitive inhibitor binding in the myristate site (GNF-2, *red*).

may have several advantages over ATP-site inhibitors, including better selectivity and slower off-rates which increase the residence time of the inhibitor bound to the kinase (106, 111). However, the paucity of available structures for the inactive, unliganded protein kinases (apo-form) represents a major hurdle in designing inhibitors targeting the inactive conformations. Methods that have been developed recently use active kinase domain structures as a basis for developing models of the DFG-out conformation that are useful for ligand screening, ligand docking, and ligand activity profiling studies (112).

The allosteric kinase inhibitors known thus far include compounds such as CI-1040, which inhibits MEK by occupying a pocket adjacent to the ATP binding site (100) (Fig. 5b), GNF2, which binds to the myristate binding site of ABL (11, 38, 40) (Fig. 6), the pleckstrin homology domain-dependent AKT inhibitors (101, 102), BMS-345541, which inhibits the IKK (103), the rapamycin derivatives targeting mTOR (53), and the recently discovered CHK1 inhibitor (105) (Fig. 5a). In addition, targeting the allosteric sites on protein kinases may provide means to identify activators rather than inhibitors which could be useful for therapeutic intervention (113–116).

4. Major Challenges in Kinase Drug Discovery

One of the major challenges in future kinase drug discovery is to better understand the cancer dependence of the target kinase and anticipate the emerging resistance to kinase inhibitor treatment. In most cases, the cancer dependence either is not known or displays a high degree of complexity that often makes the selection of patients most likely to respond (patient stratification) to a given kinase inhibitor treatment an impossible task. Understanding and predicting the cross-reactivity of kinase inhibitors in conjunction with the knowledge about the cancer dependency of the target kinase would allow a more rapid proof-of-concept and the better use of kinase inhibitors. The selectivity of kinase inhibitors as well as the knowledge about the on- and off-target pharmacology (side effects) are still poorly understood. Finally, novel approaches aimed at targeting protein kinases outside the ATP-binding pocket warranting new unexplored kinase space and improving the selectivity of kinase inhibitors are in their infancy.

4.1. Protein and Lipid Kinases and Cancer Dependence

Protein and lipid kinases that are involved in the development of cancer have a deregulated activity due to gene amplification, mutations, and/or gene rearrangements (1–10). Over time, cancer cells acquire intracellular wiring that differ from that of normal cells and usually become more dependent on the activity of a specific oncogene because, during the multistage carcinogenic process, they have lost the function of another gene that normally performs a similar function (4, 117, 118). Based on the concept of "synthetic lethality," inhibiting the activity of an oncogene could selectively target the cancer cells and spare the normal cells (117). This may be one of the reasons why only the subset of patients that have specific activating gain of function mutations in the kinase domain of EGFR and/or amplification of the EGFR often display impressive clinical responses to the EGFR inhibitors (24, 28, 119–121).

Lipid and protein kinases appear to be involved in almost every cellular signaling responsible for development, maintenance, and spreading of cancer. Amplification, overexpression and mutational activation of tyrosine kinases play a major role in development, progression, and maintenance of various cancers (1, 8, 16, 25, 34, 61, 72, 122, 123). In addition, the lipid modifying PI3K together with the Ras-Raf-MAPK which represents one of the most mutated pathways in cancer are at the receiving end of the receptor tyrosine kinases (1, 20, 21, 35, 124). While some protein and lipid kinases regulate the proliferation of cancer cells, others play a pivotal role in cell cycle regulation and cell survival, DNA damage repair as well as in the maintenance of telomeres (5–7, 22). Another important process underlying tumor growth involves the growth of new blood vessels from preexisting ones. Although a number of factors contribute to this growth, the VEGFR and FGFR kinase inhibitors have been found to be of potential value in the treatment malignancies that are dependent on angiogenesis (125–127).

The involvement of many protein and lipid kinases in the development of cancers is further complicated by the plethora of mutations that have been recently identified in different kinases (1–3, 8–10). In many instances, these mutations can be linked to specific cancers through genomic studies, as has been recently highlighted (9, 10). However, the results obtained from these large efforts leading to the compilation of the cancer "kinase mutatome" have been rather sobering. Although many activating mutations in various kinases have been found in a variety of cancers, it will take another large effort to unambiguously identify the dependence of tumor growth on a particular kinase or its pathway(s). The major difficulty is the intrinsic heterogeneity of cancers, in particular the late stage forms of cancer that harbor multiple mutations, chromosomal aberrations and display genomic instability. Demonstrating the cancer dependence of the kinase target not only will lead to the identification of inhibitors of the kinase but may also accelerate the proof-of-concept in clinical trials allowing a better selection of patients most likely to respond to the targeted therapy.

Imatinib currently serves as a paradigm for targeting dominant oncogenes. The success of imatinib has initiated debates as to whether this paradigm can be translated to other cancers. It may well be that the efficacy of imatinib in CML is an exception rather than the rule because it is caused by the single aberration (the BCR-ABL1 fusion protein), which is absent in normal cells. CML can be viewed as a genetically simple neoplasm compared to the common epithelial carcinoma of the lung, breast, colon, and prostate. Therefore, cancers caused by mutations at multiple different genetic loci may in theory require, in the worst case, a multitude of different therapeutic agents. Inhibitors of oncogenic protein and lipid kinase pathways may still have activity as single agents if their mutational activation leads to a state of "oncogene addiction," possibly due to genetic or epigenetic changes at other loci (4, 128). Thus, genetic interactions and genetic complexity may decrease rather than increase the number of agents required for the treatment of cancers. As a matter of fact, single-agent activity of imatinib, albeit not very durable, was noted against accelerated and blast-phase CML, which, in contrast to the early phase CML, are clearly associated with multiple genetic abnormalities in addition to the canonical BCR-ABL1 translocation (23, 25). Impressive and durable single-agent activity of imatinib has also been observed in GIST a multigenic cancer that develops over decades due to recurrent chromosomal abnormalities including activating mutations in the KIT or PDGF receptors (27, 34, 61, 128). The common denominator between BCR-ABL1 in CML and KIT/PDGFR in GIST is that they both represent the earliest recognizable causal mutations in their respective diseases. Therefore, targeting early causal changes is likely to be the most successful strategy in the future. To date, these considerations have not always been included in the design of clinical trials of, for example, inhibitors of EGFR or MEK (129).

On the contrary, clinical responses have also been noted with many other kinase inhibitors without a clear rationale, offering encouragement that single agents can be active in genetically complex neoplasms, although it is formally possible that the "single-agent" activity may be due to its fortuitous ability to inhibit multiple kinases. The recent introduction of the concept of individualized cancer therapy along with the development of selective drugs targeting specific alteration in tumors has provided hope for the development of more effective treatment strategies.

4.2. Multikinase Versus Selective Kinase Inhibitors

Because protein and lipid kinases mediate many of the signaling pathways by which cancer cells promote proliferation and survival, the design of drugs targeting a unique kinase with high specificity may not seem appropriate in this indication. The current focus is on the development of drugs with multiple effects to overcome many, and often overlapping biological pathways that tumors utilize to grow, resist death, and spread. A broad spectrum of target kinase inhibition appears to be a desirable property to treat cancers either by combining selective kinase inhibitors or using so-called multikinase inhibitors that display a lower selectivity. However, an unbalanced potency against one but not all targets may limit its clinically achievable inhibitory spectrum resulting in suboptimal inhibition, which in turn may lead to emergence of resistance. Multikinase inhibitors targeting the VEGF-R and/or FGF-R kinase families as single agent or in combination appear to perform better in clinical trials than the EGF-R kinase inhibitors (129). Although combination is the mainstay of cancer therapy, it is still not understood how to successfully combine these novel targeted therapies. While the combination of the VEGF targeted monoclonal antibody with conventional chemotherapy has demonstrated significant survival advantage in breast, colon, and lung cancers, the combination of the EGFR kinase inhibitor gefitinib with conventional chemotherapy did not show significant benefit in NSCLC (129).

Apart from the fact that the use of two uniquely targeted agents should avoid off-target and combination toxicities, allowing maximal dosing of each agent at the optimal schedule, the clinical benefits of combinations of various kinase inhibitors, or kinase inhibitors with other molecularly targeted agents such as inhibitors of Histone Deacetylases, hsp90, or aromatase inhibitors remain to be established (129).

On the contrary, the single-agent efficacy of highly selective kinase inhibitors such as imatinib in CML where the other kinase inhibited by imatinib do not to play important roles, lapatinib in metastatic breast cancer and everolimus in metastatic renal cancer demonstrate that the genetic complexity of tumors appears to be overcome by targeting specific pathogenic pathway nodes (4, 117, 128). In diseases where pathogenic activating mutations have been identified such as those in the EGFR gene, uniquely targeted agents such as gefitinib or erlotinib might be useful (24, 28). However, the 10% response rate to gefitinib in advanced stage NSCLC contrasts unfavorably with the 90% response rate to imatinib in CML indicating a lack of a therapeutic modality for the remaining 90% of the NSCLC patients (129). Alternatively, an appropriate selection of patients likely to respond, in particular in the NSCLC setting, may significantly increase the therapeutic benefit with the caveat that the number of overall patients treated will become smaller.

The choice of single agent versus combination therapy should be driven by the need to minimize the emergence of resistance rather than assuming that cancer is a multigenic disorder. Cancer genetics will guide the integration of conventional therapies (surgery, radiation, chemotherapy) with protein kinase inhibitors and other "molecularly targeted" therapies for treating cancer in the future. The weight of evidence in the field of kinase inhibitors in solid tumors suggests that inhibiting multiple targets produces greater benefit over single target inhibition, when no specific pathway drives tumor proliferation and survival. Therefore, targeted therapies should only be applied to patient populations where the epidemiology and molecular pathophysiology of the diseases is genetically well understood. Thus, it is of no therapeutic benefit to use targeted kinase inhibitor therapies in advanced cancer patients without a well defined genetic rationale, in particular in those patients that have been heavily pretreated with chemotherapeutic agents (129).

4.3. On- and Off-Target Pharmacology or Selectivity of Protein Kinase Inhibitors

One of the issues that is perceived as major challenge in kinase drug discovery is the selectivity for the target kinases, which defines the on- and off-target pharmacology (2, 11–14, 16, 17, 87). While development of selective kinase inhibitors is likely to be extremely important from the standpoint of minimizing drug side effects, inhibitors with exquisite selectivity are a must for chronic administration in non-life-threatening diseases such as many immunological dysfunctions (2, 11–14, 16, 87).

Thus, a good understanding of the on- and off-target pharmacology in particular with respect to side effects is paramount for the design of kinase inhibitors. Unfortunately, there are neither clear guidelines nor a general consensus about which kinases of the human kinome are "off limits." The selection of the so-called "kinase anti-targets" is rather arbitrary and biased by the availability of knockout animal and human genetic data as well as the fact that the knowledge of individual kinases is rather anecdotal than comprehensive. It should be noted that the function of most of the members of the human kinome has to date remained largely unexplored. In addition, the potency in biochemical and cellular assays of kinase inhibitors, which represents a good starting point, may not be translated directly to in vivo downregulation of the kinase target and its signaling pathway. Also, the information linking adverse side effects of protein and lipid kinase inhibitors with a particular protein kinase selectivity profile is only now beginning to emerge (130, 131). Moreover, we are still trying to understand the side effects that are generated by inhibiting multiple "antitarget kinases." Recent data suggest that simultaneous inhibition of ATM, ATR, DNAPK, Aurora, and/or other kinases involved in mitosis may be genotoxic (130, 131).

The recent systematic profiling of kinase inhibitors, in broad arrays of biochemical (and cellular) assays that offer a coverage of more than 80% of the human kinome, has provided ways to better define the selectivity profile of drug candidates including the potential for the discovery of novel mechanisms of actions (78, 80, 132). Despite of all of these efforts, we still poorly understand the selectivity profiles with respect to their liabilities regarding preclinical toxicity findings and their relevance to patients in the clinic. It is hoped that the recent progresses made in molecular profiling will further our understanding toward a better assessment and prediction of efficacy versus toxicity. So far, the selectivity of the launched small-molecular-weight kinase inhibitors (Table 1) seems not to compromise their clinical utility in cancer indications. Comparing, for example, the selectivity profile of sunitinib with that of lapatinib (see Fig. 1 in ref. 79) shows that sunitinib is less selective and presumably less well tolerated than lapatinib. Nonetheless, sunitinib is being used for the treatment of various late-stage cancers, although its selectivity profile would preclude its use in non-life-threatening clinical conditions. On the contrary, imatinib, which has been shown to have multiple kinase targets, has recently been registered also for a nononcology indication (64), suggesting that kinase inhibitors could have a more widespread use once their long-term use and safety is better understood.

Members of one protein kinase subfamily can be phylochemically more different than kinases from another class (79). For example, imatinib binds very weakly to the more closely related SRC, which has a domain structure and regulatory mechanism similar to ABL1, while it binds with high affinity to PDGFR, KIT, and DDR (17, 133, 134). The possibility that SRC is unable to bind imatinib because it cannot adopt the DFG-out conformation has been excluded recently showing that hat inhibitors including imatinib can indeed bind to a DFG-out conformation of SRC (133, 135). However, it is likely that the energy required for SRC to adopt this conformation is greater than for ABL1, and the structure of imatinib does not compensate for this as well as inhibitors that are less hydrophobic in the region that is exposed to the P-loop in ABL1. SRC prefers to adopt an inactive conformation where helix-C swings out and is stabilized by a short helix in the N-terminal part of the A-loop (136). This conformation has also been observed in Hck (107), ABL (108) and EGFR (106).

There are now plenty of examples to create more selective inhibitors that take advantage of either a particular inactive conformation such as lapatinib for EGFR (106) or other particular hallmarks in the kinase domain that can confer selectivity.

4.4. Resistance to Protein Kinase Inhibitors

Drug resistance can either occur by extrinsic compensatory mechanisms or intrinsically by reducing the affinity of the kinase inhibitor to its target (137). Mutation of single amino acids in the kinase domain resulting in the abrogation of the inhibitory potency concomitant with relapses has been documented for inhibitors of BCR–ABL1, EGFR, FLT3, KIT, and PDGFR (11, 23–25, 30, 138, 139). The most commonly found point mutation leading to resistance is the one targeting the gatekeeper residue of the kinase, whose size and shape regulates the properties of the hydrophobic pocket located at the back of the ATP binding site (11, 23–25, 30, 138, 139). The gatekeeper residue has no contact to ATP but is often in close contact with type I and type II kinase inhibitors because it is located in the hinge (87). This is the reason why gatekeeper mutations such as T315I in BCR–ABL1 (23, 25, 29), T670I in Kit (27, 138), T674I in PDGFRα (140), G697R in FLT3 (139), V561M in FGFR1 (141), T681I of PDGFRβ (142), and T341M in SRC (143) cause little or no change in kinase activity but confer inhibitor resistance to a wide spectrum of kinase inhibitors (141). In most cases, the gatekeeper mutation sterically impedes inhibitor binding (141). By contrast, the gatekeeper mutation T790M in EGFR induces resistance to gefitinib and erlotinib by significantly increasing the affinity for ATP and thereby reducing the affinity for the kinase inhibitors (24, 30).

Apart from the usual mechanisms of drug inactivation in cancer (137) as well as the findings that quiescent tumor stem cells are refractory to kinase inhibitors (144) there are additional target related mechanisms for resistance that are not based on mutations of the target kinase. These include amplification of the target like in the case of BCR–ABL1 in CML (145) and/or upregulation of alternative kinase pathways such as the receptors for hepatocyte growth factor (MET) or insulin-like growth factor (IGF1R) in the acquisition of resistance to EGFR kinase inhibitors (32). Of course, any activation of effectors downstream of receptor protein tyrosine kinases such as the Ras-Raf-MAPK and/or PI3K/Akt pathway override the effects of a receptor tyrosine kinase inhibitor.

Target dependent drug resistance has presented new therapeutic challenges, leading to the development of "second-generation" kinase inhibitors that can form covalent bonds with the target and, therefore, increase their effectiveness. In attempts to overcome resistance to the EGFR inhibitors gefitinib and erlotinib, kinase inhibitors that bind covalently to the ATP-binding site of EGFR have been developed (90, 93, 94) (Fig. 3a). Another approach is to develop noncovalent inhibitors that can tolerate various amino acids at the gatekeeper position. Several ATP-site directed inhibitors active against the T315I ABL1 gatekeeper mutant have been reported, but thus far only AP24534 has progressed to the stage of Phase I clinical trials (146). A further approach is to target the kinase with inhibitors that bind to alternative binding sites such as On012380 that is presumed to inhibit the ABL1 substrate binding site (147). A more remote binding site on the kinase domain is addressed by the GNF-2 compound which targets the myristate binding site of ABL1 and ABL2 (11, 38, 148). Finally, inhibiting pathways or pathway nodes that are utilized by the target kinase with alternative approaches targeting the chaperone function of Hsp90 (149) or farnesyl-transferase activity (150) have been demonstrated to work in cell culture, and efforts are currently underway to apply them clinically.

5. Novel Approaches to Kinase Drug Discovery

Small-molecule inhibitors such as imatinib and sorafenib inhibit the catalytic function of the kinase by binding to the adenosine part of the ATP binding pocket and by stabilizing an inactive (DGF-out in this case) conformation. Although, this ATP-competitive binding mode has improved the selectivity of kinase inhibitors due to the need for a specific inactive conformation, another potential way to gain selectivity is to identify new classes of protein kinase inhibitors that do not compete with ATP at all. These so-called type III inhibitors may potentially enable the selective regulation of specific protein kinases associated with a particular disease but without affecting other protein kinases involved in normal physiology, or without affecting other functions (structural or enzymatic) of the kinase. Therefore, targeting a pocket outside of the ATP site, also referred to as "out of the box" approaches, could add value to the so-called ATP-site-directed or "in the box" approaches (ATP mimetics) in terms of new scaffolds, intellectual property, and selectivity. Out of the box approaches may be particularly relevant for those kinase inhibitors targeting non-life-threatening diseases and which are not prone to generate resistance as has been observed in many oncology indications. In addition, these allosteric inhibitors could also be used to address the resistance caused by mutations in the ATP binding site (11, 40, 148).

Unfortunately, only a very limited number of non-ATP-competitive kinase inhibitors have thus far been identified. These include the rapamycin analogs as well as the inhibitors for ABL, IKK, AKT, CHK1, MEK, SRC, IGF1R, and others (11, 40, 53, 100–103, 105, 148, 151). In Figs. 5 and 6 only those non-ATP-competitive kinase inhibitors are shown for which there is a structure available. Even though this is only a limited number, it is surprising to see in how many ways the protein kinase activity can be inhibited (or activated as it is the case for PDK1) by occupying sites outside of the ATP pocket.

For example, recently published cocrystal structures of inhibitors bound to CHK1 have revealed an allosteric site, unique to CHK1, located in the C-terminal domain not far from the peptide substrate binding site. This site consists of a shallow groove linked to a small hydrophobic pocket (105) (Fig. 5a). Another non-ATP-competitive allosteric inhibitor has recently been developed, which targets the myristate binding-site located near the C-terminal of the ABL kinase domain, as demonstrated by genetic approaches, solution NMR, and X-ray crystallography (11, 38, 40, 148) (Fig. 6). The binding of GNF-2, like myristate, causes a conformational change that allows the SH2 and SH3 domains to clamp onto the kinase domain and hold it in an assembled inactive state in an analogous way to that observed for monophosphorylated SRC (11, 38, 40, 148). Therefore, the presence of these two domains is required to inhibit the kinase activity of ABL1 (11, 38, 40, 148) (Fig. 6). Although this type of myristate pocket is also present in SRC, it appears to serve a different function than in ABL1 (148). The potential to inhibit MEK allosterically avoiding many of the off-target activities often associated with ATP-competitive kinase inhibitors has added great value to the attractiveness of MEK as a druggable target. The allosteric MEK inhibitors bind to a unique allosteric inhibitor-binding pocket between the Mg^{2+}-ATP-binding site and helix-C (100) (Fig. 5b). The important key interactions between the bound inhibitor and the allosteric pocket have been discussed earlier (100). This allosteric site is distinct from the highly homologous ATP-binding site and is located in a region where the sequence homology to other protein kinases is low. It should be noted that these allosteric MEK inhibitors seem to work in a non-ATP-competitive, rather than an ATP-competitive, manner as they require the presence of ATP to impart inhibitory activity (100). Low-molecular-weight compounds, which target the hydrophobic motif (HM) or HM-pocket, also known as PIF-pocket of the AGC kinases, have the ability to allosterically activate PDK1 by modulating the phosphorylation-dependent conformational transition of PDK1 (116, 152) (Fig. 5c). Interaction of a low-molecular-weight compound able to mimic the phosphorylated HM within the HM/PIF-pocket activates PDK1 by stabilizing helix-C in the active form, which positions the conserved Glu from helix-C correctly to coordinate the phosphates of ATP. These data indicate the possibility of developing drugs to modulate phosphorylation-dependent conformational transitions in other AGC kinases (116, 152). Additional, less well defined pockets and substrate docking sites on protein kinases have been described which could in theory be exploited to modulate the kinase activity (153).

There are various reasons why the identification of these out of the box kinase inhibitors has been so unproductive. Traditional hit finding approaches which used recombinant highly activated catalytic domains of protein kinases (often lacking regulatory domains) have favored the identification of ATP-pocket binders. Therefore, reidentification of the same, highly promiscuous chemical matter has plagued many of these kinase screens. Only recently has it been realized that not all ATP-site directed kinase inhibitors are created alike, with some favoring the inactive over the active kinase conformation and vice versa. Approaches aimed at correcting this bias evolved from a better understanding of the molecular and structural requirements of both substrate binding sites (the ATP and protein substrate) as well as the phosphorylation state of the kinase. In addition, unbiased cell-based screening of large compound libraries, including natural compounds, using well-defined phosphorylation readouts has only been recently established (38). These cell based screens enable the use of conformations of the target kinase that cannot always be obtained in vitro in biochemical assays and may provide a head start in obtaining novel types of protein kinase inhibitors with the desired degree of selectivity. However, it may prove challenging to optimize potency and selectivity using the cellular readout only. In any case, the discovery of these novel allosteric sites provides an opportunity to design more selective protein kinase inhibitors (and activators) that are less compromised by ATP competition than typical ATP-site inhibitors.

6. Concluding Remarks

The large number of kinase inhibitors in clinical development will ensure a constant flow of novel targeted therapies to the clinic over the next 5 years. The vast majority of these kinase inhibitors are for various oncology indications that reflect not only the more acute nature of the disease but also the greater tolerability with respect to potential side effects. The future of protein kinase-targeted therapeutics in cancer appears promising, despite the fact that several protein kinase inhibitors that have entered human clinical trials are not very specific and did not achieve the anticipated results. This situation may be improved by the upcoming second generation of kinase inhibitors with a better selectivity that will be applied to a genetically better defined patient population. The development of kinase inhibitors for non-life-threatening indications where chronic regimens are being used will require a priori a better target selectivity to minimize side effects.

It should be mentioned that all of the mentioned advanced kinase inhibitors do not cover more than 10–15% of the whole kinome. Ongoing efforts using genome-wide screening in conjunction with the use of genetic organisms will unravel new disease associations and will pave the way for the discovery of many more new protein kinase targets in the coming years. Finally, protein kinase inhibitors will be important not only for the treatment of diseases but also as reagents using a systems biology approach to better understand cellular networking. There are many specific protein kinase inhibitors that cannot be used as drugs for reasons of toxicity or solubility, but are still extremely useful as research reagents (130, 154).

References

1. Blume-Jensen, P., and Hunter, T. (2001) Oncogenic kinase signalling, *Nature* **411**, 355–365.
2. Fabbro, D., Ruetz, S., Buchdunger, E., Cowan-Jacob, S. W., Fendrich, G., Liebetanz, J., Mestan, J., O'Reilly, T., Traxler, P., Chaudhuri, B., Fretz, H., Zimmermann, J., Meyer, T., Caravatti, G., Furet, P., and Manley, P. W. (2002) Protein kinases as targets for anticancer agents: from inhibitors to useful drugs, *Pharmacol. Ther.* **93**, 79–98.
3. Hunter, T. (2000) Signaling--2000 and beyond, *Cell* **100**, 113–127.
4. Weinstein, I. B. (2002) Cancer. Addiction to oncogenes--the Achilles heal of cancer, *Science* **297**, 63–64.
5. Luo, J., Solimini, N. L., and Elledge, S. J. (2009) Principles of cancer therapy: oncogene and non-oncogene addiction, *Cell* **136**, 823–837.
6. Hahn, W. C., and Weinberg, R. A. (2002) Modelling the molecular circuitry of cancer, *Nat. Rev. Cancer* **2**, 331–341.
7. Hanahan, D., and Weinberg, R. A. (2000) The hallmarks of cancer, *Cell* **100**, 57–70.
8. Bardelli, A., Parsons, D. W., Silliman, N., Ptak, J., Szabo, S., Saha, S., Markowitz, S., Willson, J. K., Parmigiani, G., Kinzler, K. W., Vogelstein, B., and Velculescu, V. E. (2003) Mutational analysis of the tyrosine kinome in colorectal cancers, *Science* **300**, 949.
9. Greenman, C., Stephens, P., Smith, R., Dalgliesh, G. L., Hunter, C., Bignell, G., Davies, H., Teague, J., Butler, A., Stevens, C., Edkins, S., O'Meara, S., Vastrik, I., Schmidt, E. E., Avis, T., Barthorpe, S., Bhamra, G., Buck, G., Choudhury, B., Clements, J., Cole, J., Dicks, E., Forbes, S., Gray, K., Halliday, K., Harrison, R., Hills, K., Hinton, J., Jenkinson, A., Jones, D., Menzies, A., Mironenko, T., Perry, J., Raine, K., Richardson, D., Shepherd, R., Small, A., Tofts, C., Varian, J., Webb, T., West, S., Widaa, S., Yates, A., Cahill, D. P., Louis, D. N., Goldstraw, P., Nicholson, A. G., Brasseur, F., Looijenga, L., Weber, B. L., Chiew, Y. E., DeFazio, A., Greaves, M. F., Green, A. R., Campbell, P., Birney, E., Easton, D. F., Chenevix-Trench, G., Tan, M. H., Khoo, S. K., Teh, B. T., Yuen, S. T., Leung, S. Y., Wooster, R., Futreal, P. A., and Stratton, M. R. (2007) Patterns of somatic mutation in human cancer genomes, *Nature* **446**, 153–158.
10. Thomas, R. K., Baker, A. C., Debiasi, R. M., Winckler, W., Laframboise, T., Lin, W. M., Wang, M., Feng, W., Zander, T., MacConaill, L., Lee, J. C., Nicoletti, R., Hatton, C., Goyette, M., Girard, L., Majmudar, K.,

Ziaugra, L., Wong, K. K., Gabriel, S., Beroukhim, R., Peyton, M., Barretina, J., Dutt, A., Emery, C., Greulich, H., Shah, K., Sasaki, H., Gazdar, A., Minna, J., Armstrong, S. A., Mellinghoff, I. K., Hodi, F. S., Dranoff, G., Mischel, P. S., Cloughesy, T. F., Nelson, S. F., Liau, L. M., Mertz, K., Rubin, M. A., Moch, H., Loda, M., Catalona, W., Fletcher, J., Signoretti, S., Kaye, F., Anderson, K. C., Demetri, G. D., Dummer, R., Wagner, S., Herlyn, M., Sellers, W. R., Meyerson, M., and Garraway, L. A. (2007) High-throughput oncogene mutation profiling in human cancer, *Nat. Genet.* **39**, 347–351.

11. Zhang, J., Yang, P. L., Gray, N. S. (2009) Targeting cancer with small molecule kinase inhibitors, *Nat. Rev. Cancer* **9**, 28–39.

12. Cohen, P. (2002) Protein kinases--the major drug targets of the twenty-first century?, *Nat. Rev. Drug Discov.* **1**, 309–315.

13. Vieth, M., Higgs, R. E., Robertson, D. H., Shapiro, M., Gragg, E. A., and Hemmerle, H. (2004) Kinomics-structural biology and chemogenomics of kinase inhibitors and targets, *Biochim. Biophys. Acta* **1697**, 243–257.

14. Vieth, M., Sutherland, J. J., Robertson, D. H., and Campbell, R. M. (2005) Kinomics: characterizing the therapeutically validated kinase space, *Drug Discov. Today* **10**, 839–846.

15. Levitzki, A. (2003) Protein kinase inhibitors as a therapeutic modality, *Acc. Chem. Res.* **36**, 462–469.

16. Fabbro, D., and Garcia-Echeverria, C. (2002) Targeting protein kinases in cancer therapy, *Curr. Opin. Drug Discov. Devel* **.5**, 701–712.

17. Cowan-Jacob, S. W. (2006) Structural biology of protein tyrosine kinases, *Cell. Mol. Life Sci.* **63**, 2608–2625.

18. Garcia-Echeverria, C. (2009) Protein and lipid kinase inhibitors as targeted anticancer agents of the Ras/Raf/MEK and PI3K/PKB pathways, *Purinergic Signal.* **5**, 117–125.

19. Garcia-Echeverria, C., and Sellers, W. R. (2008) Drug discovery approaches targeting the PI3K/Akt pathway in cancer, *Oncogene* **27**, 5511–5526.

20. Maira, S. M., Voliva, C., and Garcia-Echeverria, C. (2008) Class IA phosphatidylinositol 3-kinase: from their biologic implication in human cancers to drug discovery, *Expert Opin. Ther. Targets* **12**, 223–238.

21. Yuan, T. L., and Cantley, L. C. (2008) PI3K pathway alterations in cancer: variations on a theme, *Oncogene* **27**, 5497–5510.

22. Malumbres, M., and Barbacid, M. (2009) Cell cycle, CDKs and cancer: a changing paradigm, *Nat. Rev. Cancer* **9**, 153–166.

23. Fabbro, D., Fendrich, G., Guez V., Meyer T., Furet, P., Mestan, P., Griffin, J.D. Manley, P.W., and Cowan-Jacob, S.W. (2005) Targeted therapy with imatinib: An exception or a rule? *Handbook of Experimental Pharmacology, Inhibitors of Protein Kinases and Protein Phosphates* **167**, 361–389. .

24. Pao, W., Miller, V. A., Politi, K. A., Riely, G. J., Somwar, R., Zakowski, M. F., Kris, M. G., and Varmus, H. (2005) Acquired resistance of lung adenocarcinomas to gefitinib or erlotinib is associated with a second mutation in the EGFR kinase domain, *PLoS Med.* **2**, e73.

25. Sawyers, C. (2004) Targeted cancer therapy, *Nature* **432**, 294–297.

26. Wolf-Yadlin, A., Kumar, N., Zhang, Y., Hautaniemi, S., Zaman, M., Kim, H. D., Grantcharova, V., Lauffenburger, D. A., and White, F. M. (2006) Effects of HER2 overexpression on cell signaling networks governing proliferation and migration, *Mol Syst Biol* **2**, 54.

27. Heinrich, M. C., Corless, C. L., Demetri, G. D., Blanke, C. D., von Mehren, M., Joensuu, H., McGreevey, L. S., Chen, C. J., Van den Abbeele, A. D., Druker, B. J., Kiese, B., Eisenberg, B., Roberts, P. J., Singer, S., Fletcher, C. D., Silberman, S., Dimitrijevic, S., and Fletcher, J. A. (2003) Kinase mutations and imatinib response in patients with metastatic gastrointestinal stromal tumor, *J. Clin. Oncol* .**21**, 4342–4349.

28. Lynch, T. J., Bell, D. W., Sordella, R., Gurubhagavatula, S., Okimoto, R. A., Brannigan, B. W., Harris, P. L., Haserlat, S. M., Supko, J. G., Haluska, F. G., Louis, D. N., Christiani, D. C., Settleman, J., and Haber, D. A. (2004) Activating mutations in the epidermal growth factor receptor underlying responsiveness of non-small-cell lung cancer to gefitinib, *N. Engl. J. Med.* **350**, 2129–2139.

29. Gorre, M. E., Mohammed, M., Ellwood, K., Hsu, N., Paquette, R., Rao, P. N., and Sawyers, C. L. (2001) Clinical resistance to STI-571 cancer therapy caused by BCR-ABL gene mutation or amplification, *Science* **293**, 876–880.

30. Kobayashi, S., Boggon, T. J., Dayaram, T., Janne, P. A., Kocher, O., Meyerson, M., Johnson, B. E., Eck, M. J., Tenen, D. G., and Halmos, B. (2005) EGFR mutation and resistance of non-small-cell lung cancer to gefitinib, *N. Engl. J. Med.* **352**, 786–792.

31. Ventura, J. J., and Nebreda, A. R. (2006) Protein kinases and phosphatases as therapeutic targets in cancer, *Clin. Transl. Oncol.* **8**, 153–160.

32. Engelman, J. A., Zejnullahu, K., Mitsudomi, T., Song, Y., Hyland, C., Park, J. O., Lindeman, N., Gale, C. M., Zhao, X., Christensen, J.,

Kosaka, T., Holmes, A. J., Rogers, A. M., Cappuzzo, F., Mok, T., Lee, C., Johnson, B. E., Cantley, L. C., and Janne, P. A. (2007) MET amplification leads to gefitinib resistance in lung cancer by activating ERBB3 signaling, *Science* **316**, 1039–1043.
33. Takano, T., Ohe, Y., Sakamoto, H., Tsuta, K., Matsuno, Y., Tateishi, U., Yamamoto, S., Nokihara, H., Yamamoto, N., Sekine, I., Kunitoh, H., Shibata, T., Sakiyama, T., Yoshida, T., and Tamura, T. (2005) Epidermal growth factor receptor gene mutations and increased copy numbers predict gefitinib sensitivity in patients with recurrent non-small-cell lung cancer, *J. Clin. Oncol.* **23**, 6829–6837.
34. Ali, S., and Ali, S. (2007) Role of c-kit/SCF in cause and treatment of gastrointestinal stromal tumors (GIST), *Gene* **401**, 38–45.
35. Engelman, J. A., Chen, L., Tan, X., Crosby, K., Guimaraes, A. R., Upadhyay, R., Maira, M., McNamara, K., Perera, S. A., Song, Y., Chirieac, L. R., Kaur, R., Lightbown, A., Simendinger, J., Li, T., Padera, R. F., Garcia-Echeverria, C., Weissleder, R., Mahmood, U., Cantley, L. C., and Wong, K. K. (2008) Effective use of PI3K and MEK inhibitors to treat mutant Kras G12D and PIK3CA H1047R murine lung cancers, *Nat. Med.* **14**, 1351–1356.
36. Weisberg, E., Manley, P. W., Breitenstein, W., Bruggen, J., Cowan-Jacob, S. W., Ray, A., Huntly, B., Fabbro, D., Fendrich, G., Hall-Meyers, E., Kung, A. L., Mestan, J., Daley, G. Q., Callahan, L., Catley, L., Cavazza, C., Azam, M., Neuberg, D., Wright, R. D., Gilliland, D. G., and Griffin, J. D. (2005) Characterization of AMN107, a selective inhibitor of native and mutant Bcr-Abl, *Cancer Cell* **7**, 129–141.
37. Quintas-Cardama, A., Kantarjian, H., and Cortes, J. (2007) Flying under the radar: the new wave of BCR-ABL inhibitors, *Nat. Rev. Drug Discov.* **6**, 834–848.
38. Adrian, F. J., Ding, Q., Sim, T., Velentza, A., Sloan, C., Liu, Y., Zhang, G., Hur, W., Ding, S., Manley, P., Mestan, J., Fabbro, D., and Gray, N. S. (2006) Allosteric inhibitors of Bcr-abl-dependent cell proliferation, *Nat. Chem. Biol.* **2**, 95–102.
39. Lombardo, L. J., Lee, F. Y., Chen, P., Norris, D., Barrish, J. C., Behnia, K., Castaneda, S., Cornelius, L. A., Das, J., Doweyko, A. M., Fairchild, C., Hunt, J. T., Inigo, I., Johnston, K., Kamath, A., Kan, D., Klei, H., Marathe, P., Pang, S., Peterson, R., Pitt, S., Schieven, G. L., Schmidt, R. J., Tokarski, J., Wen, M. L., Wityak, J., and Borzilleri, R. M. (2004) Discovery of N-(2-chloro-6-methyl- phenyl)-2-(6-(4-(2-hydroxyethyl)- piperazin-1-yl)-2-methylpyrimidin-4- ylamino)thiazole-5-carboxamide (BMS-354825), a dual Src/Abl kinase inhibitor with potent antitumor activity in preclinical assays, *J. Med. Chem.* **47**, 6658–6661.
40. Zhang, J., Adrian, F.J., Jahnke, W., Cowan-Jacob, S.W., Li, A.G., Iacob, R.E., Sim, T.,Powers, J. , Dierks, C. , Sun, F., Guo, G.R., Ding, Q., Okram, B. , Choi, Y.,Wojciechowski, A., Deng, X., Liu, G., Fendrich, G., Strauss, A., Vajpai, N., Grzesiek, S., Tuntland, T., Liu, Y., Bursulaya, B., Azam, M., Manley, P.W., Engen, J.R., Daley, G.Q., Warmuth, M., Gray, N.S. (2010) Targeting wild-type and T315I Bcr-Abl by combining allosteric with ATP-site inhibitors, *Nature* **463**, 501–506.
41. Noble, M. E., Endicott, J. A., and Johnson, L. N. (2004) Protein kinase inhibitors: insights into drug design from structure, *Science* **303**, 1800–1805.
42. Bogoyevitch, M. A., and Fairlie, D. P. (2007) A new paradigm for protein kinase inhibition: blocking phosphorylation without directly targeting ATP binding, *Drug Discov. Today* **12**, 622–633.
43. Druker, B. J., Tamura, S., Buchdunger, E., Ohno, S., Segal, G. M., Fanning, S., Zimmermann, J., and Lydon, N. B. (1996) Effects of a selective inhibitor of the Abl tyrosine kinase on the growth of Bcr-Abl positive cells, *Nat. Med.* **2**, 561–566.
44. Barker, A. J., Gibson, K. H., Grundy, W., Godfrey, A. A., Barlow, J. J., Healy, M. P., Woodburn, J. R., Ashton, S. E., Curry, B. J., Scarlett, L., Henthorn, L., and Richards, L. (2001) Studies leading to the identification of ZD1839 (IRESSA): an orally active, selective epidermal growth factor receptor tyrosine kinase inhibitor targeted to the treatment of cancer, *Bioorg. Med. Chem. Lett.* **11**, 1911–1914.
45. Perez-Soler, R. (2004) The role of erlotinib (Tarceva, OSI 774) in the treatment of non-small cell lung cancer, *Clin. Cancer Res.* **10**, 4238s–4240s.
46. Moyer, J. D., Barbacci, E. G., Iwata, K. K., Arnold, L., Boman, B., Cunningham, A., DiOrio, C., Doty, J., Morin, M. J., Moyer, M. P., Neveu, M., Pollack, V. A., Pustilnik, L. R., Reynolds, M. M., Sloan, D., Theleman, A., and Miller, P. (1997) Induction of apoptosis and cell cycle arrest by CP-358,774, an inhibitor of epidermal growth factor receptor tyrosine kinase, *Cancer Res.* **57**, 4838–4848.
47. Gaul, M. D., Guo, Y., Affleck, K., Cockerill, G. S., Gilmer, T. M., Griffin, R. J., Guntrip,

S., Keith, B. R., Knight, W. B., Mullin, R. J., Murray, D. M., Rusnak, D. W., Smith, K., Tadepalli, S., Wood, E. R., and Lackey, K. (2003) Discovery and biological evaluation of potent dual ErbB-2/EGFR tyrosine kinase inhibitors: 6-thiazolylquinazolines, *Bioorg. Med. Chem. Lett.* **13**, 637–640.

48. Lowinger, T. B., Riedl, B., Dumas, J., and Smith, R. A. (2002) Design and discovery of small molecules targeting raf-1 kinase, *Curr. Pharm. Des.* **8**, 2269–2278.

49. Sun, L., Liang, C., Shirazian, S., Zhou, Y., Miller, T., Cui, J., Fukuda, J. Y., Chu, J. Y., Nematalla, A., Wang, X., Chen, H., Sistla, A., Luu, T. C., Tang, F., Wei, J., and Tang, C. (2003) Discovery of 5-(5-fluoro-2-oxo-1,2-dihydroindol-(3Z)-ylidenemethyl)-2,4- dimethyl-1H-pyrrole-3-carboxylic acid (2-diethylaminoethyl)amide, a novel tyrosine kinase inhibitor targeting vascular endothelial and platelet-derived growth factor receptor tyrosine kinase, *J. Med. Chem.* **46**, 1116–1119.

50. Sternberg, C.N., Szcylik, C. Lee, E., Salman, P.V., Mardiak, J., Davis, I.D., Pandite, L., Chen M., McCann,L. and Hawkins, R. (2009) A Randomized, Double-blind Phase III Study of Pazopanib in Treatment-naive and Cytokine-pretreated Patients with Advanced Renal Cell Carcinoma (RCC), *J. Clin. Oncol.* **27**, Abstract #5021.

51. Galanis, E., Buckner, J. C., Maurer, M. J., Kreisberg, J. I., Ballman, K., Boni, J., Peralba, J. M., Jenkins, R. B., Dakhil, S. R., Morton, R. F., Jaeckle, K. A., Scheithauer, B. W., Dancey, J., Hidalgo, M., and Walsh, D. J. (2005) Phase II trial of temsirolimus (CCI-779) in recurrent glioblastoma multiforme: a North Central Cancer Treatment Group Study, *J. Clin. Oncol.* **23**, 5294–5304.

52. Escudier, B. (2008) Phase-3 randomized trial of everolimus (RAD001) vs. placebo in metastatic renal cell carcinoma, *European Society for Medical Oncology (ESMO) 33rd Congress.*

53. Wang, X., and Sun, S. Y. (2009) Enhancing mTOR-targeted cancer therapy, *Expert Opin. Ther. Targets* **13**, 1193–1203.

54. Pascual, J. (2006) Everolimus in clinical practice--renal transplantation, *Nephrol. Dial. Transplant.* **21** Suppl 3, iii18–23.

55. Trials. (2009) http://www.clinicaltrials.gov/.

56. Druker, B. J., Talpaz, M., Resta, D. J., Peng, B., Buchdunger, E., Ford, J. M., Lydon, N. B., Kantarjian, H., Capdeville, R., Ohno-Jones, S., and Sawyers, C. L. (2001) Efficacy and safety of a specific inhibitor of the BCR-ABL tyrosine kinase in chronic myeloid leukemia, *N. Engl. J. Med.* **344**, 1031–1037.

57. Van Etten, R. A., and Shannon, K. M. (2004) Focus on myeloproliferative diseases and myelodysplastic syndromes, *Cancer Cell* **6**, 547–552.

58. Demetri, G. D., von Mehren, M., Blanke, C. D., Van den Abbeele, A. D., Eisenberg, B., Roberts, P. J., Heinrich, M. C., Tuveson, D. A., Singer, S., Janicek, M., Fletcher, J. A., Silverman, S. G., Silberman, S. L., Capdeville, R., Kiese, B., Peng, B., Dimitrijevic, S., Druker, B. J., Corless, C., Fletcher, C. D., and Joensuu, H. (2002) Efficacy and safety of imatinib mesylate in advanced gastrointestinal stromal tumors, *N. Engl. J. Med.* **347**, 472–480.

59. Siehl, J., and Thiel, E. (2007) C-kit, GIST, and imatinib, *Recent Results Cancer Res.* **176**, 145–151.

60. Buchdunger, E., Cioffi, C. L., Law, N., Stover, D., Ohno-Jones, S., Druker, B. J., and Lydon, N. B. (2000) Abl protein-tyrosine kinase inhibitor STI571 inhibits in vitro signal transduction mediated by c-kit and platelet-derived growth factor receptors, *J. Pharmacol. Exp. Ther.* **295**, 139–145.

61. Heinrich, M. C., Corless, C. L., Duensing, A., McGreevey, L., Chen, C. J., Joseph, N., Singer, S., Griffith, D. J., Haley, A., Town, A., Demetri, G. D., Fletcher, C. D., and Fletcher, J. A. (2003) PDGFRA activating mutations in gastrointestinal stromal tumors, *Science* **299**, 708–710.

62. McArthur, G. A., Demetri, G. D., van Oosterom, A., Heinrich, M. C., Debiec-Rychter, M., Corless, C. L., Nikolova, Z., Dimitrijevic, S., and Fletcher, J. A. (2005) Molecular and clinical analysis of locally advanced dermatofibrosarcoma protuberans treated with imatinib: Imatinib Target Exploration Consortium Study B2225, *J. Clin. Oncol.* **23**, 866–873.

63. Apperley, J. F., Gardembas, M., Melo, J. V., Russell-Jones, R., Bain, B. J., Baxter, E. J., Chase, A., Chessells, J. M., Colombat, M., Dearden, C. E., Dimitrijevic, S., Mahon, F. X., Marin, D., Nikolova, Z., Olavarria, E., Silberman, S., Schultheis, B., Cross, N. C., and Goldman, J. M. (2002) Response to imatinib mesylate in patients with chronic myeloproliferative diseases with rearrangements of the platelet-derived growth factor receptor beta, *N. Engl. J. Med.* **347**, 481–487.

64. Antoniu, S. A. (2009) Targeting platelet-derived growth factor with imatinib in idiopathic pulmonary arterial hypertension, *Expert. Opin. Ther. Targets* **13**, 381–383.

65. Steinberg, M. (2007) Dasatinib: a tyrosine kinase inhibitor for the treatment of chronic

myelogenous leukemia and philadelphia chromosome-positive acute lymphoblastic leukemia, *Clin. Ther.* **29**, 2289–2308.
66. Motzer, R. J., Hoosen, S., Bello, C. L., and Christensen, J. G. (2006) Sunitinib malate for the treatment of solid tumours: a review of current clinical data, *Expert Opin. Investig. Drugs* **15**, 553–561.
67. Motzer, R. J., Rini, B. I., Bukowski, R. M., Curti, B. D., George, D. J., Hudes, G. R., Redman, B. G., Margolin, K. A., Merchan, J. R., Wilding, G., Ginsberg, M. S., Bacik, J., Kim, S. T., Baum, C. M., and Michaelson, M. D. (2006) Sunitinib in patients with metastatic renal cell carcinoma, *Jama* **295**, 2516–2524.
68. Faivre, S., Demetri, G., Sargent, W., and Raymond, E. (2007) Molecular basis for sunitinib efficacy and future clinical development, *Nat. Rev. Drug Discov.* **6**, 734–745.
69. Wilhelm, S., Carter, C., Lynch, M., Lowinger, T., Dumas, J., Smith, R. A., Schwartz, B., Simantov, R., and Kelley, S. (2006) Discovery and development of sorafenib: a multikinase inhibitor for treating cancer, *Nat. Rev. Drug Discov.* **5**, 835–844.
70. Keating, G. M., and Santoro, A. (2009) Sorafenib: a review of its use in advanced hepatocellular carcinoma, *Drugs* **69**, 223–240.
71. Hynes, N. E., and Lane, H. A. (2005) ERBB receptors and cancer: the complexity of targeted inhibitors, *Nat. Rev. Cancer* **5**, 341–354.
72. Citri, A., and Yarden, Y. (2006) EGF-ERBB signalling: towards the systems level, *Nat. Rev. Mol. Cell Biol.* **7**, 505–516.
73. Muhsin, M., Graham, J., and Kirkpatrick, P. (2003) Gefitinib, *Nat. Rev. Drug Discov.* **2**, 515–516.
74. Dowell, J., Minna, J. D., and Kirkpatrick, P. (2005) Erlotinib hydrochloride, *Nat. Rev. Drug Discov.* **4**, 13–14.
75. Moy, B., Kirkpatrick, P., Kar, S., and Goss, P. (2007) Lapatinib, *Nat. Rev. Drug Discov.* **6**, 431–432.
76. Ma, W. W. J., A. (2007) Temsirolimus, *Drugs Today* **43**, 659–669.
77. Atkins, M. B., Yasothan, U., and Kirkpatrick, P. (2009) Everolimus, *Nat. Rev. Drug Discov.* **8**, 535–536.
78. Fabian, M. A., Biggs, W. H., 3rd, Treiber, D. K., Atteridge, C. E., Azimioara, M. D., Benedetti, M. G., Carter, T. A., Ciceri, P., Edeen, P. T., Floyd, M., Ford, J. M., Galvin, M., Gerlach, J. L., Grotzfeld, R. M., Herrgard, S., Insko, D. E., Insko, M. A., Lai, A. G., Lelias, J. M., Mehta, S. A., Milanov, Z. V., Velasco, A. M., Wodicka, L. M., Patel, H. K., Zarrinkar, P. P., and Lockhart, D. J. (2005) A small molecule-kinase interaction map for clinical kinase inhibitors, *Nat. Biotechnol.* **23**, 329–336.
79. Karaman, M. W., Herrgard, S., Treiber, D. K., Gallant, P., Atteridge, C. E., Campbell, B. T., Chan, K. W., Ciceri, P., Davis, M. I., Edeen, P. T., Faraoni, R., Floyd, M., Hunt, J. P., Lockhart, D. J., Milanov, Z. V., Morrison, M. J., Pallares, G., Patel, H. K., Pritchard, S., Wodicka, L. M., and Zarrinkar, P. P. (2008) A quantitative analysis of kinase inhibitor selectivity, *Nat. Biotechnol.* **26**, 127–132.
80. Melnick, J. S., Janes, J., Kim, S., Chang, J. Y., Sipes, D. G., Gunderson, D., Jarnes, L., Matzen, J. T., Garcia, M. E., Hood, T. L., Beigi, R., Xia, G., Harig, R. A., Asatryan, H., Yan, S. F., Zhou, Y., Gu, X. J., Saadat, A., Zhou, V., King, F. J., Shaw, C. M., Su, A. I., Downs, R., Gray, N. S., Schultz, P. G., Warmuth, M., and Caldwell, J. S. (2006) An efficient rapid system for profiling the cellular activities of molecular libraries, *Proc. Natl. Acad. Sci. USA* **103**, 3153–3158.
81. Aklilu, M., Kindler, H. L., Donehower, R. C., Mani, S., and Vokes, E. E. (2003) Phase II study of flavopiridol in patients with advanced colorectal cancer, *Ann. Oncol.* **14**, 1270–1273.
82. Morris, D. G., Bramwell, V. H., Turcotte, R., Figueredo, A. T., Blackstein, M. E., Verma, S., Matthews, S., and Eisenhauer, E. A. (2006) A Phase II Study of Flavopiridol in Patients With Previously Untreated Advanced Soft Tissue Sarcoma, *Sarcoma* **2006**, 64374.
83. Scott, E. N., Meinhardt, G., Jacques, C., Laurent, D., and Thomas, A. L. (2007) Vatalanib: the clinical development of a tyrosine kinase inhibitor of angiogenesis in solid tumours, *Expert Opin. Investig. Drugs* **16**, 367–379.
84. Tyagi, P. (2005) Vatalanib (PTK787/ZK 222584) in combination with FOLFOX4 versus FOLFOX4 alone as first-line treatment for colorectal cancer: preliminary results from the CONFIRM-1 trial, *Clin. Colorectal Cancer* **5**, 24–26.
85. Cohen, P. (2001) The role of protein phosphorylation in human health and disease. The Sir Hans Krebs Medal Lecture, *Eur. J. Biochem.* **268**, 5001–5010.
86. Nolen, B., Taylor, S., and Ghosh, G. (2004) Regulation of protein kinases; controlling activity through activation segment conformation, *Mol. Cell.* **15**, 661–675.
87. Liu, Y., Gray, N. S. (2006) Rational design of inhibitors that bind to inactive kinase conformations, *Nat. Chem. Biol.* **2**, 358–364.

88. Scapin, G. (2006) Protein kinase inhibition: different approaches to selective inhibitor design, *Curr. Drug Targets* 7, 1443–1454.

89. Traxler, P., Bold, G., Buchdunger, E., Caravatti, G., Furet, P., Manley, P., O'Reilly, T., Wood, J., and Zimmermann, J. (2001) Tyrosine kinase inhibitors: from rational design to clinical trials, *Med. Res. Rev.* 21, 499–512.

90. Kwak, E. L., Sordella, R., Bell, D. W., Godin-Heymann, N., Okimoto, R. A., Brannigan, B. W., Harris, P. L., Driscoll, D. R., Fidias, P., Lynch, T. J., Rabindran, S. K., McGinnis, J. P., Wissner, A., Sharma, S. V., Isselbacher, K. J., Settleman, J., and Haber, D. A. (2005) Irreversible inhibitors of the EGF receptor may circumvent acquired resistance to gefitinib, *Proc. Natl. Acad. Sci. USA* 102, 7665–7670.

91. Rabindran, S. K., Discafani, C. M., Rosfjord, E. C., Baxter, M., Floyd, M. B., Golas, J., Hallett, W. A., Johnson, B. D., Nilakantan, R., Overbeek, E., Reich, M. F., Shen, R., Shi, X., Tsou, H. R., Wang, Y. F., and Wissner, A. (2004) Antitumor activity of HKI-272, an orally active, irreversible inhibitor of the HER-2 tyrosine kinase, *Cancer Res.* 64, 3958–3965.

92. Rastelli, G., Rosenfeld, R., Reid, R., and Santi, D. V. (2008) Molecular modeling and crystal structure of ERK2-hypothemycin complexes, *J. Struct. Biol.* 164, 18–23.

93. Heymach, J. V., Nilsson, M., Blumenschein, G., Papadimitrakopoulou, V., and Herbst, R. (2006) Epidermal growth factor receptor inhibitors in development for the treatment of non-small cell lung cancer, *Clin. Cancer Res.* 12, 4441s-4445s.

94. Felip, E., Santarpia, M., and Rosell, R. (2007) Emerging drugs for non-small-cell lung cancer, *Expert Opin. Emerg. Drugs* 12, 449–460.

95. Filippakopoulos, P., Kofler, M., Hantschel, O., Gish, G. D., Grebien, F., Salah, E., Neudecker, P., Kay, L. E., Turk, B. E., Superti-Furga, G., Pawson, T., and Knapp, S. (2008) Structural coupling of SH2-kinase domains links Fes and Abl substrate recognition and kinase activation, *Cell* 134, 793–803.

96. Wissner, A., Fraser, H. L., Ingalls, C. L., Dushin, R. G., Floyd, M. B., Cheung, K., Nittoli, T., Ravi, M. R., Tan, X., and Loganzo, F. (2007) Dual irreversible kinase inhibitors: quinazoline-based inhibitors incorporating two independent reactive centers with each targeting different cysteine residues in the kinase domains of EGFR and VEGFR-2, *Bioorg. Med. Chem.* 15, 3635–3648.

97. Pan, Z., Scheerens, H., Li, S. J., Schultz, B. E., Sprengeler, P. A., Burrill, L. C., Mendonca, R. V., Sweeney, M. D., Scott, K. C., Grothaus, P. G., Jeffery, D. A., Spoerke, J. M., Honigberg, L. A., Young, P. R., Dalrymple, S. A., and Palmer, J. T. (2007) Discovery of selective irreversible inhibitors for Bruton's tyrosine kinase, *ChemMedChem.* 2, 58–61.

98. Cohen, M. S., Hadjivassiliou, H., and Taunton, J. (2007) A clickable inhibitor reveals context-dependent autoactivation of p90 RSK, *Nat. Chem. Biol.* 3, 156–160.

99. Wymann, M. P., Bulgarelli-Leva, G., Zvelebil, M. J., Pirola, L., Vanhaesebroeck, B., Waterfield, M. D., and Panayotou, G. (1996) Wortmannin inactivates phosphoinositide 3-kinase by covalent modification of Lys-802, a residue involved in the phosphate transfer reaction, *Mol. Cell. Biol.* 16, 1722–1733.

100. Ohren, J. F., Chen, H., Pavlovsky, A., Whitehead, C., Zhang, E., Kuffa, P., Yan, C., McConnell, P., Spessard, C., Banotai, C., Mueller, W. T., Delaney, A., Omer, C., Sebolt-Leopold, J., Dudley, D. T., Leung, I. K., Flamme, C., Warmus, J., Kaufman, M., Barrett, S., Tecle, H., and Hasemann, C. A. (2004) Structures of human MAP kinase kinase 1 (MEK1) and MEK2 describe novel noncompetitive kinase inhibition, *Nat. Struct. Mol. Biol.* 11, 1192–1197.

101. Barnett, S. F., Defeo-Jones, D., Fu, S., Hancock, P. J., Haskell, K. M., Jones, R. E., Kahana, J. A., Kral, A. M., Leander, K., Lee, L. L., Malinowski, J., McAvoy, E. M., Nahas, D. D., Robinson, R. G., and Huber, H. E. (2005) Identification and characterization of pleckstrin-homology-domain-dependent and isoenzyme-specific Akt inhibitors, *Biochem. J.* 385, 399–408.

102. Lindsley, C. W., Zhao, Z., Leister, W. H., Robinson, R. G., Barnett, S. F., Defeo-Jones, D., Jones, R. E., Hartman, G. D., Huff, J. R., Huber, H. E., and Duggan, M. E. (2005) Allosteric Akt (PKB) inhibitors: discovery and SAR of isozyme selective inhibitors, *Bioorg. Med. Chem. Lett.* 15, 761–764.

103. McIntyre, K. W., Shuster, D. J., Gillooly, K. M., Dambach, D. M., Pattoli, M. A., Lu, P., Zhou, X. D., Qiu, Y., Zusi, F. C., and Burke, J. R. (2003) A highly selective inhibitor of I kappa B kinase, BMS-345541, blocks both joint inflammation and destruction in collagen-induced arthritis in mice, *Arthritis Rheum.* 48, 2652–2659.

104. Vanderpool, D., Johnson, T. O., Ping, C., Bergqvist, S., Alton, G., Phonephaly, S., Rui, E., Luo, C., Deng, Y. L., Grant, S., Quenzer, T., Margosiak, S., Register, J., Brown, E., and Ermolieff, J. (2009) Characterization of the CHK1 allosteric inhibitor binding site, *Biochemistry* 48, 9823–9830.

105. Converso, A., Hartingh, T., Garbaccio, R. M., Tasber, E., Rickert, K., Fraley, M. E., Yan, Y., Kreatsoulas, C., Stirdivant, S., Drakas, B., Walsh, E. S., Hamilton, K., Buser, C. A., Mao, X., Abrams, M. T., Beck, S. C., Tao, W., Lobell, R., Sepp-Lorenzino, L., Zugay-Murphy, J., Sardana, V., Munshi, S. K., Jezequel-Sur, S. M., Zuck, P. D., and Hartman, G. D. (2009) Development of thioquinazolinones, allosteric Chk1 kinase inhibitors, *Bioorg. Med. Chem. Lett.* **19**, 1240–1244.

106. Wood, E. R., Truesdale, A. T., McDonald, O. B., Yuan, D., Hassell, A., Dickerson, S. H., Ellis, B., Pennisi, C., Horne, E., Lackey, K., Alligood, K. J., Rusnak, D. W., Gilmer, T. M., and Shewchuk, L. (2004) A unique structure for epidermal growth factor receptor bound to GW572016 (Lapatinib): relationships among protein conformation, inhibitor off-rate, and receptor activity in tumor cells, *Cancer Res.* **64**, 6652–6659.

107. Schindler, T., Sicheri, F., Pico, A., Gazit, A., Levitzki, A., and Kuriyan, J. (1999) Crystal structure of Hck in complex with a Src family-selective tyrosine kinase inhibitor, *Mol. Cell* **3**, 639–648.

108. Levinson, N. M., Kuchment, O., Shen, K., Young, M. A., Koldobskiy, M., Karplus, M., Cole, P. A., and Kuriyan, J. (2006) A Src-like inactive conformation in the abl tyrosine kinase domain, *PLoS Biol.* **4**, e144.

109. Hodous, B. L., Geuns-Meyer, S. D., Hughes, P. E., Albrecht, B. K., Bellon, S., Bready, J., Caenepeel, S., Cee, V. J., Chaffee, S. C., Coxon, A., Emery, M., Fretland, J., Gallant, P., Gu, Y., Hoffman, D., Johnson, R. E., Kendall, R., Kim, J. L., Long, A. M., Morrison, M., Olivieri, P. R., Patel, V. F., Polverino, A., Rose, P., Tempest, P., Wang, L., Whittington, D. A., and Zhao, H. (2007) Evolution of a highly selective and potent 2-(pyridin-2-yl)-1,3,5-triazine Tie-2 kinase inhibitor, *J. Med. Chem.* **50**, 611–626.

110. Schroeder, G. M., Chen, X. T., Williams, D. K., Nirschl, D. S., Cai, Z. W., Wei, D., Tokarski, J. S., An, Y., Sack, J., Chen, Z., Huynh, T., Vaccaro, W., Poss, M., Wautlet, B., Gullo-Brown, J., Kellar, K., Manne, V., Hunt, J. T., Wong, T. W., Lombardo, L. J., Fargnoli, J., and Borzilleri, R. M. (2008) Identification of pyrrolo(2,1-f)(1,2,4)triazine-based inhibitors of Met kinase, *Bioorg. Med. Chem. Lett.* **18**, 1945–1951.

111. Tummino, P. J., and Copeland, R. A. (2008) Residence time of receptor-ligand complexes and its effect on biological function, *Biochemistry* **47**, 5481–5492.

112. Kufareva, I., and Abagyan, R. (2008) Type-II kinase inhibitor docking, screening, and profiling using modified structures of active kinase states, *J. Med. Chem.* **51**, 7921–7932.

113. Grimsby, J., Sarabu, R., Corbett, W. L., Haynes, N. E., Bizzarro, F. T., Coffey, J. W., Guertin, K. R., Hilliard, D. W., Kester, R. F., Mahaney, P. E., Marcus, L., Qi, L., Spence, C. L., Tengi, J., Magnuson, M. A., Chu, C. A., Dvorozniak, M. T., Matschinsky, F. M., and Grippo, J. F. (2003) Allosteric activators of glucokinase: potential role in diabetes therapy, *Science* **301**, 370–373.

114. Guertin, K. R., and Grimsby, J. (2006) Small molecule glucokinase activators as glucose lowering agents: a new paradigm for diabetes therapy, *Curr. Med. Chem.* **13**, 1839–1843.

115. Sanders, M. J., Ali, Z. S., Hegarty, B. D., Heath, R., Snowden, M. A., and Carling, D. (2007) Defining the mechanism of activation of AMP-activated protein kinase by the small molecule A-769662, a member of the thienopyridone family, *J. Biol. Chem.* **282**, 32539–32548.

116. Hindie, V., Stroba, A., Zhang, H., Lopez-Garcia, L. A., Idrissova, L., Zeuzem, S., Hirschberg, D., Schaeffer, F., Jorgensen, T. J., Engel, M., Alzari, P. M., and Biondi, R. M. (2009) Structure and allosteric effects of low-molecular-weight activators on the protein kinase PDK1, *Nat. Chem. Biol.* **5**, 758–764.

117. Kaelin, W. G., Jr. (2005) The concept of synthetic lethality in the context of anticancer therapy, *Nat. Rev. Cancer* **5**, 689–698.

118. Weinstein, I. B., Begemann, M., Zhou, P., Han, E. K., Sgambato, A., Doki, Y., Arber, N., Ciaparrone, M., and Yamamoto, H. (1997) Disorders in cell circuitry associated with multistage carcinogenesis: exploitable targets for cancer prevention and therapy, *Clin. Cancer Res.* **3**, 2696–2702.

119. Cappuzzo, F., Hirsch, F. R., Rossi, E., Bartolini, S., Ceresoli, G. L., Bemis, L., Haney, J., Witta, S., Danenberg, K., Domenichini, I., Ludovini, V., Magrini, E., Gregorc, V., Doglioni, C., Sidoni, A., Tonato, M., Franklin, W. A., Crino, L., Bunn, P. A., Jr., and Varella-Garcia, M. (2005) Epidermal growth factor receptor gene and protein and gefitinib sensitivity in non-small-cell lung cancer, *J. Natl. Cancer. Inst.* **97**, 643–655.

120. Mellinghoff, I. K., Wang, M. Y., Vivanco, I., Haas-Kogan, D. A., Zhu, S., Dia, E. Q., Lu, K. V., Yoshimoto, K., Huang, J. H., Chute, D. J., Riggs, B. L., Horvath, S., Liau, L. M., Cavenee, W. K., Rao, P. N., Beroukhim, R., Peck, T. C., Lee, J. C., Sellers, W. R., Stokoe, D., Prados, M., Cloughesy, T. F., Sawyers, C. L., and Mischel, P. S. (2005) Molecular determinants of the response of glioblastomas to EGFR kinase inhibitors, *N. Engl. J. Med.* **353**, 2012–2024.

121. Taron, M., Ichinose, Y., Rosell, R., Mok, T., Massuti, B., Zamora, L., Mate, J. L., Manegold, C., Ono, M., Queralt, C., Jahan, T., Sanchez, J. J., Sanchez-Ronco, M., Hsue, V., Jablons, D., Sanchez, J. M., and Moran, T. (2005) Activating mutations in the tyrosine kinase domain of the epidermal growth factor receptor are associated with improved survival in gefitinib-treated chemorefractory lung adenocarcinomas, *Clin. Cancer Res.* **11**, 5878–5885.

122. Riedemann, J., and Macaulay, V. M. (2006) IGF1R signalling and its inhibition, *Endocr. Relat. Cancer* **13 Suppl 1**, S33-43.

123. Zwick, E., Bange, J., and Ullrich, A. (2002) Receptor tyrosine kinases as targets for anticancer drugs, *Trends Mol. Med.* **8**, 17–23.

124. Fruman, D. A., Meyers, R. E., and Cantley, L. C. (1998) Phosphoinositide kinases, *Annu. Rev. Biochem.* **67**, 481–507.

125. Chen, H. X., and Cleck, J. N. (2009) Adverse effects of anticancer agents that target the VEGF pathway, *Nat. Rev. Clin. Onco.l* **6**, 465–477.

126. Ivy, S. P., Wick, J. Y., and Kaufman, B. M. (2009) An overview of small-molecule inhibitors of VEGFR signaling, *Nat. Rev. Clin. Oncol.* **6**, 569–579.

127. Murakami, M., and Simons, M. (2008) Fibroblast growth factor regulation of neovascularization, *Curr. Opin. Hematol.* **15**, 215–220.

128. Kaelin, W. G., Jr. (2004) Gleevec: prototype or outlier?, *Sci. STKE 2004*, pe12.

129. Dancey, J. E., and Chen, H. X. (2006) Strategies for optimizing combinations of molecularly targeted anticancer agents, *Nat. Rev. Drug. Discov.* **5**, 649–659.

130. Force, T., Krause, D. S., and Van Etten, R. A. (2007) Molecular mechanisms of cardiotoxicity of tyrosine kinase inhibition, *Nat. Rev. Cancer.* **7**, 332–344.

131. Olaharski, A. J., Gonzaludo, N., Bitter, H., Goldstein, D., Kirchner, S., Uppal, H., and Kolaja, K. (2009) Identification of a kinase profile that predicts chromosome damage induced by small molecule kinase inhibitors, *PLoS Comput. Biol.* **5**, e1000446.

132. Goldstein, D. M., Gray, N. S., and Zarrinkar, P. P. (2008) High-throughput kinase profiling as a platform for drug discovery, *Nat. Rev. Drug Discov.* **7**, 391–397.

133. Seeliger, M. A., Nagar, B., Frank, F., Cao, X., Henderson, M. N., and Kuriyan, J. (2007) c-Src binds to the cancer drug imatinib with an inactive Abl/c-Kit conformation and a distributed thermodynamic penalty, *Structure* **15**, 299–311.

134. Nagar, B., Hantschel, O., Young, M. A., Scheffzek, K., Veach, D., Bornmann, W., Clarkson, B., Superti-Furga, G., and Kuriyan, J. (2003) Structural basis for the autoinhibition of c-Abl tyrosine kinase, *Cell* **112**, 859–871.

135. Dar, A. C., Lopez, M. S., and Shokat, K. M. (2008) Small molecule recognition of c-Src via the Imatinib-binding conformation, *Chem. Biol.* **15**, 1015–1022.

136. Xu, W., Harrison, S. C., and Eck, M. J. (1997) Three-dimensional structure of the tyrosine kinase c-Src, *Nature* **385**, 595–602.

137. Szakacs, G., Paterson, J. K., Ludwig, J. A., Booth-Genthe, C., and Gottesman, M. M. (2006) Targeting multidrug resistance in cancer, *Nat. Rev. Drug Discov.* **5**, 219–234.

138. Fletcher, J. A., and Rubin, B. P. (2007) KIT mutations in GIST, *Curr. Opin. Genet. Dev.* **17**, 3–7.

139. Cools, J., Mentens, N., Furet, P., Fabbro, D., Clark, J. J., Griffin, J. D., Marynen, P., and Gilliland, D. G. (2004) Prediction of resistance to small molecule FLT3 inhibitors: implications for molecularly targeted therapy of acute leukemia, *Cancer Res.* **64**, 6385–6389.

140. Cools, J., Stover, E. H., Boulton, C. L., Gotlib, J., Legare, R. D., Amaral, S. M., Curley, D. P., Duclos, N., Rowan, R., Kutok, J. L., Lee, B. H., Williams, I. R., Coutre, S. E., Stone, R. M., DeAngelo, D. J., Marynen, P., Manley, P. W., Meyer, T., Fabbro, D., Neuberg, D., Weisberg, E., Griffin, J. D., and Gilliland, D. G. (2003) PKC412 overcomes resistance to imatinib in a murine model of FIP1L1-PDGFRalpha-induced myeloproliferative disease, *Cancer Cell* **3**, 459–469.

141. Blencke, S., Zech, B., Engkvist, O., Greff, Z., Orfi, L., Horvath, Z., Keri, G., Ullrich, A., and Daub, H. (2004) Characterization of a conserved structural determinant controlling protein kinase sensitivity to selective inhibitors, *Chem. Biol.* **11**, 691–701.

142. Daub, H., Specht, K., and Ullrich, A. (2004) Strategies to overcome resistance to targeted protein kinase inhibitors, *Nat. Rev. Drug Discov.* **3**, 1001–1010.

143. Bishop, A. C. (2004) A hot spot for protein kinase inhibitor sensitivity, *Chem. Biol.* **11**, 587–589.

144. Graham, S. M., Jorgensen, H. G., Allan, E., Pearson, C., Alcorn, M. J., Richmond, L., and Holyoake, T. L. (2002) Primitive, quiescent, Philadelphia-positive stem cells from patients with chronic myeloid leukemia are insensitive to STI571 in vitro, *Blood* **99**, 319–325.

145. le Coutre, P., Tassi, E., Varella-Garcia, M., Barni, R., Mologni, L., Cabrita, G., Marchesi, E.,

Supino, R., and Gambacorti-Passerini, C. (2000) Induction of resistance to the Abelson inhibitor STI571 in human leukemic cells through gene amplification, *Blood* **95**, 1758–1766.

146. O'Hare, T., Shakespeare, W. C., Zhu, X., Eide, C. A., Rivera, V. M., Wang, F., Adrian, L. T., Zhou, T., Huang, W. S., Xu, Q., Metcalf, C. A., 3rd, Tyner, J. W., Loriaux, M. M., Corbin, A. S., Wardwell, S., Ning, Y., Keats, J. A., Wang, Y., Sundaramoorthi, R., Thomas, M., Zhou, D., Snodgrass, J., Commodore, L., Sawyer, T. K., Dalgarno, D. C., Deininger, M. W., Druker, B. J., and Clackson, T. (2009) AP24534, a pan-BCR-ABL inhibitor for chronic myeloid leukemia, potently inhibits the T315I mutant and overcomes mutation-based resistance, *Cancer Cell* **16**, 401–412.

147. Gumireddy, K., Reddy, M. V., Cosenza, S. C., Boominathan, R., Baker, S. J., Papathi, N., Jiang, J., Holland, J., and Reddy, E. P. (2005) ON01910, a non-ATP-competitive small molecule inhibitor of Plk1, is a potent anticancer agent, *Cancer Cell* **7**, 275–286.

148. Fabbro, D., Manley, P.W., Jahnke, W., Liebetanz, J., Szyttenholm, A., Fendrich, G., Strauss, A., Zhang, J., Gray, N.S., Adrian, F., Warmuth, M. , Pelle, X., Grotzfeld, R., Berst, F., Marzinzik, A., Furet, P., Cowan-Jacob, S.W., Mestan, J. (2010) Inhibitors of the Abl kinase directed at either the ATP- or myristate-binding site *Biochem. Biophys. Acta* **1804**, 454–462.

149. Gorre, M. E., Ellwood-Yen, K., Chiosis, G., Rosen, N., and Sawyers, C. L. (2002) BCR-ABL point mutants isolated from patients with imatinib mesylate-resistant chronic myeloid leukemia remain sensitive to inhibitors of the BCR-ABL chaperone heat shock protein 90, *Blood* **100**, 3041–3044.

150. Copland, M., Pellicano, F., Richmond, L., Allan, E. K., Hamilton, A., Lee, F. Y., Weinmann, R., and Holyoake, T. L. (2008) BMS-214662 potently induces apoptosis of chronic myeloid leukemia stem and progenitor cells and synergizes with tyrosine kinase inhibitors, *Blood* **111**, 2843–2853.

151. Steiner, L., Blum, G., Friedmann, Y., and Levitzki, A. (2007) ATP non-competitive IGF-1 receptor kinase inhibitors as lead antineoplastic and anti-papilloma agents, *European Journal of Pharmacology* **562**, 1–11.

152. Biondi, R. M., and Nebreda, A. R. (2003) Signalling specificity of Ser/Thr protein kinases through docking-site-mediated interactions, *Biochem. J.* **372**, 1–13.

153. Sheridan, D. L., Kong, Y., Parker, S. A., Dalby, K. N., and Turk, B. E. (2008) Substrate discrimination among mitogen-activated protein kinases through distinct docking sequence motifs, *J. Biol. Chem.* **283**, 19511–19520.

154. Robert, C., Soria, J. C., Spatz, A., Le Cesne, A., Malka, D., Pautier, P., Wechsler, J., Lhomme, C., Escudier, B., Boige, V., Armand, J. P., and Le Chevalier, T. (2005) Cutaneous side-effects of kinase inhibitors and blocking antibodies, *Lancet Oncol.* **6**, 491–500.

155. Hur, W., Velentza, A., Kim, S., Flatauer, L., Jiang, X., Valente, D., Mason, D. E., Suzuki, M., Larson, B., Zhang, J., Zagorska, A., Didonato, M., Nagle, A., Warmuth, M., Balk, S. P., Peters, E. C., and Gray, N. S. (2008) Clinical stage EGFR inhibitors irreversibly alkylate Bmx kinase, *Bioorg Med. Chem. Lett.* **18**(22), 5916–5919.

156. Walker, E. H., Pacold, M. E., Perisic, O., Stephens, L., Hawkins, P. T., Wymann, M. P., and Williams, R. L. (2000) Structural determinants of phosphoinositide 3-kinase inhibition by wortmannin, LY294002, quercetin, myricetin, and staurosporine, *Mol. Cell.* **6**(4), 909–919.

157. Wood, E. R., Shewchuk, L. M., Ellis, B., Brignola, P., Brashear, R. L., Caferro, T. R., Dickerson S. H., Dickson, H. D., Donaldson, K. H., Gaul, M., Griffin, R. J., Hassell A. M., Keith, B., Mullin, R., Petrov, K. G., Reno, M. J., Rusnak, D. W., Tadepalli, S. M., Ulrich, J. C., Wagner, C. D., Vanderwall, D. E., Waterson, A. G., Williams, J. D., White, W. L., and Uehling, D. E. (2008) 6-Ethynylthieno[3,2-d]- and 6-ethynylthieno[2,3-d]pyrimidin-4-anilines as tunable covalent modifiers of ErbB kinases, *Proc. Natl. Acad. Sci. USA* **105**(8), 2773–2778.

158. Ohori, M., Kinoshita, T., Yoshimura, S., Warizaya, M., Nakajima, H., and Miyake, H. (2007) Role of a cysteine residue in the active site of ERK and the MAPKK family, *Biochem Biophys Res. Commun.* **353**(3), 633–637.

159. Elling, R. A., Fucini, R. V., and Romanowski, M. J. (2008) Structures of the wild-type and activated catalytic domains of Brachydanio rerio Polo-like kinase 1 (Plk1): changes in the active-site conformation and interactions with ligands, *Acta. Crystallogr. D. Biol. Crystallogr.* **64**(Pt 9), 909–918.

160. Michalczyk, A., Klüter, S., Rode, H. B., Simard, J. R., Grütter, C., Rabiller, M., and Rauh, D. (2008) Structural insights into how irreversible inhibitors can overcome drug resistance in EGFR, *Bioorg. Med. Chem.* **16**(7), 3482–3488. Epub 2008 Feb 20.

161. Blair, J. A., Rauh, D., Kung, C., Yun, C. H., Fan, Q. W., Rode, H., Zhang, C., Eck, M. J., Weiss, W. A., and Shokat, K. M. (2007) Structure-guided development of affinity probes for tyrosine kinases using chemical genetics, *Nat. Chem. Biol.* **3**(4), 229–238. Epub 2007 Mar 4.

Chapter 2

Small-Molecule Protein and Lipid Kinase Inhibitors in Inflammation and Specific Models for Their Evaluation

Matthias Gaestel and Alexey Kotlyarov

Abstract

The inflammatory response requires complex and coordinated cooperation of different signaling pathways and cell types. Therefore, more than 40 different protein or lipid kinases can be regarded as potential small-molecule inhibitor targets to approach a therapy of acute inflammation, such as septic syndrome, and especially chronic inflammation, such as rheumatoid arthritis or inflammatory bowel disease. Besides the general considerations about selectivity and potency of small-molecule kinase inhibitors, in this chapter special emphasis is put on the inflammation-specific methods and assays available for testing potential small-molecule inhibitors for their anti-inflammatory activity. Examples for human cell-based assays for characterization of the effect of inhibitors on contribution of various cell types, such as monocytes, neutrophils, mast cells, T-cells, and synovial fibroblasts, to the inflammatory scenario are given. It is further demonstrated how these assays are complemented by rodent models for septic syndrome, rheumatoid arthritis, ulcerative colitis, Crohn's disease, and systemic lupus erythematosus. Finally, it is discussed how the results obtained by these methods can be further validated and which future strategies for the treatment of chronic inflammation will exist.

Key words: Animal models, Sepsis, Rheumatoid and collagen-induced arthritis, Crohn's disease, Ulcerative colitis, Lupus erythematosis

1. Introduction

Acute and chronic inflammation is based on a complex, multicellular scenario where protein and lipid kinases are involved in many steps and places (for recent reviews see refs. 1 and 2). Hence, there is a strong potential for the use of small-molecule kinase inhibitors to interfere with inflammation and, more relevantly, to contribute to therapy of chronic inflammation such as rheumatoid arthritis (RA) or inflammatory bowel disease (IBD). After identification of the first inflammation relevant protein kinases targeted by Smith Kline Beecham compounds of the SB203580-type, the p38 MAPKs

Table 1
Kinases involved in inflammation (for details and signaling pathways see refs. 1, 4)

Kinase superfamily	Members involved in inflammation
Receptor tyrosine kinases	c-KIT (mast-stem cell growth factor receptor), recepteur d'origine nantais (RON), TYRO3, AXL, and MER (TAM) receptor family
Nonreceptor tyrosine kinases	Janus kinase (JAK)1/2/3, Tyrosine kinase 2 (TYK2), Lymphocyte cell-specific protein tyrosine kinase (LCK), T-cell-specific kinase (TSK or ITK), Zeta-chain-associated protein kinase (ZAP)70, Spleen tyrosine kinase (SYK), Bone marrow tyrosine kinase in chromosome X (BMX), Bruton's tyrosone kinase (BTK)
Protein-serine/threonine kinases	IL-1R-associated kinase (IRAK)1/2/4, TGF-β-activated protein kinase (TAK)1, MAPK kinase kinase (MEKK)3, TNFR-associated factor (TRAF) family member-associated (TANK)-binding kinase (TBK)1, inhibitor of κB (IκB) kinase (IKK) α/β/ε, Tumor progression locus 2 (Tpl2 or c-COT), Extracellular signal-regulated kinase (ERK)1/2, c-JUN N-terminal kinase (JNK)1/2, p38 MAPK α/β, MAPK-activated protein kinase (MAPKAPK or MK) 2/3, MAPK interacting kinase (MNK)1/2, Receptor-interacting serine–threonine kinase (RIP)
Dual specific protein kinases	MAPK kinase 1/2 (MEK1/2), 3/4/6/7 (MKK3/4/6/7)
Lipid kinases	Phosphoinositide 3-kinase (PI3K) γ/δ

α and β, more than 15 years ago (3), today a long list of more than 40 potential target kinases exists (see refs. 1, 4 and Table 1). Several small inhibitors against these targets are already in clinical trials, while others has to be identified, characterized, and optimized further before entering clinics.

Methods of molecular biology are mainly involved in analyzing selectivity and potency of small-molecule inhibitors by various in vitro assays. To monitor selectivity of protein kinase inhibitors, a screen of in vitro activity over a panel of recombinant protein kinases (5), competitive binding assays against a kinase expression library (6), or a proteomic analysis of the competitive affinity purification of kinases in the presence of inhibitor molecules (7) are carried out. Although some small-molecule inhibitors show rather high selectivity, with the exception of rapamycin, which uses a completely different mechanism of action via cyclophilin-binding, there is no monospecific kinase inhibitor identified so far. To increase selectivity and potency of kinase inhibitors, there is a general trend to shift from ATP-competitive inhibitors to molecules that, in addition, confer allosteric inhibition of the kinase, such as the p38 MAPK-inhibitor BIRB 796 (8), or, to inhibitors that target activator-kinase, such as the MEK1 inhibitors of the Parke Davis-family and the U0126 compound, or kinase–substrate interaction, such as the recently described JNK-inhibitor BI-78D3 (9). Potency of inhibitors is usually characterized by the IC_{50} value – the inhibitor concentration that is necessary to reduce kinase activity in an in vitro assay to 50%. When comparing IC_{50} values, it should be taken into account that this value depends on assay conditions, such as ATP and substrate concentration, structure of the recombinant kinase, and the presence of further kinase-binding components.

Nevertheless, the above issues are not specific for targeting inflammation, but represent general considerations for all small-molecule kinase inhibitors. For targeting inflammation, the cell-based assays and the animal models, in which the inhibitory molecules has to be tested, are the specific issues and are discussed in more detail here.

2. Cell-Based Assays for Small-Molecule Inhibitors to Target Inflammation

As stated above, many cell types and cytokines are involved in the inflammatory response and, hence, the choice of the inflammatory stimulus, cell type and readout parameter for analyzing the anti-inflammatory action of an inhibitor is crucial. The cell type to be analyzed is often chosen according to the known cell-type specific function or, if the function is not known, to the expression and activity pattern of the kinase targeted by the small molecule. However, it may well be that a specific kinase is involved in regulation of inflammatory processes in more than one cell-type. At the moment, this is not reflected by the assays, which all try to use only one well-defined cell-type. Furthermore, since inhibitors are finally searched for therapeutic treatment of humans, preferential cellular assays of anti-inflammatory action should use human primary cells or cell lines to avoid effects due to structural variations of the kinase molecules between species. As a result of these considerations, only few cell-based assays seem suited. Owing to the various cellular players in inflammation, the cell-based assays always represent only a specific part of the inflammatory scenario (Table 2). Monocytes are preferred to monitor the effect of small-molecule inhibitors on TLR-mediated innate immunity. The prominent TLR4-ligand LPS is used as a sepsis-relevant stimulus and secretion of the "master"-cytokine TNF is an ideal readout parameter. In addition, sometimes the influence of the inhibitor on the phosphorylation of intracellular substrates of the kinase of choice is also monitored (10, 11). Other aspects of inflammation are better represented by mast cells (12), T-cells (13), or neutrophils (11), and appropriate assays have been developed using these cell types (Table 2). Also, disease-specific primary cells, such as synovial fibroblasts from RA patients, were used to monitor the disease-modifying properties of the compound more directly (14). IC_{50} values determined in these

Table 2
Examples of cell-based assays

Cells	Stimuli	Readout	Kinase inhibitors analyzed and IC_{50} (if available)
Cell line THP-1, human monocytic leukemia cell line	LPS	TNF	MK2, Compound 83, $IC_{50} = 1.6$ μM (32) P38, BIRB 796, $IC_{50} = 18$ nM (8)
Cell line U937, human monocytic leukemia cell line	LPS	Phospho-Hsp27, TNF	MK2, Compound 23, $IC_{50} = 4.8$ μM (10)
Primary human monocytes derived from human blood buffy coats by negative selection	LPS, IL-1b	TNF	Tpl2/C-COT, compound 1, $IC_{50} = 0.6$ μM (33)
Human embryonic kidney cells (HEK293) overexpressing TLR4	LPS	NFkB-dependent reporter gene	BTK, Effect of LFM-A13 measured (34)
Human mast cells culture derived from cord blood CD34+ progenitor cells and expanded by Flt3, SCF, and IL-6 treatment (35)	Sensitization with IgEkappa, stimulation with anti-IgE-antibodies	Degranulation by measurement of tryptase activity in supernatant	SYK, Compound 36, $IC_{50} = 70$ nM (12)
Human CD4+ T-cell purified from whole blood	Activation of TCR and CD28 by anti-CD3- and anti-CD28-antibodies	IL-2	ITK, Compound 8×, $IC_{50} = 1.6$ μM (13)
Human RA synovial fibroblasts	IL-1α	Phospho-ERK	Effect of PD184352 measured (14)
Human neutrophils purified from blood by Percoll gradient centrifugation	TNF priming, fMLP stimulation	Intracellular PIP3, Oxidative burst by oxidation of exogenous cytochrome C in the supernatant	PI3Kγ, AS-252424, $IC_{50} = 2$ μM (11)

Cells, stimuli, and readouts, kinases targeted and inhibitors

cell-based assays are usually higher than the values obtained from in vitro assays. This is mainly due to "bioavailability" of the compounds, which includes permeation to the relevant cellular compartment, intracellular solubility, competitive off-target binding to other cellular components, and intracellular stability of the compound.

3. Inflammatory Disease Models Appropriate for Testing of Small Molecules

3.1. Sepsis Model

Sepsis is a systemic response to infection that includes fever, enhanced heartbeat and respiration rate, decreased blood pressure, and multiple organ dysfunction. The septic syndrome is observed in intensive care units worldwide. It is a major cause of death, with mortality rates that range from 20% for sepsis to >60% for septic shock. Sepsis is commonly elicited by lipopolysaccharide (LPS), a constitutive component of the outer membrane of gram-negative bacteria. The part of LPS that causes septic shock is lipid A, which acts as bacterial endotoxin. The response to LPS occurs through Toll-like Receptors (TLRs) and results in the release of the proinflammatory cytokines TNF, IL-1, and IL-6 which trigger the inflammatory reactions. Overproduction of these cytokines causes pathological amplification of the inflammatory cascade leading to sepsis. For mice, two sepsis models are established, which are designated low-dose and high-dose LPS model.

In the low-dose LPS model, mice are sensitized by preceding administration of D-galactosamine, leading to severe depletion in hepatic UTP and inhibition of macromolecular synthesis, and subsequently (after 1–3 h) injected with low-dose LPS (15). Mice given 300 mg D-galactosamine/kg (typically 20 mg) have a lethal dose with 50% survival (LD_{50}) of 0.5 ng LPS per animal, with death occurring about 5–9 h later. In the low-dose model, lethality is due to massive hepatic necrosis in response to LPS by a process dependent upon TNF and IFN-γ. Sometimes, D-galactosamine is also combined with medium-dose LPS treatment (Table 3).

High-dose LPS challenge of mice is based on intraperitoneal or intravenous injection with LPS doses of 25–100 μg per animal. The LD_{50} is around 150 μg, with lethality after approximately 1.5 day. The observed mortality is due to cytokine induced endothelial cell injury and highly correlates with TNF, IL-1, and IL-6 levels. High-dose LPS is the most often used assay for analysis of inhibitory compounds and for characterization of mouse knockouts of potential target kinases (Table 3).

3.2. Models for Rheumatoid Arthritis

RA is an inflammatory polyarthritis of unknown autoimmune-based origin leading to joint deformation, destruction, and final loss of function. Its worldwide distribution has an estimated prevalence of 1–2%. In contrast to RA, the factors that induce experimental arthritis in mouse are well established. Such factors are living bacteria or bacterial components, adjuvants, cartilage specific proteins or other antigens used in different experimental models.

The collagen-induced arthritis (CIA) model (16) is the most commonly used and best described model so far. Immunization of mice with autologous or heterologous type II collagen with incomplete Freund's adjuvant leads to arthritis with a maximum severity

Table 3
Examples of animal models of inflammation for testing of inhibitors or mouse kinase knock outs

Animal model	Inhibitor application and inflammatory stimulus	Readout	References
Rat or mouse high dose LPS model	MK2- or p38-Inhibitors orally dosed prior LPS-challenge	Serum TNF measured by LC-MS or ELISA	(10, 36)
Mouse (low dose) LPS D-gal model	A combination of LPS (5–50 mg per kg body weight) and D-gal (0.4–1 g per kg body weight) simultaneously injected intraperitoneally into MK2-KO mice	Serum TNF level after 90 min measured by ELISA, Lethality between 1 and 24 h	(18, 37)
Collagen-induced arthritis in DBA/1LacJ mice	Kinase knockout (MK2) mice treated with bovine collagen type II	Arthritic score, IL-6 mRNA in paws,	(18)
Collagen-induced arthritis in DBA/1LacJ mice	Mice treated with bovine collagen type II and subsequently with daily doses of p38-inhibitor Org 48762-0	Arthritic score	(36)
Mouse DSS-induced chronic ulcerative colitis	MEK-inhibitor RDEA119 Orally dosed	Histological colonic damage score	(38)
MRL/lpr-mice spontaneously developing symptoms of SLE at about month 5	PI3Kγ-inhibitor AS605240 administered intraperitoneally every 12 h starting from month 2 until month 5	Titer of DNA-specific autoantibodies or number of CD4+ memory T-cells	(28)

around day 30. Importantly, CIA is accompanied by expression of TNF and IL-1β in the joints. Any blockade of these molecules leads to alleviation of arthritis. Accordingly, inhibition or deletion of protein kinase targets, such as p38 or MK2, results in decreased arthritic score in this model (17, 18) (Table 3).

In the serum transfer model of arthritis, mice expressing the KRN T-cell receptor transgene and the MHC class II molecule Ag7 (K/BxN mice) develop inflammatory arthritis, and serum from these mice, due to pathogenic autoantibodies to glucose-6-phosphate isomerase, causes similar arthritis in a wide range of mouse strains (19). Hence, this model could be extremely useful for the investigation of the development of autoimmune-induced arthritis.

3.3. Models for Crohn's Disease and Ulcerative Colitis

CD and UC are the two major forms of chronic inflammatory bowel disease (IBD). The clinical appearance of IBD is heterogeneous, which may reflect an uneven impact of genetic factors, microbial factors in the enteric environment and altered immune response in the etiology of IBD. So far, there is no animal model which exactly reproduces human IBD. However, some animal models resemble certain aspects of IBD and can be used for both, further investigation of the underlying pathophysiological mechanisms and validation of therapeutic strategies.

The first suited model is dextran sodium sulfate (DSS)-induced colitis. Here, feeding of mice with DSS polymers (30–60 kDa) in the drinking water for several days induces an acute colitis characterized by bloody diarrhea, ulcerations and infiltrations with granulocytes (20). DSS is directly toxic to gut epithelial cells of the basal crypts and, hence, affects the integrity of the mucosal barrier. The DSS colitis model is particularly useful for studying the contribution of innate immune mechanisms of colitis.

Other models are trinitrobenzene sulfonate (TNBS)- and oxazolone-induced colitis. Here, in susceptible strains of mice colitis can be induced by administration of the hapten TNBS (21) or the organic compound oxazolone (22) in ethanol. As a result, modifications of otherwise nonimmunogenic autologous or microbial proteins transform them immunogenic to the host and causes autoimmune colitis with high lethality. In addition, various mouse knockouts (KOs) and transgenic mice develop IBD spontaneously due to direct or indirect modulation of T-cell function, such as IL-2- and IL-10-KO (23, 24), to TNF upregulation by a targeted TNF mRNA stabilizing mutation (ΔARE, (25)) or perturbations in the gut epithelium, such as keratin 8-KO (26).

3.4. A Model for Systemic Lupus Erythematosis

SLE is a chronic autoimmune disease with deregulated T-cell mediated B-cell activation resulting in inflammation and tissue damage. This disease, which is nine times more frequent in women than in men and affects around 0.1% of the population, often harms skin, joints, heart, kidney, and nervous system. Owing to symptomatic treatment with corticosteroids, the mortality was decreased to around 20% after 20 years. A genetic model that reflects many aspects of SLE is the mouse inbred strain MRL/*lpr* (lymph proliferation), which carries a homozygote recessive Fas-antigen mutation (27). Together with an additional autosomal dominant mutation, which affects the induction of macroscopic skin lesions, the *lpr* mutation accelerates the progression of skin lesions to a severe systemic disease similar to SLE.

Male MRL/*lpr*-mice spontaneously develop symptoms of SLE at 5–6 month of age, while females develop SLE 1 month earlier. Hence, to analyze the effect of a small-molecule inhibitor of SLE, mice have to be treated repeatedly with the compound beginning between month 2 and 3.5. As disease-relevant readout, DNA-specific autoantibodies or CD4+ memory T-cells can be quantified after 5 months in these animals (28).

4. Conclusions

There are various cell-based and animal models of inflammation available for testing efficiency of small-molecule kinase inhibitors in inflammation. While the cell-based models of human origin represent only specific parts of the complex multicellular inflammatory scenario, the animal models mirrors the complex scenario much better – but 70 million years of divergent evolution between rodents and humans make direct transfer of the result to humans sometimes problematic. However, a combination of human cell-based and animal models in evaluation of small-molecule kinase inhibitors could be sufficient for characterization of compounds of interest before entering clinics. However, inhibitor studies should be complemented with studies using mouse knockouts or catalytic-dead knockins of the target kinase and target knockdown approaches in human cells.

Future developments of small-molecule inhibitors in inflammation should take into account that intracellular signaling proceeds in networks including feedback control (cf. refs. 1, 29). Hence, inhibition of a specific kinase target can even increase the long-term inflammatory response leading to adverse effects. Better understanding of signaling networks will facilitate the combination of targets and use of inhibitor cocktails for a specific anti-inflammatory therapy. Finally, since signaling involves kinase cascades with specific kinase–kinase and kinase–substrate interaction often based on docking motifs, which can be targeted by peptides as well (reviewed in refs. 30, 31), the targeting of catalytic activity and allosteric properties of protein or lipid kinases should be complemented with targeting specific protein–protein interaction.

Together, there is a strong need and a realistic perspective for orally available small-molecule inhibitors for the therapy of inflammation. However, in contrast to the use of small-molecule inhibitors for the treatment of cancer, the treatment of chronic inflammation by such molecules will be more difficult, since higher efficacy compared with classical treatments, fewer side effects, and extraordinary low toxicity are required for the long-term treatment of usually non-life-threatening nonmalignant diseases.

References

1. Gaestel, M., Kotlyarov, A., and Kracht, M. (2009) Targeting innate immunity protein kinase signaling in inflammation. *Nat. Rev. Drug Discov.* **8**, 480–499.
2. Rommel, C., Camps, M., and Ji, H. (2007) PI3K delta and PI3K gamma: partners in crime in inflammation in rheumatoid arthritis and beyond? *Nat. Rev. Immunol.* **7**, 191–201.
3. Lee, J. C., Laydon, J. T., McDonnell, P. C., Gallagher, T. F., Kumar, S., Green, D., McNulty, D., Blumenthal, M. J., Heys, J. R., Landvatter, S. W., and et al. (1994) A protein kinase involved in the regulation of inflammatory cytokine biosynthesis. *Nature* **372**, 739–746.
4. Gaestel, M., Mengel, A., Bothe, U., and Asadullah, K. (2007) Protein kinases as small

molecule inhibitor targets in inflammation. *Curr. Med. Chem.* **14**, 2214–2234.

5. Bain, J., Plater, L., Elliott, M., Shpiro, N., Hastie, C. J., McLauchlan, H., Klevernic, I., Arthur, J. S., Alessi, D. R., and Cohen, P. (2007) The selectivity of protein kinase inhibitors: a further update. *Biochem J.* **408**, 297–315.

6. Karaman, M. W., Herrgard, S., Treiber, D. K., Gallant, P., Atteridge, C. E., Campbell, B. T., Chan, K. W., Ciceri, P., Davis, M. I., Edeen, P. T., Faraoni, R., Floyd, M., Hunt, J. P., Lockhart, D. J., Milanov, Z. V., Morrison, M. J., Pallares, G., Patel, H. K., Pritchard, S., Wodicka, L. M., and Zarrinkar, P. P. (2008) A quantitative analysis of kinase inhibitor selectivity. *Nat. Biotechnol.* **26**, 127–132.

7. Bantscheff, M., Eberhard, D., Abraham, Y., Bastuck, S., Boesche, M., Hobson, S., Mathieson, T., Perrin, J., Raida, M., Rau, C., Reader, V., Sweetman, G., Bauer, A., Bouwmeester, T., Hopf, C., Kruse, U., Neubauer, G., Ramsden, N., Rick, J., Kuster, B., and Drewes, G. (2007) Quantitative chemical proteomics reveals mechanisms of action of clinical ABL kinase inhibitors. *Nat. Biotechnol.* **25**, 1035–1044.

8. Pargellis, C., Tong, L., Churchill, L., Cirillo, P. F., Gilmore, T., Graham, A. G., Grob, P. M., Hickey, E. R., Moss, N., Pav, S., and Regan, J. (2002) Inhibition of p38 MAP kinase by utilizing a novel allosteric binding site. *Nat. Struct. Biol.* **9**, 268–272.

9. Stebbins, J. L., De, S. K., Machleidt, T., Becattini, B., Vazquez, J., Kuntzen, C., Chen, L. H., Cellitti, J. F., Riel-Mehan, M., Emdadi, A., Solinas, G., Karin, M., and Pellecchia, M. (2008) Identification of a new JNK inhibitor targeting the JNK-JIP interaction site. *Proc. Natl. Acad. Sci. USA* **105**, 16809–16813.

10. Anderson, D. R., Meyers, M. J., Vernier, W. F., Mahoney, M. W., Kurumbail, R. G., Caspers, N., Poda, G. I., Schindler, J. F., Reitz, D. B., and Mourey, R. J. (2007) Pyrrolopyridine Inhibitors of Mitogen-Activated Protein Kinase-Activated Protein Kinase 2 (MK-2). *J. Med. Chem.* **50**, 2647–2654.

11. Condliffe, A. M., Davidson, K., Anderson, K. E., Ellson, C. D., Crabbe, T., Okkenhaug, K., Vanhaesebroeck, B., Turner, M., Webb, L., Wymann, M. P., Hirsch, E., Ruckle, T., Camps, M., Rommel, C., Jackson, S. P., Chilvers, E. R., Stephens, L. R., and Hawkins, P. T. (2005) Sequential activation of class IB and class IA PI3K is important for the primed respiratory burst of human but not murine neutrophils. *Blood* **106**, 1432–1440.

12. Farmer, L. J., Bemis, G., Britt, S. D., Cochran, J., Connors, M., Harrington, E. M., Hoock, T., Markland, W., Nanthakumar, S., Taslimi, P., Ter Haar, E., Wang, J., Zhaveri, D., and Salituro, F. G. (2008) Discovery and SAR of novel 4-thiazolyl-2-phenylaminopyrimidines as potent inhibitors of spleen tyrosine kinase (SYK). *Bioorg. Med. Chem. Lett.* **18**, 6231–6235.

13. Lo, H. Y., Bentzien, J., Fleck, R. W., Pullen, S. S., Khine, H. H., Woska, J. R., Jr., Kugler, S. Z., Kashem, M. A., and Takahashi, H. (2008) 2-Aminobenzimidazoles as potent ITK antagonists: trans-stilbene-like moieties targeting the kinase specificity pocket. *Bioorg. Med. Chem. Lett.* **18**, 6218–6221.

14. Thiel, M. J., Schaefer, C. J., Lesch, M. E., Mobley, J. L., Dudley, D. T., Tecle, H., Barrett, S. D., Schrier, D. J., and Flory, C. M. (2007) Central role of the MEK/ERK MAP kinase pathway in a mouse model of rheumatoid arthritis: potential proinflammatory mechanisms. *Arthritis Rheum.* **56**, 3347–3357.

15. Galanos, C., Freudenberg, M. A., and Reutter, W. (1979) Galactosamine-induced sensitization to the lethal effects of endotoxin. *Proc. Natl. Acad. Sci. USA* **76**, 5939–5943.

16. Trentham, D. E., Townes, A. S., and Kang, A. H. (1977) Autoimmunity to type II collagen an experimental model of arthritis. *J. Exp. Med.* **146**, 857–868.

17. Mihara, K., Almansa, C., Smeets, R. L., Loomans, E. E., Dulos, J., Vink, P. M., Rooseboom, M., Kreutzer, H., Cavalcanti, F., Boots, A. M., and Nelissen, R. L. (2008) A potent and selective p38 inhibitor protects against bone damage in murine collagen-induced arthritis: a comparison with neutralization of mouse TNFalpha. *Br. J. Pharmacol.* **154**, 153–164. Epub 2008 Feb 2025.

18. Hegen, M., Gaestel, M., Nickerson-Nutter, C. L., Lin, L. L., and Telliez, J. B. (2006) MAPKAP kinase 2-deficient mice are resistant to collagen-induced arthritis. *J. Immunol.* **177**, 1913–1917.

19. Korganow, A. S., Ji, H., Mangialaio, S., Duchatelle, V., Pelanda, R., Martin, T., Degott, C., Kikutani, H., Rajewsky, K., Pasquali, J. L., Benoist, C., and Mathis, D. (1999) From systemic T cell self-reactivity to organ-specific autoimmune disease via immunoglobulins. *Immunity* **10**, 451–461.

20. Okayasu, I., Hatakeyama, S., Yamada, M., Ohkusa, T., Inagaki, Y., and Nakaya, R. (1990) A novel method in the induction of reliable experimental acute and chronic ulcerative colitis in mice. *Gastroenterology* **98**, 694–702.

21. Morris, G. P., Beck, P. L., Herridge, M. S., Depew, W. T., Szewczuk, M. R., and Wallace, J. L. (1989) Hapten-induced model of chronic inflammation and ulceration in the rat colon. *Gastroenterology* **96**, 795–803.

22. Boirivant, M., Fuss, I. J., Chu, A., and Strober, W. (1998) Oxazolone colitis: A murine model of T helper cell type 2 colitis treatable with antibodies to interleukin 4. *J. Exp. Med.* **188**, 1929–1939.

23. Sadlack, B., Merz, H., Schorle, H., Schimpl, A., Feller, A. C., and Horak, I. (1993) Ulcerative colitis-like disease in mice with a disrupted interleukin-2 gene. *Cell.* **75**, 253–261.

24. Kuhn, R., Lohler, J., Rennick, D., Rajewsky, K., and Muller, W. (1993) Interleukin-10-deficient mice develop chronic enterocolitis. *Cell.* **75**, 263–274.

25. Kontoyiannis, D., Pasparakis, M., Pizarro, T. T., Cominelli, F., and Kollias, G. (1999) Impaired on/off regulation of TNF biosynthesis in mice lacking TNF AU-rich elements: implications for joint and gut-associated immunopathologies. *Immunity* **10**, 387–398.

26. Baribault, H., Penner, J., Iozzo, R. V., and Wilson-Heiner, M. (1994) Colorectal hyperplasia and inflammation in keratin 8-deficient FVB/N mice. *Genes Dev.* **8**, 2964–2973.

27. Furukawa, F., and Yoshimasu, T. (2005) Animal models of spontaneous and drug-induced cutaneous lupus erythematosus. *Autoimmunity Reviews* **4**, 345–350.

28. Barber, D. F., Bartolome, A., Hernandez, C., Flores, J. M., Redondo, C., Fernandez-Arias, C., Camps, M., Ruckle, T., Schwarz, M. K., Rodriguez, S., Martinez, A. C., Balomenos, D., Rommel, C., and Carrera, A. C. (2005) PI3Kgamma inhibition blocks glomerulonephritis and extends lifespan in a mouse model of systemic lupus. *Nat. Med.* **11**, 933–935.

29. Cohen, P. (2009) Targeting protein kinases for the development of anti-inflammatory drugs. *Curr. Opin. Cell Biol.* **21**, 317–324.

30. Gaestel, M. (2008) Specificity of signaling from MAPKs to MAPKAPKs: kinases' tango nuevo. *Front. Biosci.* **13**, 6050–6059.

31. Gaestel, M., and Kracht, M. (2009) Peptides as signaling inhibitors for mammalian MAPK kinase cascades. *Curr. Pharm. Des.* **15**, 2471–2480.

32. Wu, J. P., Wang, J., Abeywardane, A., Andersen, D., Emmanuel, M., Gautschi, E., Goldberg, D. R., Kashem, M. A., Lukas, S., Mao, W., Martin, L., Morwick, T., Moss, N., Pargellis, C., Patel, U. R., Patnaude, L., Peet, G. W., Skow, D., Snow, R. J., Ward, Y., Werneburg, B., and White, A. (2007) The discovery of carboline analogs as potent MAPKAP-K2 inhibitors. *Bioorg. Med. Chem Lett.* **17**, 4664–4669.

33. Hall, J. P., Kurdi, Y., Hsu, S., Cuozzo, J., Liu, J., Telliez, J. B., Seidl, K. J., Winkler, A., Hu, Y., Green, N., Askew, G. R., Tam, S., Clark, J. D., and Lin, L. L. (2007) Pharmacologic inhibition of tpl2 blocks inflammatory responses in primary human monocytes, synoviocytes, and blood. *J. Biol. Chem.* **282**, 33295–33304.

34. Doyle, S. L., Jefferies, C. A., and O'Neill, L. A. (2005) Bruton's tyrosine kinase is involved in p65-mediated transactivation and phosphorylation of p65 on serine 536 during NFkappaB activation by lipopolysaccharide. *J. Biol. Chem.* **280**, 23496–23501.

35. Braselmann, S., Taylor, V., Zhao, H., Wang, S., Sylvain, C., Baluom, M., Qu, K., Herlaar, E., Lau, A., Young, C., Wong, B. R., Lovell, S., Sun, T., Park, G., Argade, A., Jurcevic, S., Pine, P., Singh, R., Grossbard, E. B., Payan, D. G., and Masuda, E. S. (2006) R406, an orally available spleen tyrosine kinase inhibitor blocks fc receptor signaling and reduces immune complex-mediated inflammation. *J. Pharmacol. Exp. Ther.* **319**, 998–1008.

36. Mihara, K., Almansa, C., Smeets, R. L., Loomans, E. E., Dulos, J., Vink, P. M., Rooseboom, M., Kreutzer, H., Cavalcanti, F., Boots, A. M., and Nelissen, R. L. (2008) A potent and selective p38 inhibitor protects against bone damage in murine collagen-induced arthritis: a comparison with neutralization of mouse TNFalpha. *Br. J. Pharmacol.* **154**, 153–164.

37. Kotlyarov, A., Neininger, A., Schubert, C., Eckert, R., Birchmeier, C., Volk, H. D., and Gaestel, M. (1999) MAPKAP kinase 2 is essential for LPS-induced TNF-alpha biosynthesis. *Nat. Cell. Biol.* **1**, 94–97.

38. Miampamba, M., Larson, G., Lai, C., Johansen, A., Miner, J., Vernier, J., Girardet, J., and Quart, B. (2008) RDEA119, a Potent and Highly Selective MEK1/2 Inhibitor is Beneficial in Dextran Sulfate Sodium (DSS)-Induced Chronic Colitis in Mice. *The ACG Annual Scientific Meeting and Postgraduate Course, October 3–8, 2008, Orlando, Florida.*

Chapter 3

Measuring the Activity of Leucine-Rich Repeat Kinase 2: A Kinase Involved in Parkinson's Disease

Byoung Dae Lee, Xiaojie Li, Ted M. Dawson, and Valina L. Dawson

Abstract

Mutations in the *LRRK2* (Leucine-Rich Repeat Kinase 2) gene are the most common cause of autosomal dominant Parkinson's disease. LRRK2 has multiple functional domains including a kinase domain. The kinase activity of LRRK2 is implicated in the pathogenesis of Parkinson's disease. Developing an assay to understand the mechanisms of LRRK2 kinase activity is important for the development of pharmacologic and therapeutic applications. Here, we describe how to measure in vitro LRRK2 kinase activity and its inhibition.

Key words: Parkinson's disease, LRRK2, In vitro kinase assay

1. Introduction

Parkinson's disease (PD) is the second most common neurodegenerative disease in the world. It affects approximately 1–2% of the US population above the age of 65. The pathological hallmark of PD is the presence of cytoplasmic inclusions known as Lewy bodies and the degeneration of dopaminergic neurons in the nigrostriatal pathway (1). Although the majority of PD cases are sporadic, there are familial cases of PD in which mutations in a variety of genes have been linked to PD. This suggests an unambiguous role of genetic component in the development of PD (2, 3). Previous studies provide us various clues for the pathogenesis of PD. The identification of the *Leucine-Rich Repeat Kinase 2 (LRRK2)*-linked PD has opened up new opportunities for the study of etiology of PD and the discovery of novel therapeutic targets for PD.

LRRK2 mutations are very common in Parkinson's disease (PD) patients, both sporadic and familial. *LRRK2*-linked PD patients showed very similar clinical and neuropathologic features as idiopathic PD (4, 5). Familial mutations within the *LRRK2* gene have been found to cause the alterations of amino acid throughout the entire LRRK2 protein (5–11). LRRK2 contains multiple functional domains, including two enzymatic domains (GTPase domain and kinase domain) and two protein–protein interacting domains (N-terminal LRR domain and C-terminal WD40 domain) (12). The exact physiological function of LRRK2 protein is still not yet clear. However, genetic and biochemical studies suggest that LRRK2 mutations most likely cause disease through a dominant gain-of-function mechanism. Many disease-associated LRRK2 mutant proteins showed enhanced kinase activity in the in vitro kinase assay. Expression of LRRK2 protein can lead to cytotoxicity in cultured cells and primary neurons. Toxicity is dependent on kinase activity and GTP binding activity of LRRK2 (13–16). To further study kinase activity and toxicity of LRRK2 protein, an optimized in vitro kinase assay was developed. We show that exogenously overexpressed LRRK2 protein can autophosphorylate itself and the generic substrate, myelin basic protein (MBP).

2. Materials

2.1. Cell Culture

1. Human Embryonic Kidney (HEK) 293 FT cells.
2. Opti-MEM I Reduced–Serum Media (1×) liquid.
3. Fetal bovine serum.
4. TrypLE™ Express with Phenol Red.
5. Fugene HD Transfection Reagent.
6. LRRK2: a plasmid containing GST-tagged LRRK2 is available from the authors on request.

2.2. Cell Lysis and Preparation of LRRK2

1. Phosphate-buffered Saline (PBS, 10× stock): 1.37 mM NaCl, 27 mM KCl, 100 mM Na_2HPO_4, and 18 mM KH_2PO_4. Adjust to pH 7.4 with HCl.
2. Cell lysis buffer: 50 mM HEPES, 150 mM NaCl, 5 mM EGTA, 0.5% NP-40. Adjust to pH 7.4 with HCl.
3. Washing buffer: 1× PBS with 0.5% NP-40 and 150 mM NaCl.
4. Gluthathione-Sepharose 4B.
5. Protein G Sepharose, Protein A Sepharose, or protein G Dynabead (see Note 1).

2.3. In Vitro Kinase assay

1. Kinase assay buffer: 20 mM HEPES, 150 mM NaCl, 5 mM EGTA, and 20 mM b-Glycerol phosphate. Adjust pH to 7.4.

Make 2 M b-glycerol phosphate and freeze single-use aliquots (500 μl) at −20°C.

2. MgCl$_2$ (2 M stock): Store at room temperature.
3. Adenosine 5′-triphosphate disodium salt (ATP, ≥99% purity, 100 mM stock): freeze single-use aliquots (10 μl) at −80°C.
4. Adenosine 5′-triphosphate, [g-^{32}P]: 6,000 Ci/mmol 10 mCi/ml EasyTide. Store at 4°C (see Note 2).
5. Myelin Basic Protein (MBP, 5 μg/μl stock): The assay described in this protocol used MBP, dephosphorylated, produced from bovine brain. Freeze single-use aliquots (20 μl) at −20°C (see Note 3).
6. Laemmli sample buffer (5× stock): 0.25 M Tris–HCl, pH 6.8, 6% (w/v) SDS, 40% (w/v) glycerol, 0.04% (w/v) bromophenol blue, 12.5% (v/v) β-mercaptoethanol. Freeze in 1 ml aliquots at −20°C.

2.4. SDS-Polyacrylamide Gel Electrophoresis

1. Separate gel buffer (4× stock): 1.5 M Tris–HCl, pH 8.8, 0.4% SDS.
2. Stacking gel buffer (4× stock): 0.5 M Tris–HCl, pH 6.8, 0.4% SDS.
3. 30% acrylamide/bisacrylamide solution (see Note 4).
4. N,N,N′,N′-tetramethyl-ethylenediamine (TEMED).
5. Ammonium persulfate: 10% (w/v) solution in water. Freeze single-use aliquots (200 μl) at −20°C.
6. Isobutanol.
7. Precision plus protein dual-color standards.
8. Running buffer (10× stock): 250 mM Tris (do not adjust pH), 1.92 M glycine, 1% (w/v) SDS.

2.5. Coomassie Brilliant Staining

1. Fixing solution: 10% (v/v) acetic acid, 40% (v/v) methanol in water. Prepare fresh solution every time.
2. Colloidal Blue Staining Kit: any such kit may be used.

2.6. Western Blotting for LRRK2

1. Transfer buffer (10× stock): 250 mM Tris (do not adjust pH), 1.92 M glycine. Prepare working solution by diluting one part of stock with seven parts water and adding two parts of methanol.
2. Nitrocellulose membrane and 3 MM chromatography paper.
3. Tris-buffered saline with Tween20 (TBST, 10× stock): 200 mM Tris–HCl, pH 7.4, 1.37 M NaCl, 0.5% Tween20.
4. Blocking buffer: 5% (w/v) nonfat dry milk in 1× TBST.
5. Antibody dilution buffer: 5% (w/v) nonfat dry milk in 1× TBST.
6. Enhanced chemiluminescent (ECL) reagent and X-ray film.
7. Horseradish peroxidase (HRP) conjugated anti-GST antibody.

2.7. Radiography

1. Storage Phosphor Screen and Cassette.
2. Phosphoimager: Typhoon 9410 and ImageQuant 6.0 software.

3. Methods

LRRK2 encodes a kinase domain with highest similarity to the mixed lineage kinase (MLK) motif found in proteins that commonly have both Ser/Thr and Tyr kinase activities. The most convenient method to detect the active form of the kinase is using the phosphospecific antibodies, such as phospho-p38 MAPK (Thr180/Tyr182) and phospho-AKT (S473) antibodies. However, because the phosphospecific antibody that detects active LRRK2 is not available yet, West et al. (17) developed an assay that measures the ability of LRRK2 to phosphorylate generic substrate of kinases, myelin basic protein (MBP) by measuring the incorporation of [^{32}P] radioisotope-labeled phosphate to the kinase substrates. This assay also detects autophosphorylation of recombinant LRRK2 in the absence of any potential cofactor or activators (17). Here, we describe how to prepare recombinant LRRK2 and how to measure its activity by checking its autophosphorylation and MBP phosphorylation.

Because of technical difficulty in expressing LRRK2 protein, sufficient amount of the protein cannot be prepared. Currently, the most effective method for preparation of full length LRRK2 protein is by using mammalian expression systems. Several epitope-tagged LRRK2 proteins have been developed including myc-LRRK2 (17), V5-LRRK2 (13), HA-LRRK2 (18), flag-LRRK2 (14), and GST-LRRK2 (19). By using these epitope-tagged LRRK2 systems, recombinant LRRK2 protein can be prepared after transiently expression in HEK293 cells. Prepared recombinant LRRK2 protein is incubated with inhibitor and/or activator in the presence of [γ-^{32}P] ATP and MBP. LRRK2 autophosphorylation and MBP phosphorylation can be estimated using a Phosphoimager and suitable software (e.g., ImageQuant 6.0). Input levels of protein present on the gel are determined by coomassie brilliant blue staining.

3.1. Preparation of Recombinant LRRK2 Protein

3.1.1. Transfection for Transient Expression of LRRK2 Protein in HEK293 FT Cells

1. HEK293 FT cells are cultured in Opti-MEM I medium supplemented with 10% FBS. Cells are passaged every 3 or 4 days when approaching confluence with TrypLE™ Express to new culture dishes. For the transfection, confluent cells are split into 60-mm culture dish for a single experiment data point.

2. Fugene HD is used as a transfection reagent to transiently express LRRK2 in HEK293 FT cells. Transfection is performed 1 day after plating the cells. First, dilute 4 μg DNA to 0.2 ml Opti-MEM I without serum and then add 12 μl Fugene HD to DNA-diluted medium. Briefly vortex the transfection mixture

and incubate for 15 min at room temperature. After incubation, add the transfection mixture to the cells in a drop-wise manner on the medium. Before collecting the cells, incubate for 48 h at 37°C in a CO_2 incubator.

3.1.2. Preparation of Epitope-Tagged LRRK2 Proteins from HEK293 FT Cells

1. 1 day before collecting the transfected cells, the immune complex of antibody and protein G or protein A has to be prepared. To prepare the immune complex, resuspend protein G sepharose or protein A sepharose thoroughly to obtain a homogeneous suspension. Transfer 30 μl protein G sepharose or protein A sepharose to a microcentrifuge tube. Wash with 1 ml PBS and sediment the resin by centrifugation at $1,000 \times g$ for 5 min. Discard the supernatant and repeat this wash step. Add 30 μl PBS and 1–2 μg antibody. Rotate this complex at 4°C overnight.

2. Sediment the immune complex by centrifugation at $1,000 \times g$ for 5 min. Remove the supernatant and wash the resin with 1 ml lysis buffer. Sediment the resin by centrifugation at $1,000 \times g$ for 5 min. The pellet contains the immune complex.

3. Prepare cold PBS and lysis buffer containing protease inhibitors. After aspirating the medium, add 4 ml of cold PBS to the culture dish and place culture dish on ice. After aspirating PBS, add 0.5 ml of cold lysis buffer to culture dish. Scrape cells with a cell scraper and transfer the lysate to a microcentrifuge tube. Vigorously vortex the lysate and rotate at 4°C for 30 min followed by centrifugation at $20,000 \times g$ for 15 min.

4. Take 20 μl supernatant to check LRRK2 expression. Mix the immune complex (prepared in step 1–2) and cell lysate and rotate at 4°C overnight.

5. Collect the resin by centrifugation at $1,000 \times g$ for 5 min and discard the supernatant. Resuspend the resin with 0.5 ml washing buffer and sediment the resin by centrifugation at $1,000 \times g$ for 5 min. Discard the supernatant and repeat the wash three more times.

6. After the last washing step, discard the supernatant and wash the resin with 0.5 ml kinase assay buffer. Sediment by centrifugation at $1,000 \times g$ for 5 min and add 20 μl kinase assay buffer (see Note 5).

3.1.3. Preparation of GST-Fusion LRRK2 Proteins from HEK293 FT Cells

1. Prepare cold PBS and lysis buffer containing protease inhibitors. After aspirating the medium from HEK293 FT cells transfected with GST-fusion LRRK2, add 4 ml of cold PBS to culture dish and place culture dish on ice. After aspirating PBS, add 0.5 ml of cold lysis buffer to the culture dish. Scrape the cells with a cell scraper and transfer to a microcentrifuge tube. Vigorously vortex the lysate and rotate at 4°C for 30 min followed by centrifugation at $20,000 \times g$ for 15 min.

2. Resuspend Gluthathione-Sepharose thoroughly to obtain a homogeneous suspension. Transfer 30 μl slurry to a microcentrifuge tube. Wash the slurry with 1 ml PBS and sediment the slurry by centrifugation at $1,000 \times g$ for 5 min. Discard the supernatant and repeat this wash step.

3. Take 20 μl supernatant from step 1 to check LRRK2 expression. Mix the washed slurry and supernatant from step 1. Rotate the mixture at 4°C overnight.

4. Collect the resin by centrifugation at $1,000 \times g$ for 5 min and discard the supernatant. Resuspend the resin with 0.5 ml washing buffer and sediment by centrifugation at $1,000 \times g$ for 5 min. Discard the supernatant and repeat the washing step three more times (see Note 5).

5. After washing the resin, resuspend the resin with 0.5 ml of elution buffer without glutathione. After centrifugation at $1,000 \times g$ for 5 min, discard the supernatant and add 30 μl elution buffer with 20 mM glutathione to the resin. Rotate the mixture at 4°C for 30 min. Eluted protein is obtained after centrifugation at $1,000 \times g$ for 5 min. Transfer 20 μl of eluted LRRK2 protein to a microcentrifuge tube.

3.2. In Vitro Kinase Assay of LRRK2

1. Prepare 20 μl of reaction volume by adding kinase assay buffer to recombinant LRRK2 protein.

2. Inhibitors or activators to be tested can be added at an appropriate concentration. The volume of inhibitor/activator must not exceed 0.5 μl. Preincubate recombinant LRRK2 protein and inhibitor/activator mixture for 5 min at 30°C. When immunoprecipitated recombinant LRRK2 is used in the kinase assay, the reaction tube has to be stirred to prevent sedimentation of resin. An orbital mixing heating plate will be helpful. However, stirring is not necessary when using purified GST-fusion LRRK2 protein.

3. The kinase reaction is initiated with addition of 5 μl of kinase reaction buffer containing 10 mM ATP, 20 mM $MgCl_2$, 2.5 μg MBP, and 0.5 μCi [g-^{32}P] ATP after preincubation of recombinant LRRK2 protein and inhibitor/activator. Incubate the reaction for 15 min at 30°C with gentle rocking.

4. Stop the reaction by adding 6.25 μl of 5× Laemmli sample buffer. Heat the sample at 75°C for 10 min (see Note 6). Sediment the resin at $1,000 \times g$ for 5 min and the supernatant is resolved onto a SDS-PAGE gel.

3.3. SDS-PAGE

1. These instructions are for the Mini-PROTEAN Electrophoresis System from Bio-Rad Laboratories. Other minigel systems may also be used. Prepare two different percentages of SDS-PAGE gels. Use a 12% gel to detect phosphorylation of LRRK2 and MBP and a 6% gel to confirm LRRK2 expression.

2. Prepare a 12% separation gel solution by mixing 4 ml (2 ml for 6%) 30% acrylamide/bis solution, 2.5 ml 4× separation gel buffer, 3.5 ml (5.5 ml for 6%) water, 50 ml 10% (w/v) ammonium persulfate solution, and 10 µl TEMED per a 1.5-mm thick gel. Pour the mixture in a glass gel plate, leaving space for stacking gel, and overlay with isobutanol. Polymerization will take about 20 min (see Note 7).

3. Remove the isobutanol and rinse the top of the gel three times with water.

4. Prepare stacking gel solution by mixing 0.5 ml 30% acrylamide/bis solution, 1 ml 4× stacking gel buffer, 2.5 ml water, 30 µl 10% (w/v) ammonium persulfate solution, and 5 µl TEMED per a 1.5-mm thick gel. Pour the mixture to top of the separate gel and insert a 15-well comb. Polymerization will take about 20 min.

5. Prepare running buffer by diluting one part of 10× running buffer with nine parts of water.

6. Set the gel to running chamber and pour the running buffer to the upper and lower chambers. Load 35 µl of each sample in a well and add 3 ml of prestained protein standard.

7. After completing assembly of units, run the gel at 100 V. When dye front is close to bottom of the gel (this will take about 2 h), stop and proceed to next step (see Note 8).

3.4. Detection of Phosphorylated LRRK2 and MBP

1. The amount of LRRK2 and MBP that has been loaded on the gel can be visualized by staining with coomassie brilliant blue. For staining, fix the gel with 10% (v/v) acetic acid and 50% (v/v) methanol for 30 min on low-speed shaker.

2. Prepare coomassie brilliant blue solution as described in user manual. Briefly, mix 55 ml water, 20 ml methanol, 20 ml stainer A, and 5 ml stainer B for two gels. Pour the staining solution to gel and shake the gel for 1–2 h.

3. Decant staining solution when LRRK2 and MBP proteins clearly appear on the gel and rinse the gel with water. Shake the gel and replace water until background is clear.

4. Place the gel between sheet protectors and seal with sealer.

5. Place the sealed gel on the Storage Phosphor Screen Cassette and cover it with Storage Phosphor Screen. Expose gel to Storage Phosphor Screen overnight.

6. Read the Storage Phosphor Screen with a Phosphoimager and analyze by the ImageQuant 6.0 software.

3.5. Western Blotting for LRRK2 Expression

1. These instructions are for the Mini-Trans Blot Cell from Bio-Rad Laboratories. Other western blotting equipment may also be used. Prepare 1 L of 1× transfer buffer containing 20% methanol and hold ready a tray that is large enough to submerge

transfer cassette. Cut two sheets of Whatman 3 MM paper to the size of the transfer cassette foam pad and a sheet of the nitrocellulose membrane larger than the size of the separating gel.

2. Pour the transfer buffer to the tray and place the transfer cassette with a piece of foam pad and a sheet of Whatman 3 MM paper on one side of the cassette.

3. Disassemble the gel units and remove the stacking gel. After rinsing the gel with water, place it on a sheet of wet Whatman 3 MM paper and lay the wet nitrocellulose membrane on top of the gel. A further sheet of wet Whatman 3 MM paper is laid on the nitrocellulose membrane. Be careful that no bubbles are trapped in the resulting sandwich. The second wet foam pad is laid on the top and the transfer cassette is closed.

4. The cassette is placed in the transfer tank such that the nitrocellulose membrane is between the gel and the anode. Place a cooling unit in the tank and fill it with transfer buffer. To maintain a low buffer temperature, a refrigerated/circulating water bath can be used. Alternatively, the tank can be placed on ice.

5. Transfer can be accomplished at either 100 V for 2 h or 25 V overnight.

6. Once the transfer is done, disassemble the units and rinse the nitrocellulose membrane with water. Incubate the nitrocellulose membrane with blocking solution for 30 min on low-speed shaker.

7. Discard the blocking solution and then rinse the nitrocellulose membrane with TBST.

8. Horseradish peroxidase (HRP) conjugated antibodies against most of epitope-tags are available. By using these antibodies, you can save incubation times for secondary antibody (see step 11). Dilute the antibody by 1:5,000 in antibody dilution buffer and incubate the nitrocellulose for 1–2 h at room temperature on a low-speed shaker.

9. The antibody is then removed and the membrane is washed four times for 10 min with TBST on low-speed shaker.

10. If you used HRP-conjugated antibodies, skip this step (and step 12). Otherwise, prepare the secondary antibody is as a 1:10,000 dilution in antibody dilution buffer and incubate with the nitrocellulose membrane for 30 min at room temperature on low-speed shaker.

11. Discard the secondary antibody and wash the membrane four times for 10 min with TBST on low-speed shaker.

12. Prepare ECL reagent (e.g., Thermo Scientific) by mixing one part of luminol/enhancer solution and one part of stable peroxide solution. Be careful not to contaminate each solution. Place the membrane on sheet protector, blotted with Kim-Wipes, and

then add ECL reagent on the membrane. After covering the membrane with the other side of sheet protector, blot the excess ECL reagent with Kim-Wipes.

13. This step is done in a dark room under safe light conditions. The sheet protector containing the membrane is placed in an X-ray film cassette with X-ray film for a suitable exposure time. The film can be developed using a standard X-ray film processor.

4. Notes

1. Protein A sepharose can also be used if your antibody comes from rabbit (total Ig) or mouse (total Ig) serum (see Subheading 2.2).
2. The physical half-life of ^{32}P is 14.3 days. Use isotope within 1 month after manufacture for kinase assay. Take all precautions required by your local authorities when working with radioactive isotopes (see Subheading 2.3).
3. Because purified MBP is usually basally phosphorylated, dephosphorylated MBP (commercially available) is better to use as a kinase substrate in the kinase assay (see Subheading 2.3).
4. Acrylamide is neurotoxic when unpolymerized, so care should be taken (see Subheading 2.4).
5. After final washing step, supernatant has to be completely removed. Using a 1-ml syringe with a 26 gauge needle will be helpful (see Subheading 3.1.2).
6. LRRK2 may be degraded if boiled at 100°C (see Subheading 3.2).
7. The protein sizes of LRRK2 and MBP are around 280 and 22 kDa, respectively. To resolve these two proteins on a single gel, a 12% SDS-PAGE gel or a 8–16% SDS-PAGE gradient gel must be used (*see* Subheading 3.3).
8. Because unincorporated radioisotopes are located at the dye front on the gel, be careful that the dye is not run off the gel. Before staining the gel, cut off dye front to avoid high background signals on X-ray films (*see* Subheading 3.3).

Acknowledgments

This work was supported by the USPHS P50NS038377 and R01NS048206. T.M.D. is the Leonard and Madlyn Abramson Professor in Neurodegenerative Diseases at Johns Hopkins.

References

1. Braak, H., Del Tredici, K., Rub, U., de Vos, R. A., Jansen Steur, E. N., and Braak, E. (2003) Staging of brain pathology related to sporadic Parkinson's disease. *Neurobiol Aging* **24**, 197–211.
2. Morris, H. R. (2005) Genetics of Parkinson's disease. *Ann Med* **37**, 86–96.
3. Lesage, S., and Brice, A. (2009) Parkinson's disease: from monogenic forms to genetic susceptibility factors. *Hum. Mol. Genet.* **18**, R48–59.
4. Elbaz, A. (2008) LRRK2: bridging the gap between sporadic and hereditary Parkinson's disease. *Lancet Neurol.* **7**, 562–564.
5. Haugarvoll, K., Rademakers, R., Kachergus, J. M., Nuytemans, K., Ross, O. A., Gibson, J. M., Tan, E. K., Gaig, C., Tolosa, E., Goldwurm, S., Guidi, M., Riboldazzi, G., Brown, L., Walter, U., Benecke, R., Berg, D., Gasser, T., Theuns, J., Pals, P., Cras, P., De Deyn, P. P., Engelborghs, S., Pickut, B., Uitti, R. J., Foroud, T., Nichols, W. C., Hagenah, J., Klein, C., Samii, A., Zabetian, C. P., Bonifati, V., Van Broeckhoven, C., Farrer, M. J., and Wszolek, Z. K. (2008) Lrrk2 R1441C parkinsonism is clinically similar to sporadic Parkinson disease. *Neurology* **70**, 1456–1460.
6. Change, N., Mercier, G., and Lucotte, G. (2008) Genetic screening of the G2019S mutation of the LRRK2 gene in Southwest European, North African, and Sephardic Jewish subjects. *Genet. Test.* **12**, 333–339.
7. Tan, E. K., Tan, L. C., Lim, H. Q., Li, R., Tang, M., Yih, Y., Pavanni, R., Prakash, K. M., Fook-Chong, S., and Zhao, Y. (2008) LRRK2 R1628P increases risk of Parkinson's disease: replication evidence. *Hum. Genet.* **124**, 287–288.
8. Tomiyama, H., Mizuta, I., Li, Y., Funayama, M., Yoshino, H., Li, L., Murata, M., Yamamoto, M., Kubo, S., Mizuno, Y., Toda, T., and Hattori, N. (2008) LRRK2 P755L variant in sporadic Parkinson's disease. *J. Hum. Genet.* **53**, 1012–1015.
9. Floris, G., Cannas, A., Solla, P., Murru, M. R., Tranquilli, S., Corongiu, D., Rolesu, M., Cuccu, S., Sardu, C., Marrosu, F., and Marrosu, M. G. (2009) Genetic analysis for five LRRK2 mutations in a Sardinian parkinsonian population: Importance of G2019S and R1441C mutations in sporadic Parkinson's disease patients. *Parkinsonism Relat. Disord.* **15**, 277–280.
10. Gorostidi, A., Ruiz-Martinez, J., Lopez de Munain, A., Alzualde, A., and Marti Masso, J. F. (2009) LRRK2 G2019S and R1441G mutations associated with Parkinson's disease are common in the Basque Country, but relative prevalence is determined by ethnicity. *Neurogenetics* **10**, 157–159.
11. Patra, B., Parsian, A. J., Racette, B. A., Zhao, J. H., Perlmutter, J. S., and Parsian, A. (2009) LRRK2 gene G2019S mutation and SNPs [haplotypes] in subtypes of Parkinson's disease. *Parkinsonism Relat. Disord.* **15**, 175–180.
12. Zimprich, A., Biskup, S., Leitner, P., Lichtner, P., Farrer, M., Lincoln, S., Kachergus, J., Hulihan, M., Uitti, R. J., Calne, D. B., Stoessl, A. J., Pfeiffer, R. F., Patenge, N., Carbajal, I. C., Vieregge, P., Asmus, F., Muller-Myhsok, B., Dickson, D. W., Meitinger, T., Strom, T. M., Wszolek, Z. K., and Gasser, T. (2004) Mutations in LRRK2 cause autosomal-dominant parkinsonism with pleomorphic pathology. *Neuron* **44**, 601–607.
13. Greggio, E., Jain, S., Kingsbury, A., Bandopadhyay, R., Lewis, P., Kaganovich, A., van der Brug, M. P., Beilina, A., Blackinton, J., Thomas, K. J., Ahmad, R., Miller, D. W., Kesavapany, S., Singleton, A., Lees, A., Harvey, R. J., Harvey, K., and Cookson, M. R. (2006) Kinase activity is required for the toxic effects of mutant LRRK2/dardarin. *Neurobiol. Dis.* **23**, 329–341.
14. Smith, W. W., Pei, Z., Jiang, H., Dawson, V. L., Dawson, T. M., and Ross, C. A. (2006) Kinase activity of mutant LRRK2 mediates neuronal toxicity. *Nat. Neurosci.* **9**, 1231–1233.
15. Cookson, M. R., Dauer, W., Dawson, T., Fon, E. A., Guo, M., and Shen, J. (2007) The roles of kinases in familial Parkinson's disease. *J. Neurosci.* **27**, 11865–11868.
16. West, A. B., Moore, D. J., Choi, C., Andrabi, S. A., Li, X., Dikeman, D., Biskup, S., Zhang, Z., Lim, K. L., Dawson, V. L., and Dawson, T. M. (2007) Parkinson's disease-associated mutations in LRRK2 link enhanced GTP-binding and kinase activities to neuronal toxicity. *Hum. Mol. Genet.* **16** pp. 223–232.
17. West, A. B., Moore, D. J., Biskup, S., Bugayenko, A., Smith, W. W., Ross, C. A., Dawson, V. L., and Dawson, T. M. (2005) Parkinson's disease-associated mutations in leucine-rich repeat kinase 2 augment kinase activity. *Proc. Natl. Acad. Sci. USA* **102**, 16842–16847.
18. Gloeckner, C. J., Kinkl, N., Schumacher, A., Braun, R. J., O'Neill, E., Meitinger, T., Kolch, W., Prokisch, H., and Ueffing, M. (2006) The Parkinson disease causing LRRK2 mutation I2020T is associated with increased kinase activity. *Hum. Mol. Genet.* **15**, 223–232.
19. Covy, J. P., and Giasson, B. I. (2009) Identification of compounds that inhibit the kinase activity of leucine-rich repeat kinase 2. *Biochem. Biophys. Res. Commun.* **378**, 473–477.

Chapter 4

Measuring PI3K Lipid Kinase Activity

Elisa Ciraolo, Alessia Perino, and Emilio Hirsch

Abstract

Class IA phosphoinositide-3 kinases (PI3Ks) signaling has recently emerged as a key element in cancer development because of its ability to trigger a complex panoply of cellular responses controlling survival and proliferation. Many cancers show inappropriately activated PI3K pathway, and tumors with high PI3K activity are frequently resistant to traditional chemotherapy. Indeed, preclinical studies demonstrated a prominent role for the PI3K pathway in cancer cell survival and growth, thus validating PI3K as a potential drug target in cancer. The emerging interest in inhibiting PI3Ks in cancer have prompted the aggressive development of new selective PI3K pathway inhibitors as cancer therapy, and many of these molecules are currently in early-phase clinical trials. In this chapter, we describe methods to measure the PI3K lipid kinase activity in vitro, which is the standard procedure to test the efficacy of inhibitors.

Key words: PI3K, PI3K lipid kinase activity, Phosphatidylinositol 3,4,5-trisphosphate, Phosphatidylinositol, PI3K inhibitors

1. Introduction

Signal transduction downstream of tyrosine kinase receptors (RTKs) needs lipid production to activate the intracellular signaling cascade (1). Among them, membrane lipids such as phosphatidylinositol 3,4,5-trisphosphate ($PI(3,4,5)P_3$), act as a docking site for cytoplasmic signaling proteins. PI3Ks are lipid kinases that trigger the production of $PI(3,4,5)P_3$. While the unique member of class IB, PI3Kγ, is mainly activated by G protein-coupled receptors (GPCRs), class IA PI3K signaling is clearly triggered by activated RTKs (2). Upon receptor activation, the PI3K regulatory subunit p85 is recruited to the tyrosine-phosphorylated motifs on the receptor, and this event triggers the lipid kinase activity of PI3K. At the same time, this localizes the enzyme next to the plasma membrane, in proximity of its lipid substrate phosphatidylinositol 4,5-bisphosphate ($PI(4,5)P_2$).

RTKs have emerged as important targets for drug design in cancer, and many RTK inhibitors are now used as new pharmacological agents such as Gleevec for the treatment of chronic myeloid leukemia (3) or Iressa for lung cancer (4). Nevertheless, the administration of these drugs often causes the development of resistance that usually compromises the response to therapy and the prognosis. One of the most common events that contribute to the establishment of drug resistance is the propensity of the cell to activate the PI3K/AKT pathway (5). Indeed, since the PI3K signaling pathway is strictly controlled by RTKs, an ideal RTK inhibitor should be effective in downregulating at the same time the RTK activity and the PI3K-Akt pathway. On the contrary, in human cancer another mechanism of PI3K activation, independent from RTKs has emerged. Indeed, PI3K was found to be mutated and overexpressed in many tumors (6). The simple overexpression of wild-type class IA PI3K is sufficient to induce an oncogenic phenotype in cultured cells (6). More recently, somatic activating mutations have been identified in the class IA PI3K catalytic subunit p110α, these mutations occur in up to 30% of common epithelial cancers including colon, breast, prostate and endometrial cancers (7). All these findings have encouraged the development of new PI3K inhibitors and several small molecules that inhibit PI3K are now in clinical trials. These molecules differ in their selectivity, ability to inhibit a specific PI3K isoform, and potency. The in vitro measurement of PI3K lipid kinase activity provides a measurement of both selectivity and potency.

Herein, we describe the method to measure the lipid kinase activity of these enzymes in vitro. Many antibodies against the different PI3K isoforms are now commercially available, which allows the analysis of the activity of each PI3K isoform in different contexts. In addition, several companies offer recombinant enzymes that are ready to use. We first describe how to measure the lipid kinase activity of PI3Ks isolated from cells in the presence or absence of stimuli. Second, we describe how to measure the lipid kinase activity of recombinant proteins in the presence or absence of inhibitors.

2. Materials

2.1. Cell Culture and Lysis

1. Phosphate Buffered Saline (PBS): 137 mM NaCl, 2.7 mM KCl, 10 mM Na_2HPO_4, and 1.76 mM KH_2PO_4 pH 7.4 in bidistilled water. Sterilize by autoclaving.
2. Trypsin/EDTA solution (10×): 5.0 g/l porcine trypsin and 2 g/l EDTA in 0.9% sodium chloride. Sterilize and filter prior to use.

3. Lysis Buffer for protein extraction: 20 mM Tris–HCl pH 8.0, 138 mM NaCl, 5 mM EDTA, 2.7 mM KCl, 1 mM MgCl$_2$, 1 mM CaCl$_2$, 5% glycerol, 1 mM sodium-o-vanadate, 1 μg/ml aprotinin, 1 μg/ml leupeptin, 1 μg/ml pepstatin, 1%, Nonidet P-40 (NP40), 20 mM NaF, 10 mM Sodium Pyrophosphate.

4. Bradford protein assay: The methods described here use a commercial kit. Any assay measuring protein content may be used.

5. Cell culture medium: Dulbecco's modified Eagle's medium (DMEM) supplemented with 10% FBS, 2 mM glutamine, 100 μg/ml streptomycin, and 100 units/ml penicillin.

6. Growth factors: 1 μM insulin in DMEM; 1 μM IGF-1 in DMEM.

2.2. Immunoprecipitation of PI3K

1. Washing Buffer: 0.1 M Tris–HCl pH 7.4, 0.5 M LiCl.
2. Kinase Buffer: 20 mM HEPES–HCl pH 7.4, 5 mM MgCl$_2$.
3. p85 Antibody: The methods described here have been tried and tested with the commercially available p85 antibodies from Cell Signaling Technology and Upstate.
4. IRS-1 antibody: The methods described here have been tried and tested with the commercially available IRS-1 antibodies from Cell Signaling Technology, Upstate and Santa Cruz Biotechnology.
5. Protein G-coupled sepharose beads: available from several commercial sources.

2.3. PI3K Lipid Kinase Assay

The methods described here have been tried and tested with the commercially available lipids and recombinant enzymes from Jena Bioscience.

1. Phosphatidylinositol (PI) stock solution: 1 mg/ml L-α-PI Phosphatidylinositol from bovine liver in CHCl$_3$–MetOH (2:1 v/v). Store aliquots (300 μl) at −80°C.
2. Phosphatidylserine (PS) stock solution: 1 mg/ml L-α-Phosphatidylserine from porcine brain in CHCl$_3$–MetOH (9:1 v/v). Store aliquots (300 μl) at −80°C.
3. TGX-221 inhibitor: 200 μM stock in 100% DMSO (see Note 1).
4. Recombinant proteins: p110α/p85α, p110β/p85α, p110δ/p85α, and p110γ.
5. Cold ATP: 6 mM ATP in bidistilled water. Store single-use aliquots at −20°C. Do not freeze and thaw aliquots to avoid hydrolysis.
6. Radioactive ATP: ^{32}P-γATP, specific activity 6,000 Ci/mmol.

2.4. Thin Layer Chromatography

1. Thin Layer Chromatography (TLC) plates.
2. TLC Buffer: 45%:35%:8.5%:1.5% (v/v) $CHCl_3$–MetOH–H_2O–25% NH_4OH.

3. Methods

Class IA PI3K are heterodimeric enzymes constituted by a regulatory and a catalytic subunit. Five regulatory subunits exist (p85α, p55α, p50α, p85β, and p55γ), which interact with three catalytic subunits (p110α, p110β, and p110δ) (8). While p110α and p110β are ubiquitously expressed in mammals, p110δ expression is predominant in leukocytes. In vitro, class IA PI3Ks are able to generate three different inositols: the phosphatidylinositol 3-phosphate (PI(3)P), phosphatidylinositol (3,4)-bisphosphate (PI(3,4)P2), and phosphatidylinositol (3,4,5)-trisphosphate (PI(3,4,5)P3) (Fig. 1) (9). Here, we describe how to measure the production of PI(3)P by PI3K. In particular, we first describe the methods to assay the lipid kinase activity associated to the p85 regulatory subunits and to the activated RTKs. Second, we describe how to measure the lipid kinase activity by using PI3K recombinant proteins.

3.1. Immunoprecipitation of PI3K Activity from Cells Using an Anti-p85 Antibody

1. Grow NIH-3T3 cells in 10-cm cell-culture dishes in Dulbecco's modified Eagle's medium (DMEM) supplemented with 10% FBS, 2 mM glutamine, 100 μg/ml streptomycin and 100 units/ml penicillin at 37°C in a 5% CO_2 atmosphere. When cells are confluent, they are passaged with 1× trypsin/EDTA onto either a new 10-cm dish to maintain the culture or to a 15 cm dish to perform the experiment. Cells usually grow very fast, reach confluence after 48 h, and can be split 1:4 or 1:5.
2. When a 15-cm dish is confluent, transfer the dish on ice and wash twice with ice-cold PBS. Discard PBS carefully.
3. Add 500 μl of ice-cold Lysis Buffer to the dish and incubate for 10–15 min at 4°C with moderate shaking. Scrape lysed cells from the dish and centrifuge at 8,000×g for 10 min at 4°C in a 1.5-ml tube (see Note 2).
4. Collect supernatant in a new tube and measure protein concentration with the Bradford Protein Assay as follows. Dilute the concentrated Bradford Protein Assay Dye Reagent 1:5 in bidistilled water and transfer 1 ml of this reagent into a 1 ml polystyrene cuvette. Add to the cuvette 5 μl of the cell lysate and mix until the solution changes color completely. Read the absorbance in a visible light spectrophotometer at 595 nm. Compare the absorbance value with a standard curve (see Note 3).
5. Incubate 1–2 mg of protein extract with 5 μg of anti-p85 antibody, followed by the addition of protein G-coupled sepharose beads. Incubate the sample for 2 h at 4°C with rotation.

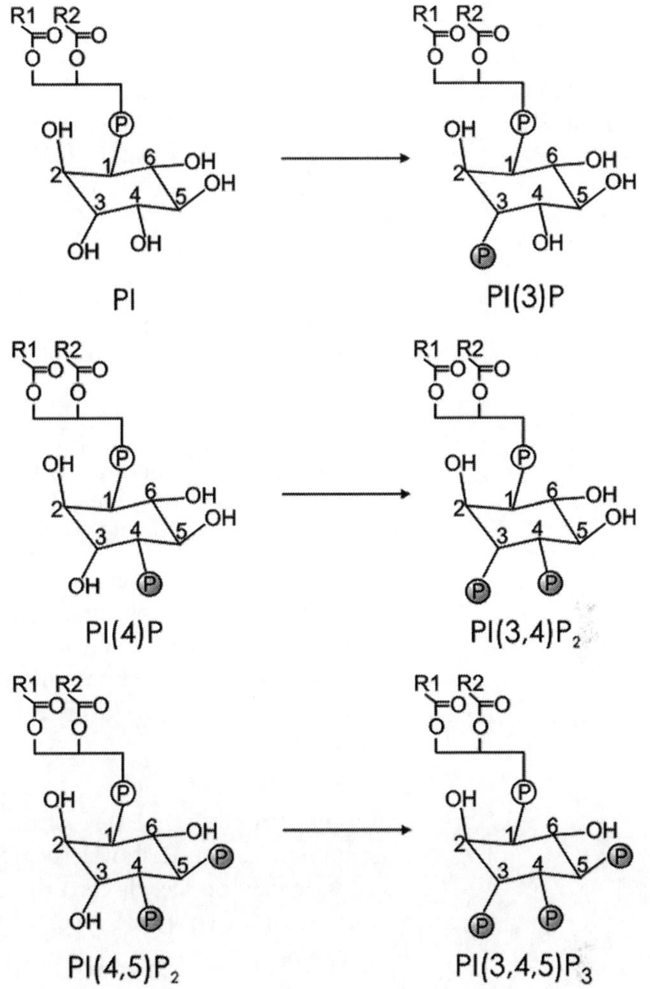

Fig. 1. PI3K substrates and products. While in vivo class I PI3Ks are able to phosphorylate only Phosphatidylinositol 4,5-bisphosphate (PI(4,5)P$_3$) to produce Phosphatidylinositol 3,4,5-trisphosphate (PI(3,4,5)P$_3$), in vitro they also use the Phosphatidylinositol (PI) and Phosphatidylinositol 4-phosphate (PI(4)P) to generate Phosphatidylinositol 3-phosphate (PI(3)P) and Phosphatidylinositol 3,4-bisphosphate (PI(3,4)P$_2$).

6. After incubation, immune complexes bound to the beads are centrifuged for 4 min at 2,000×*g* at 4°C. Discard the supernatant and keep the beads.
7. Wash the beads two times with 1 ml of Lysis Buffer, two times with 1 ml of Washing Buffer, and two times with 1 ml of Kinase Buffer (see Note 4).
8. After the last wash step, carefully remove all of the supernatant using a flat-end syringe. Take care not to disrupt the protein G Sepharose bead pellet. Resuspend beads with 40 µl of Kinase Buffer.
9. Proceed as described in Subheading 3.3.

3.2. Immunoprecipitation of PI3K Activity from Stimulated Cells Using the Anti-IRS-1 Antibody

The insulin receptor (IR) and the insulin-like growth factor-1 receptor (IGF-1R) are RTKs that transmit the signal to intracellular pathway via an adaptor such as the insulin receptor substrate IRS. To date, four members of the IRS family (IRS-1, IRS-2, IRS-3, and IRS-4) have been identified. Upon extracellular ligand binding, tyrosine-phosphorylated motifs on the RTK function as docking sites for IRS proteins. Subsequently, the IRS itself is directly phosphorylated by the receptor. This event enables the IRS proteins to activate PI3K though the direct interaction with p85. Thus, in this section we describe the method to measure the PI3K activity associated to IRS-1 after stimulation with insulin or IGF-1 (10).

1. Grow NIH-3T3 cells in 15-cm cell culture dishes in Dulbecco's modified Eagle's medium (DMEM) supplemented with 10% FBS, 2 mM glutamine, 100 µg/ml streptomycin and 100 units/ml penicillin at 37°C in a 5% CO_2 atmosphere.

2. When cells are confluent, split cells so that each dish contains $2-4 \times 10^6$ cells. The day after, two dishes are washed twice with PBS and then maintained serum-starved overnight in DMEM supplemented with 2 mM glutamine, 100 µg/ml streptomycin, and 100 units/ml penicillin at 37°C in a 5% CO_2 atmosphere.

3. After starvation, stimulate one plate for 5 min with DMEM supplemented with 1 µM of insulin or 1 µM of IGF-1. After stimulation, transfer both plates (stimulated and unstimulated) very quickly on ice, discard the stimulus and then wash plates once with ice-cold PBS (see Note 5). Remove all the PBS.

4. Add 500 µl of Lysis Buffer to each plate and incubate for 10 min at 4°C with moderate shaking. Scrape lysed cells from the dish, collect in a 1.5-ml tube and centrifuge at $8,000 \times g$ for 10 min at 4°C. Transfer the supernatant to a new tube and use all protein extract for the immunoprecipitation (next step).

5. Incubate proteins with 5 µg anti-IRS-1 antibody, followed by addition of protein G sepharose beads. Incubate sample for 2 h at 4°C with rotation (see Note 6).

6. After incubation, centrifuge immune complexes bound to the beads for 4 min at $2,000 \times g$ at 4°C. Discard the supernatant and keep the beads.

7. Wash the beads twice with 1 ml of Lysis Buffer, twice with 1 ml of Washing Buffer, and twice with 1 ml Kinase Buffer.

8. After the last washing step, carefully remove all the supernatant using a flat-end syringe and resuspend the beads with 40 µl of Kinase Buffer.

9. Proceed as described in Subheading 3.3.

3.3. Lipid Kinase Assay to Measure PI3K Lipid Kinase Activity

1. Determine the specific activity (S_A) of the commercial radioactive ATP. The specific activity is specified as of the calibration date (provided by the supplier). This must be taken into consideration when calculated concentrations in mass-dependent applications. The specific activity on any day prior to the calibration date can be calculating using the formula shown in Fig. 2a. The specific activity on any day after the calibration date can be calculated using the formula shown in Fig. 2b.

2. To prepare Substrate Solution I (at least 300 μl), add 300 μl of 1 mg/ml PS stock solution and 300 μl of 1 mg/ml PI stock solution to a 1.5-ml tube. Dry the lipids very carefully under a stream of nitrogen gas. Resuspend dried lipids in 300 μl of Kinase Buffer and sonicate for 15 sec at moderate amplitude prior to use (see Note 7). Keep lipids on ice.

3. To prepare Substrate Solution II (10 μl for each sample), mix 0.1 μl of the 6 mM cold ATP stock solution and 5 μCi of radioactive ^{32}P-ATP with Kinase Buffer to reach a final volume of 10 μl.

a
$$S_A = \frac{S_{Acal}}{D_F + \frac{S_{Acal}*(1-D_F)}{S_{Atheo}}}$$

b
$$S_A = \frac{D_F}{\frac{1}{S_{Acal}} - \frac{1-D_F}{S_{Atheo}}}$$

Fig. 2. Formulas to calculate the specific activity (S_A) of commercial radioactive ATP. SA_{cal} is the specific activity on the calibration date. DF is the fraction of current radioactivity that will remain on the calibration date (see Table 1). For example, for a date 8 days prior to the calibration date DF=0,678. SA_{theo} is 9120 for the theoretical specific activity of carrier free ^{32}P.

Table 1
Decay chart

day	0	1	2	3	4	5	6	7	8	9
0	1.000	0.953	0.906	0.865	0.824	0.785	0.748	0.712	0.678	0.646
10	0.616	0.587	0.559	0.532	0.507	0.483	0.460	0.436	0.418	0.396
20	0.379	0.361	0.344	0.328	0.312	0.297	0.283	0.270	0.257	0.245
30	0.233	0.222	0.212	0.202	0.192	0.183	0.174	0.166	0.158	0.151
40	0.144	0.137	0.130	0.124	0.118	0.113	0.107	0.102	0.096	0.093
50	0.088	0.084	0.080	0.077	0.073	0.069	0.066	0.063	0.060	0.057
60	0.054	0.052	0.049	0.047	0.045	0.043	0.041	0.039	0.037	0.035

This table is used to calculate the specific activity of ^{32}P-γATP at a date different from the assay date

4. Add 10 µl of the Substrate Solution I and 10 µl of the Substrate Solution II to the immunoprecipitates (see Subheadings 3.1 and 3.2).

5. Allow the kinase reaction to proceed at 30°C for 10 min under constant mixing.

6. Stop the reaction by adding 100 µl of 1 N HCl.

7. Extract lipids by adding 200 µl of $CHCl_3$/MetOH (1:1 v/v). Vortex and centrifuge for 4 min at $2,000 \times g$. After centrifugation, two liquid phases are present. Collect the lower phase (the organic phase containing the phosphorylated lipids) and transfer to a new 1.5-ml tube (see Note 8).

8. Make three holes in the lid of each tube and dry lipids in a vacuum concentrator for 30 min at room temperature (see Note 9).

9. Continue to Subheading 3.5.

3.4. Measurement of PI3K Lipid Kinase Activity Using Recombinant Protein, in the Presence or Absence of PI3K Inhibitors

1. Dilute 100 ng of recombinant p110β in 10 µl of Kinase Buffer to obtain a concentration of 10 µg/ml (see Note 10).

2. Dilute the PI3K inhibitor TGX221 in Kinase Buffer to a concentration of 200 nM.

3. Prepare Substrate Solution I and Substrate Solution II as described in Subheading 3.3.

4. Using a 1.5-ml tube, mix 10 µl of recombinant protein, 30 µl of 200 nM TGX221, 10 µl of Substrate Solution I, and finally 10 µl of the Substrate solution II.

5. Allow the kinase reaction to proceed at 30°C for 10 min under constant mixing.

6. Stop the reaction by adding 100 µl of 1 N HCl.

7. Extract lipids by adding 200 µl of $CHCl_3$/MetOH solution (1:1 v/v). Vortex and centrifuge for 4 min at $2,000 \times g$. After centrifugation, two phases are present. Collect the lower phase (the organic phase containing the phosphorylated lipids) and transfer to a new 1.5-ml tube (see Note 8).

8. Make three holes in the lid of each tube and dry lipids in a vacuum concentrator for 30 min at room temperature (see Note 9).

9. Continue with Subheading 3.5.

3.5. Thin Layer Chromatography

1. Handle the TLC plate carefully and always wear gloves to avoid contamination of the silica gel layer.

2. Heat the TLC plate in an oven at 57°C for 15–30 min. The TLC plate needs to be dried carefully because humidity on the silica gel interferes with chromatography.

3. Sample should be spotted on the TLC plate at 1.5 cm distance (or more) from the base of the plate. Using a pencil and a ruler, trace a line at 1.5 cm distance from the base. Take care

when you use the pencil since the silica gel is delicate and scratches should be avoided.

4. Resuspend dried lipids in 30–40 µl of a $CHCl_3$–MetOH solution (2:1, v/v). Mix by flicking the tube with a finger to resuspend the lipids.

5. By using a glass syringe, collect the resuspended lipids and apply 5–10 µl drops of the sample on the TLC plate following the line traced with the pencil and allow the sample to dry at room temperature (see Note 11).

6. Clean the glass syringe with $CHCl_3$–MetOH solution (2:1, v/v) between samples to avoid carry-over of material from one sample to the other.

7. Following the last sample application, allow the TLC plate to dry for 5–10 min at room temperature.

8. Develop the TLC plate using the Chromatographic Buffer in a glass chromatography tank. Dip the sample side of the TLC plate into the buffer (see Note 12). The buffer will be absorbed by the silica gel and it will drag lipid along by capillary action. Because different analytes ascend the TLC plate at different rates, separation of lipids is achieved. In this case, since only the Phosphatidylinositol 3-phosphate (PI(3)P) is produced, the TLC chromatography separates the lipids from unbound ^{32}P-ATP, which remains at the traced start line.

9. Remove the TLC plate from the tank when the solvent front has reached 3 cm from the top.

10. Dry the TLC plate for 10–15 min at 37°C and expose it to radiographic film for different time points. The time of exposure will depend on the intensity of the signal and has to be determined empirically (see Note 13).

4. Notes

1. Do not dissolve the TGX-221 powder in less than 100% DMSO, since this may lead to the formation of aggregates in water (see Subheading 2.3, step 3).

2. It is critical to keep cell lysate, PBS and Lysis Buffer on ice during all manipulations to minimize the risk of protease and phosphatase activity (see Subheading 3.1, step 3).

3. Prepare a standard curve of absorbance versus micrograms of albumin and determine amounts from the curve. Determine concentrations of original samples from the amount protein, volume/sample, and dilution factor, if any. Consider that the Bradford method is sensitive to about 5–100 µg of protein (see Subheading 3.1, step 4).

4. Keep all solutions and samples in ice to minimize risk of protease and phosphatase activity. In addition, many lipid kinases are sensitive to detergents. Do not use sodium dodecyl sulfate (SDS) in the lysis buffer, since SDS kills lipid kinase activity and causes protein denaturation. On the contrary, NP40 inhibits PI3K activity and it is, therefore, crucial to remove all the detergent solution by careful wash with WB and KB solutions. Immunoprecipitates are generally washed by pelletting protein G beads by centrifugation (4 min at $2,000 \times g$), aspirating 90% of the supernatant and adding 1 ml of the next washing solution (see Subheading 3.1, step 7).

5. It is important to transfer very quickly the plates on ice and keep them on it during all passages to block at the same time the stimulation and any phosphatase activity (see Subheading 3.2, step 3).

6. Since phosphotyrosine are not stable for long time at 4°C and hydrolysis may occur, do not incubate the immune complexes for more than 2 h at 4°C. In addition, do not use frozen cell lysates, since freezing destroys protein-protein interactions (see Subheading 3.2, step 5).

7. Dry lipids only with nitrogen gas. Nitrogen is an inert gas and does not hydrolyze lipids. When you dry PI and PS with nitrogen, check that chloroform and methanol are completely evaporated; otherwise, residual solvent cause PI and PS precipitation when KB is added. Sonication should be performed on ice. Moreover, resuspend lipids in at least 300 μl of KB, since a smaller volume is difficult to sonicate. The PI should appear cloudy at first and eventually clear. Excessive sonication results in oxidized, precipitated lipid. Once sonicated, the lipid mixture should not be frozen, and any excess should be discarded (see Subheading 3.3, step 2).

8. Generally, the lower phase can be removed using a 200 μl gel loading tip. By keeping the tip on the bottom of the tube, the lower phase can be removed from the bottom upward, taking care not to contaminate it with the upper phase (see Subheadings 3.3, step 7 and 3.4, step 7).

9. Dried lipids may be stored at −20°C for several days (see Subheadings 3.3, step 8 and 3.4, step 8).

10. The amount of protein used in the lipid kinase assay depends on the specific activity of the PI3K isoform. When PtdIns are used as substrate, p110 beta display less lipid kinase activity than alpha (11). Generally, the amount of p110 used in this assay is variable from 10 to 1 μg for each reaction. For example, as shown in Fig. 3, we use 100 ng of p110β recombinant protein in the presence or absence of the p110β specific inhibitor TGX221 (see Subheading 3.4, step 1).

11. If you have more samples, spot them leaving enough space between each one (at least 1.5 cm, see Subheading 3.5, step 5).

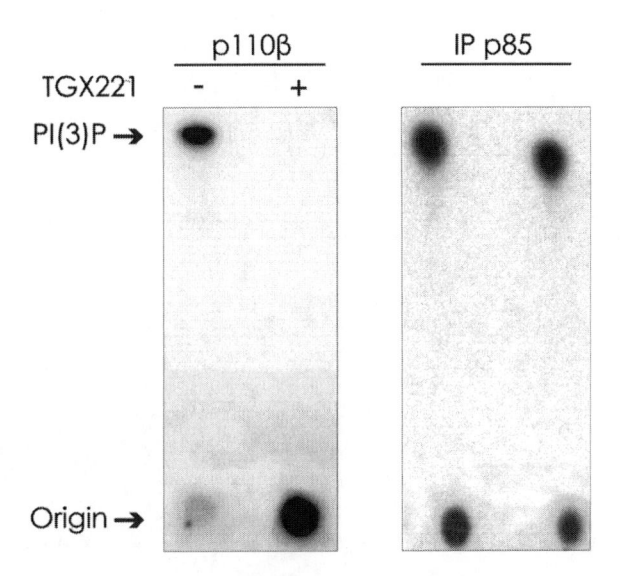

Fig. 3. Lipid kinase assay. *Left panel*: Lipid kinase assay of the p110β recombinant protein in presence or absence of specific inhibitor. The recombinant protein was incubated with 100 nM of TGX221. Samples were loaded (origin) on the TLC and run in a chromatographic chamber. In the presence of inhibitor, p110β is not able to produce PI(3)P and no signal is detectable. *Right panel*: Lipid kinase activity associated to p85. Class IA PI3Ks were immunoprecipitated with 5 μg of anti-p85 antibody. Immunocomplexes were then incubated with the appropriate amount of ^{32}P-ATP and substrate (PI) and loaded on the TLC plate (origin). The signal corresponding to the PI(3)P product is clearly detectable on the radiographic film.

12. When you dip the plate into the buffer make sure that the liquid does not cover the spotted samples. In a chromatography tank, as displayed in Fig. 4 we suggest the use of 30–40 ml of chromatography buffer (see Subheading 3.5, step 8).

13. Although the radioactive lipid kinase assay has been successfully used for many years, the use of the radioactive ^{32}P isotope has several disadvantages, including licensing restrictions, disposal costs, short shelf-life, and potential health risks associated with exposure. In addition, the screening of new potential inhibitory molecules recently has required the development of new non radioactive high-throughput screening strategies with similar sensitivity. To this day, different companies offer new methods for the in vitro measurement of the PI3K lipid kinase activity. Here, we present two examples of new lipid kinase assays. These assays are versatile, since that they can be adapted to all protein kinases including the lipid protein kinase. The Adapta® Universal Kinase Assay Kit is a fluorescence-based immunoassay for the detection of the ADP production. The ADP formed during the lipid phophorylation by PI3K is detected through a TR-FRET signal whose reduction is proportional to the ADP produced. The ADP-Glo™ Kinase Assay is a luminescent kinase assay that measures the ADP

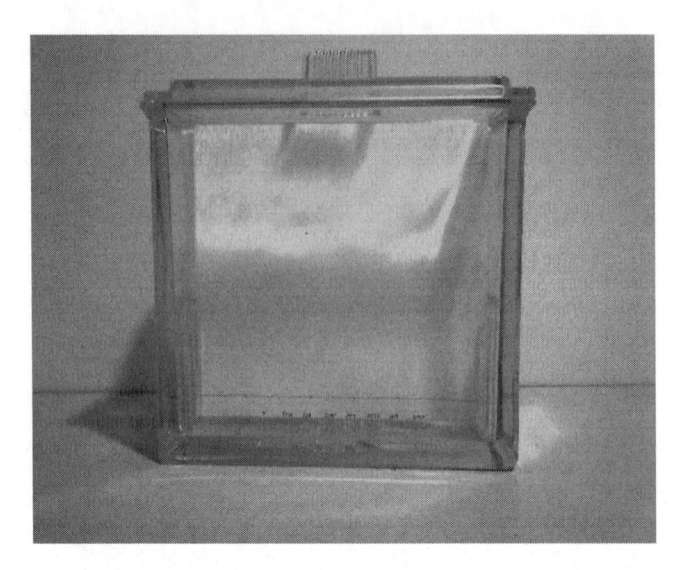

Fig. 4. TLC chromatography tank. This is an example of a TLC developing chamber able to hold and run five 20 × 20 cm TLC plates.

formed in a kinase reaction. During the assay, the ADP formed by the lipid kinase activity is converted to ATP, which is the substrate of a Luciferase, leading to the consequent production of light. In this assay, the luminescent signal directly correlates with the amount of the produced ADP (see Subheading 3.5, step 10).

References

1. Engelman, J. A., Luo, J., and Cantley, L. C. (2006) The evolution of phosphatidylinositol 3-kinases as regulators of growth and metabolism. *Nat. Rev. Genet.* 7, 606–619.
2. Hirsch, E., Ciraolo, E., Ghigo, A., and Costa, C. (2008) Taming the PI3K team to hold inflammation and cancer at bay, *Pharmacology & therapeutics 118*, 192–205.
3. Nadal, E., and Olavarria, E. (2004) Imatinib mesylate (Gleevec/Glivec) a molecular-targeted therapy for chronic myeloid leukaemia and other malignancies. *International journal of clinical practice* 58, 511–516.
4. Helfrich, B. A., Raben, D., Varella-Garcia, M., Gustafson, D., Chan, D. C., Bemis, L., Coldren, C., Baron, A., Zeng, C., Franklin, W. A., Hirsch, F. R., Gazdar, A., Minna, J., and Bunn, P. A., Jr. (2006) Antitumor activity of the epidermal growth factor receptor (EGFR) tyrosine kinase inhibitor gefitinib (ZD1839, Iressa) in non-small cell lung cancer cell lines correlates with gene copy number and EGFR mutations but not EGFR protein levels. *Clin. Cancer Res.* 12, 7117–7125.
5. McCubrey, J. A., Steelman, L. S., Abrams, S. L., Lee, J. T., Chang, F., Bertrand, F. E., Navolanic, P. M., Terrian, D. M., Franklin, R. A., D'Assoro, A. B., Salisbury, J. L., Mazzarino, M. C., Stivala, F., and Libra, M. (2006) Roles of the RAF/MEK/ERK and PI3K/PTEN/AKT pathways in malignant transformation and drug resistance. *Advances in enzyme regulation* 46, 249–279.
6. Samuels, Y., Wang, Z., Bardelli, A., Silliman, N., Ptak, J., Szabo, S., Yan, H., Gazdar, A., Powell, S. M., Riggins, G. J., Willson, J. K., Markowitz, S., Kinzler, K. W., Vogelstein, B., and Velculescu, V. E. (2004) High frequency of

mutations of the PIK3CA gene in human cancers. *Science* **304**, 554.

7. Engelman, J. A. (2009) Targeting PI3K signalling in cancer: opportunities, challenges and limitations. *Nat. Rev. Cancer* **9**, 550–562.

8. Geering, B., Cutillas, P. R., Nock, G., Gharbi, S. I., and Vanhaesebroeck, B. (2007) Class IA phosphoinositide 3-kinases are obligate p85-p110 heterodimers. *Proc. Natl. Acad. Sci.USA* **104**, 7809–7814.

9. Vanhaesebroeck, B., and Waterfield, M. D. (1999) Signaling by distinct classes of phosphoinositide 3-kinases. *Exp. Cell Res.* **253**, 239–254.

10. Kahn, C. R., White, M. F., Shoelson, S. E., Backer, J. M., Araki, E., Cheatham, B., Csermely, P., Folli, F., Goldstein, B. J., Huertas, P., and et al. (1993) The insulin receptor and its substrate: molecular determinants of early events in insulin action. *Rec. Prog. Horm. Res.* **48**, 291–339.

11. Beeton, C. A., Chance, E. M., Foukas, L. C., and Shepherd, P. R. (2000) Comparison of the kinetic properties of the lipid- and protein-kinase activities of the p110alpha and p110beta catalytic subunits of class-Ia phosphoinositide 3-kinases. *Biochem J*. 350 Pt 2, 353–359.

Chapter 5

A Fluorescence Polarization Assay for the Discovery of Inhibitors of the Polo-Box Domain of Polo-Like Kinase 1

Wolfgang Reindl, Klaus Strebhardt, and Thorsten Berg

Abstract

Polo-like kinase 1 (Plk1) is a key player in mitosis and has been widely recognized as a therapeutic target for many human cancer types. Apart from its kinase domain, Plk1 harbors a protein–protein interaction domain dubbed "polo-box domain" (PBD), by which the enzyme binds to its intracellular anchorage sites and to at least a fraction of its substrates. Recent evidence indicates that the inhibition of the PBD by small molecules is feasible and might allow for the discovery of highly specific inhibitors of the enzyme. This chapter details the practical work necessary to set up an assay based on fluorescence polarization for the discovery of inhibitors of the Plk1 PBD, which can be used for high-throughput screening in a 384-well format.

Key words: Binding assay, Fluorescence polarization, High-throughput screening, Polo-box domain, Polo-like kinase 1

1. Introduction

The serine/threonine kinase Plk1 (1–3) is of crucial importance for several steps in mitosis and is generally considered to be a target for antitumor therapy. Apart from its catalytic domain, Plk1 has a protein–protein interaction domain termed "polo-box domain" (PBD), which is required for proper intracellular localization of the enzyme and for docking to at least a subset of the enzyme's substrates (4, 5). The PBD binds to peptide motifs bearing a core S-(pT/pS)-(P/X) motif. Because the PBD is unique to the family of polo-like kinases, it has been hypothesized that inhibitors of the Plk1 PBD could be more specific than ATP-competitive inhibitors (3, 5). In fact, small molecules that target the function of the Plk1 PBD have already been shown to effectively induce mitotic arrest in cancer cells (6–8). In this chapter, we describe a detailed experimental procedure for a previously reported assay system based on fluorescence polarization (9) that can be used in high-throughput screening campaigns to identify small-molecule inhibitors of the Plk1 PBD (6, 8).

Fluorescence polarization assays monitor the increase in rotational mobility of a relatively small molecule upon separation from a larger binding partner (10). The small binding partner is represented by a peptide known to bind to the Plk1 PBD. It is labeled with 5-carboxyfluorescein at its N-terminus (6, 9). Excitation of the fluorophores with linearly polarized light leads to excitation of only those fluorophores which have the proper orientation relative to the plane of polarization of the light. Thus, at the time of excitation, all excited fluorophores (whether their attached peptides are protein-bound or not) are orientated in a uniform manner. If the peptide is bound to the Plk1 PBD, it rotates relatively slowly as part of the high-molecular weight complex, which results in a relatively uniform spatial orientation of the peptide/protein complex at the time of fluorescence emission. This is recorded as a high value of the fluorescence polarization. Small molecules that are able to inhibit the function of the Plk1 PBD liberate the fluorophore-labeled peptide, which in turn rotates more rapidly, leading to a lower degree of spatial orientation at the time of fluorescence emission, and thereby to a lower value of the fluorescence polarization.

2. Materials

2.1. Protein Expression

1. Kanamycin (200× stock): 500 mg kanamycin in 50 mL water. Sterile filter and store at −20°C in 5 mL aliquots. Working concentration: 50 μg/mL.

2. Chloramphenicol (1,000× stock): 340 mg chloramphenicol in 10 mL ethanol. Sterile filter and store at −20°C in 1 mL aliquots. Working concentration: 34 μg/mL.

3. LB medium is supplemented with kanamycin and chloramphenicol at the indicated final concentrations briefly before use.

4. LB agar is supplemented with kanamycin and chloramphenicol at the indicated final concentrations briefly before pouring.

5. Isopropyl-β-D-thiogalactopyranoside (IPTG, 1 M, 1,000× stock): 5 g IPTG in 21 mL of water. Sterile filter and store at −20°C in 2 mL aliquots. Working concentration: 1 mM.

6. Binding buffer (8× stock): 4 M NaCl, 160 mM Tris–HCl, 40 mM imidazole, pH 7.9. Sterile filter and store at room temperature. Dilute 125 mL of 8× binding buffer with 875 mL water to obtain the working concentration and store at 4°C.

2.2. Protein Purification

1. Phenylmethanesulfonyl fluoride (PMSF, 100 mM, 200× stock, Sigma-Aldrich): 0.87 g PMSF in 50 mL ethanol. Store at 4°C. Working concentration: 0.5 mM.

2. Aprotinin (200× stock, Calbiochem): 5,000 K.I.U (Kallikrein Inhibitory Units)/mL water. Working concentration: 25 K.I.U/mL. Store at 4°C.

3. Dithiothreitol (DTT, 1 M, 1,000× stock): 1 g DTT in 6.48 mL water. Sterile filter and store in 1 mL aliquots at −20°C. Working concentration: 1 mM.

4. Charge buffer (8× stock): 400 mM $NiSO_4$. Sterile filter and store at room temperature. Dilute 125 mL of 8× stock with 875 mL water to obtain the working concentration.

5. Wash buffer A (8× stock): 4 M NaCl, 160 mM Tris–HCl, 480 mM imidazole, pH 7.9. Sterile filter and store at room temperature. Dilute 125 mL of 8× stock with 875 mL water to obtain the working concentration and store at 4°C.

6. Wash buffer B (8× stock): 4 M NaCl, 160 mM Tris–HCl, 1.6 mM imidazole, pH 7.9. Sterile filter and store at room temperature. Dilute 125 mL of 8× stock with 875 mL water to obtain the working concentration and store at 4°C.

7. Elution buffer (4× stock): 2 M NaCl, 80 mM Tris–HCl, 4 M imidazole, pH 7.9. Sterile filter and store at room temperature. Dilute 125 mL of 4× stock with 375 mL water to obtain the working concentration and store at 4°C.

8. Dialysis buffer: 400 mM NaCl, 50 mM Tris–HCl, pH 8.0, 1 mM EDTA, 1 mM DTT, 10% glycerol, 0.1% Nonidet P-40. Add DTT immediately before use. Store at 4°C.

9. SpectraPor® dialysis membrane: Spectrum, MWCO 3,500.

10. Millex®-HA sterile syringe filters: Millipore, 0.45 μm.

11. Poly-Prep® chromatography columns: Bio-Rad, size 0.8 × 4 cm.

12. His•Bind® resin: Novagen.

2.3. Binding Assays

1. HPLC-purified peptides: 2 mg 5-carboxyfluorescein-GPMQSpTPLNG, 10 mg MAGPMQSpTPLNGAKK, and 10 mg MAGPMQSTPLNGAKK. All peptides have a free C-terminus; the latter two peptides also have a free N-terminus. Store the peptides at 4°C in the dark.

2. Assay buffer: 50 mM NaCl, 10 mM Tris–HCl, pH 8.0, 1 mM EDTA, 1 mM DTT, 0.1% Nonidet P-40, 10% DMSO. Add the DTT immediately before use. Sterile filter and store at 4°C.

3. Inhibition buffer: 50 mM NaCl, 10 mM Tris–HCl, pH 8.0, 1 mM EDTA, 1 mM DTT, 0.1% Nonidet P-40, 7.2% DMSO. Add the DTT immediately before use. Sterile filter and store at 4°C.

4. Screening buffer: 50 mM NaCl, 10 mM Tris–HCl, pH 8.0, 1 mM EDTA, 1 mM DTT, 0.1% Nonidet P-40, 9.5% DMSO. Add the DTT immediately before use. Sterile filter and store at 4°C.

5. Microtiter plates: Corning 384-well assay plate, black, non-treated, Cat. no. 3573.

3. Methods

3.1. Protein Expression and Purification

1. We have recently described the cloning of human Plk1 amino acids 326–603 into a modified pET28a vector containing an N-terminus 10× His-tag and a modified multiple cloning site consisting only of cleavage sites for FseI (F) and AscI (A) (6, 9). This plasmid (denoted pET28a-FA-Plk1PBD) was used in our studies and is available from the authors on request. Like the commercial vector, the above one carries a kanamycin resistance gene.

2. Incubate 9 µL of competent Rosetta BL21DE3 cells with pET28a-FA-Plk1PBD (10 ng dissolved in 1 µL water) for 5 min on ice. Subsequently, the sample is first incubated at 42°C for 30 s and then on ice for 2 min. After addition of 50 µL LB medium without antibiotics, the sample is spun on a rotating wheel for 1 h at 37°C. The entire sample is placed on LB plates containing kanamycin and chloramphenicol. Pick a single colony and set up a streak plate containing kanamycin and chloramphenicol. Incubate for 14 h at 37°C.

3. 10 mL of LB medium containing kanamycin and chloramphenicol are inoculated with a single colony from the streak plate and shaken for 14 h at 37°C.

4. This culture is used as a starter culture for 1 L of LB medium, which is grown at 37°C and shaken at 140 rpm in a conical flask with chicanes until an OD_{600} of 0.5–0.6 is reached.

5. At the OD_{600} of 0.5–0.6, the culture is transferred to room temperature under continued shaking. After 15 min, the liquid will have reached room temperature, and the OD_{600} will be approximately 0.8–0.9. At this point, 1 mL of a 1 M IPTG solution in water is added to induce protein expression, and the flask is continuously shaken at room temperature for 14 h.

6. The bacterial culture is transferred to centrifuge buckets and the culture is centrifuged at $1,500 \times g$ for 15 min at 4°C. The clear supernatant is removed and discarded. The pellet is frozen at –80°C to facilitate the subsequent lysis of the bacterial walls. The pellet is stable at –80°C for at least several months.

7. After thawing on ice, the pellet is re-suspended in 40 mL binding buffer by pipetting the liquid up and down repeatedly. Add 200 μL PMSF and 200 μL aprotinin.

8. The suspension is divided into four equal parts and each sample is sonificated four times on ice using a Sonoplus HD70 sonicator (Bandelin GmbH) for 2 min at 70% power level and 70/30 pulse/pause interval. The samples are placed on ice for at least 2 min in between sonifications. Because PMSF is unstable under aqueous conditions, additional 50 μL of PMSF are added to the samples after the third sonication cycle. Parallel to step 8, prepare the affinity column as described in step 10.

9. Combine the four samples and centrifuge the suspension at $40,000 \times g$ for 20 min at 4°C. The suspension is filtered through a Millex®-HA sterile filter (0.45 μm) to remove cell debris and other insoluble components.

10. Pour 2.5 mL 50% His•Bind® resin into a Poly-Prep® chromatography column and let the liquid run out through the column. Rinse first with 4 mL of autoclaved water, then apply 6.5 mL of $NiSO_4$ solution, and finally apply 4 mL of binding buffer.

11. Apply filtered supernatant to the column at 4°C. Collect the flow-through and apply it to the column for a second time. Add PMSF and aprotinin to all buffers used. Collect all fractions from this point on. Add 12.5 mL of binding buffer, 5 mL of wash buffer A, and 2.5 mL of wash buffer B. Wait for the liquid on top of the column to run through the column before adding the next buffer. Add 5 mL of elution buffer and collect two separate fractions of 2.5 mL. In case the eluted protein begins to precipitate (as indicated by clouding of the solution), add more elution buffer to the protein solutions immediately.

12. Check the purity of elution fractions by SDS-PAGE. Combine clean fractions.

13. Dialyze the combined clean protein fractions against 100-times the volume of dialysis buffer at 4°C for at least 8 h. Change the dialysis buffer and repeat the procedure twice. Determine concentration via Bradford assay. Snap-freeze 50–100 μL aliquots in liquid nitrogen, and store at −80°C until use.

3.2. Binding Assays

1. Weigh approximately 1 mg of peptide 5-carboxyfluorescein-GPMQSpTPLNG (average molecular weight: 1,438 g/mol) into a glass vial and add dry DMSO to a final concentration of 2 mM (see Note 1). This corresponds to adding 348 μL of DMSO per mg of peptide. Pipette the DMSO solution up and down repeatedly to ensure complete and homogenous solution of the peptide. Prepare 10 μL aliquots of the 2 mM peptide solution in Eppendorf tubes. Seal tops with parafilm and store aliquots at −20°C.

2. Add 1 µL of the 2 mM solution of 5-carboxyfluorescein-GPMQSpTPLNG to 4 mL assay buffer in a 15 mL Falcon tube. After mixing, add 21 µL of this solution to 329 µL assay buffer to generate a 30 nM solution of 5-carboxyfluorescein-GPMQSpTPLNG. This quantity is sufficient for generating one binding curve. All steps are carried out at room temperature. The final solution is stored in the dark on ice or at 4°C.

3. Dilute your stock of purified, dialyzed protein prepared in step 13 of Subheading 3.1 to a concentration of 3,840 nM with assay buffer. Prepare 8 twofold dilutions (1,920, 960, 480, 240, 120, 60, 30, and 15 nM) containing at least 80 µL of each concentration. These quantities are sufficient to generate a single binding curve (see Note 1).

4. Combine 66.7 µL of the protein solutions generated in step 3 with 33.3 µL of peptide solution in nine different Eppendorf tubes. As negative control, dilute 33.3 µL of peptide solution with 66.7 µL assay buffer in an additional tube. Mix the contents thoroughly.

5. Incubate the samples for 15 min at room temperature.

6. Of each tube, transfer three aliquots of 30 µL into three adjacent wells of a 384-well microtiter plate. Fill three additional wells of the microtiter plate with assay buffer for control purposes.

7. Using a microplate reader equipped for monitoring fluorescence polarization, excite the fluorophores with linearly polarized light (485 nm) and read the fluorescence emission parallel and perpendicular to the plane of excitation at 535 nm. Define wells containing assay buffer only to allow the instrument to subtract the background fluorescence before calculating the fluorescence polarization values. After reading, cover the plate with a plastic lid and store it at room temperature in the dark for additional measurements. An Ultra Evolution microplate reader (Tecan) was used for the experiments described here.

8. Plot binding curve in SigmaPlot (SPSS Science Software) or similar graph analysis software. Fit a curve through the data points (e.g., Hill four parameters). Determine the K_d-value of the peptide–protein interaction. This corresponds to the protein concentration at which half-maximal binding occurs (based on the extrapolated maximum value of fluorescence polarization for infinitely high protein concentrations) (see Fig. 1).

9. The assay must be sufficiently stable with regard to time to be used for screening. To this end, you need to verify that the binding curve does not significantly change over the time required to perform the screen, which will take approximately 1–2 h for each individual plate, but can take significantly longer for large compound collections. Thus, read the plate again

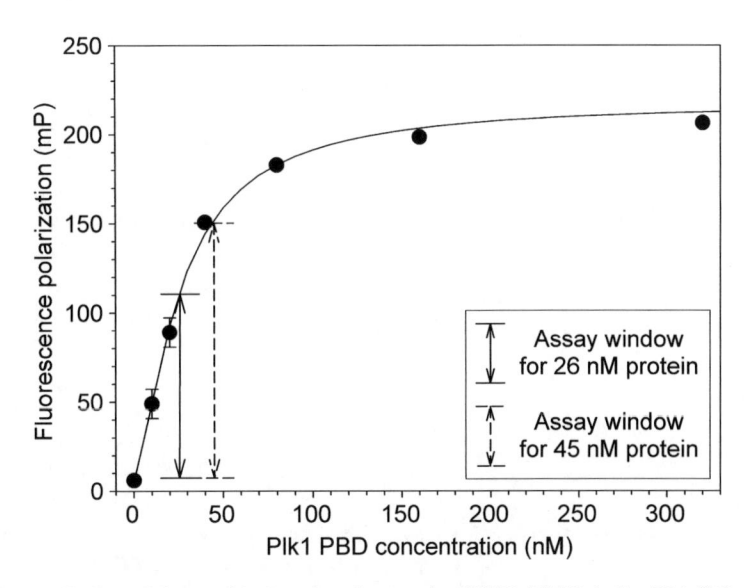

Fig. 1. Binding of the peptide 5-carboxyfluorescein-GPMQSpTPLNG to the Plk1 PBD as determined by fluorescence polarization. The figure illustrates that protein concentrations corresponding to the K_d-value or slightly exceeding it are suitable for use in the assay. In the example depicted here, the K_d-value was determined to be 26 nM, and 45 nM protein was chosen for further assay development. Assay windows obtained for Plk1 PBD concentrations of 26 nM and 45 nM are indicated by the *solid* and *dashed arrows*, respectively (9).

after an additional 1, 2, 4, 6, and 8 h starting from the time the solutions were transferred to the plate. Cover the plate with a plastic lid and store it at room temperature in the dark in between measurements. Plot the binding curves obtained at the various time points into the same diagram. Instability over time is indicated by an increase in the K_d-values. The assay should be stable over a minimum of 1 h in order to be of practical use (see Note 2).

10. From the binding curve taken after 1 h of incubation in the plates, select a protein concentration to be used in the subsequent inhibition experiments. Two effects must be carefully balanced in this respect. On the one hand, the size of the assay window (defined as the difference in fluorescence polarization between unbound fluorophore-labeled peptide and peptide in the presence of protein, see Fig. 1) increases with protein concentration, which facilitates the distinction between actual inhibition by a test compound from assay noise. On the other hand, saturation of binding will occur at higher protein concentrations, which makes it harder to detect active compounds in a screen. To balance the two counteracting effects, we recommend choosing a protein concentration corresponding to the K_d-value or slightly exceeding it. This will allow for a reasonably sized assay window (preferably larger than 100 mP),

while avoiding saturation of binding between the peptide and the protein. In the example shown in Fig. 1, the K_d-value was determined to be 26 nM, and a final protein concentration of 45 nM was chosen for assay development (9).

3.3. Inhibition Assays

In order to verify that the increase in fluorescence polarization observed upon addition of your protein construct to the fluorophore-labeled peptide comprising the PBD binding motif is in fact caused by the specific, reversible interaction between the peptide and the protein, the effects of a positive and negative control peptide must be assessed.

1. Weigh in approximately 1 mg of positive control peptide MAGPMQSpTPLNGAKK (average molecular weight: 1,611 g/mol) and negative control peptide MAGPMQSTPLNGAKK (average molecular weight: 1,531 g/mol). Generate a 10 mM stock solution in dry DMSO (to this end, add 62.1 μL DMSO per mg of positive control peptide and 65.3 μL DMSO per mg of negative control peptide). Mix thoroughly. Prepare 10 μL aliquots in Eppendorf tubes. Seal tops with parafilm and store at −20°C.

2. Prepare the following solutions of positive and negative control peptides by adding dry DMSO to the 10 mM stock solutions: 5 mM, 2.5 mM, 500 μM, 250 μM, 50 μM, 25 μM, 5 μM, 2.5 μM, 500 nM, and 50 nM. For a single inhibition curve, prepare 5 μL of each dilution (see Note 3).

3. Prepare 1 mL of a 30 nM solution of the fluorophore-labeled peptide 5-carboxyfluorescein-GPMQSpTPLNG in assay buffer and keep the solution in the dark at 4°C or on ice. This quantity will be sufficient for a single inhibition experiment with both the positive and the negative control peptides.

4. Prepare 1.7 mL of protein solution in inhibition buffer at a 1.55-fold higher concentration than the concentration chosen for assay development and keep on ice. This quantity will be sufficient for a single inhibition experiment with both the positive and the negative control peptides.

5. Add 2 μL of the dilution of the positive and negative control peptide prepared in step 2 to 64.7 μL of protein solution prepared in step 4. As control, add 2 μL of DMSO to 64.7 μL of this protein solution. Also add 2 μL of DMSO to 64.7 μL inhibition buffer without protein. Mix all samples thoroughly by pipetting at least half of the volume in the tubes up and down repeatedly, as DMSO tends to sink to the bottom of the wells. Incubate for 1 h at room temperature.

6. Add 33.3 μL of the 30 nM fluoropeptide solution prepared in step 3 to each sample, mix thoroughly, and incubate for 15 min at room temperature.

7. Transfer 30 μL aliquots of each tube into three adjacent wells of a 384-well microtiter plate. Also, fill three adjacent wells with 30 μL of assay buffer.

8. Read fluorescence polarization by excitation at 485 nm and emission at 535 nm. Define the wells containing assay buffer only as blank controls so that the instrument can subtract background fluorescence before calculating fluorescence polarization.

9. Using the binding curve for an incubation period of 1 h in the microtiter plates obtained in step 9 of Subheading 3.2, convert the fluorescence polarization values to percent binding between protein and fluorophore-labeled peptide. The fluorescence polarization obtained from the wells containing fluorophore-labeled peptide in the absence of protein should correspond to the theoretical binding value of 0% binding. The fluorescence polarization obtained from the fluorophore-labeled peptide in the presence of protein should correspond to the theoretical binding value of 100% binding. Small deviations from the theoretical values are common; larger deviations indicate that the experimental conditions used for the binding curve differ from the ones used for the inhibition curve.

10. Plot the inhibition curve and determine at what concentration a well-fitted curve (e.g., four parameters logistic curve) crosses the mark of 50% binding to determine the IC_{50} value of the positive control. The negative control is not expected to show significant inhibition at concentrations of 10 μM (Fig. 2).

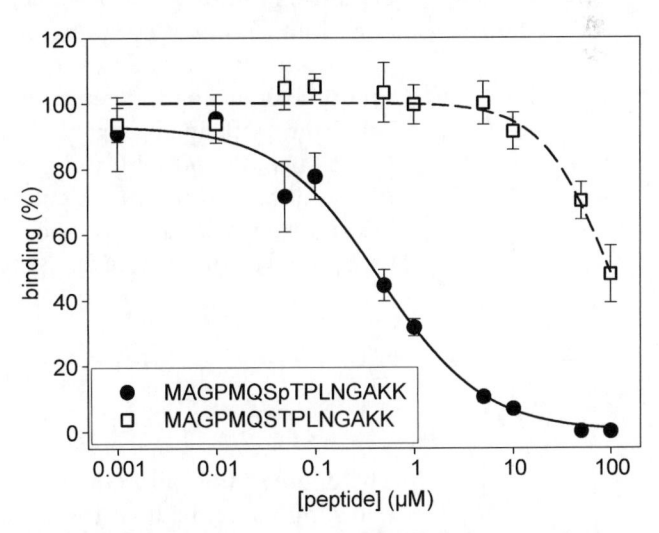

Fig. 2. Inhibition of binding between 5-carboxyfluorescein-GPMQSpTPLNG and the Plk1 PBD by the positive control peptide MAGPMQSpTPLNGAKK (*solid circles*), and the unphosphorylated negative control peptide MAGPMQSTPLNGAKK (*squares*) obtained in the presence of 10% DMSO (9).

3.4. Application of the Assay to High-Throughput Screening

1. Prepare an amount of protein solution in screening buffer sufficient for three 384-well plates with protein (≥10 mL per plate) at 1.5-times the final protein concentration chosen for assay development. Add 19.9 µL of this protein solution to columns 1–22 of a 384-well microtiter plate.
2. Add 100 nL of test compounds dissolved in DMSO into columns 1–20 using a pintool. Mix by shaking and incubate for 1 h at room temperature.
3. Add 0.5 µL of a 600 µM solution of positive control peptide in DMSO into the wells in column 22.
4. For each screening plate, prepare 4 mL of a 30 nM solution of 5-carboxyfluorescein-GPMQSpTPLNG in assay buffer. Add 10 µL of this solution to columns 1–22 of the 384-well microtiter plates. Mix by pipetting or shaking. Incubate for 15 min at room temperature. Centrifuge plate at $1,000 \times g$ for 2 min at room temperature (see Note 4).
5. Add 30 µL of a 10 nM solution of the fluorophore-labeled peptide 5-carboxyfluorescein-GPMQSpTPLNG in assay buffer into column 23.
6. Add 30 µL of assay buffer into the wells in column 24.
7. Read fluorescence polarization of the entire plate. Define the blank wells (column 24) to allow for subtraction of background fluorescence before calculation of fluorescence polarization. The values obtained from the wells containing fluorophore-labeled peptide only (column 23) are defined as 0% binding. The values obtained from the wells containing fluorophore-labeled peptide and protein (column 21) are defined as 100% binding (see Note 5). Convert the fluorescence polarization values to percent inhibition by means of the binding curve for the relevant time of incubation generated in step 9 of Subheading 3.2. The values obtained from the wells containing fluorophore-labeled peptide, protein, and positive control peptide (column 22) do not enter into the calculations, but serve as a control to assure reversibility and specificity of binding under the given experimental conditions (see Notes 6–9).

4. Notes

1. The diluted fluorophore-labeled peptide and the thawed protein aliquots can be used for up to 3 days when kept on ice or at 4°C; however, we recommend using freshly thawed aliquots and freshly prepared fluorophore-labeled peptide solutions to minimize the risk of assay variations due to deteriorated reagents (see Subheading 3.2).

2. While the presence of 1 mM dithiothreitol (DTT) in the assay buffer increases protein stability, it may interfere with the activity of some reactive test compounds. We found that the assay is almost similarly stable with respect to time in the absence of DTT (see Subheading 3.2).

3. Store diluted positive and negative control peptides in a drying cabinet or under similar conditions with reduced humidity at room temperature. Diluted peptides are stable for up to 3 days (see Subheading 3.3).

4. An alternative screening approach that would minimize addition steps during screening would be to mix the protein and the fluorescein-labeled peptide on the large scale required for screening, plate out approximately 30 µL of the mixture, and to add the test compounds afterwards. This procedure should yield virtually identical results for reversible inhibitors; however, competitive irreversible inhibitors may display lower activity under the alternative conditions (see Subheading 3.4).

5. The number of the control wells and their position on the plate in the high-throughput screens depends on the formatting of the screening library and the flexibility of the screening robot. Leaving as little as one column (e.g., column 24) free for controls would still allow be sufficient. Minimum controls are (a) three wells containing assay buffer only (blank controls for background fluorescence), (b) three wells containing fluorophore-labeled peptide and protein (defines 100% relative binding), (c) three wells containing the fluorophore-labeled peptide in assay buffer, without protein (defines 0% binding), and (d) three wells containing fluorophore-labeled peptide, protein, and 10 µM final concentration of positive control peptide (indicates the degree of reversibility of binding between fluorophore-labeled peptide and protein under the given experimental conditions) (see Subheading 3.4).

6. The assay as described here contains approximately 10% DMSO in all solutions which are ready for analysis of fluorescence polarization (9). The assay also works in the absence of any DMSO, and any intermediate concentrations of this co-solvent. Thus, the protocol can be adapted to lower DMSO concentrations under the formal condition that identical DMSO concentrations are used for the binding curves and the screening. However, in practice, the error introduced by matching data sets generated under slightly different DMSO concentrations is negligible. In this context, it should be pointed out that for practical reasons, the DMSO concentration in the control wells representing the bound state (9.7% DMSO) and the inhibited state (11.3% DMSO) slightly deviate from 10%. This can easily be improved by the aid of additional buffers and solutions, but doing so does not lead to significantly different screening results (see Subheading 3.4).

7. Before screening a large set of test compounds, it is advisable to verify that the protein batch prepared for the screen leads to the desired value of fluorescence polarization. We have noticed on several occasions that variations in the pipetting scheme used for setting up dilution series (i.e., the number of dilution steps and the concentrations of the intermediate dilutions) can influence the activity of the protein at the final dilution. Large-scale preparations of protein batches used for screening usually require less predilution steps than the small-scale preparations used for assay development; these variations in the pipetting schemes can lead to unexpected results (see Subheading 3.4).

8. We recommend screening the compound library in duplicate, and to follow-up only those compounds which show a certain inhibition in both duplicate screens. This reduces the number of hits that require follow-up. In our experience, inhibition data that occurred in only one out of two duplicate screening plates are usually not reproducible when the assay is repeated manually (see Subheading 3.4).

9. Setting the threshold percentage of inhibition in a screen is somewhat arbitrary and depends on the expectations of the experimenter regarding the activity of interesting compounds or on whether a certain hit rate has been predefined. We suggest screening at final compound concentrations between 10 and 50 µM in initial screens of nontargeted libraries, and select compounds that show ≥50% inhibition under these conditions (see Subheading 3.4).

Acknowledgments

This work was generously supported by the Department of Molecular Biology (director: Axel Ullrich) at the Max Planck Institute of Biochemistry, and the Bundesministerium für Bildung und Forschung (NGFN-2, grant 01GS0453 to K.S. and grant 01GS0451 to T.B.).

References

1. Barr, F. A., Sillje, H. H., and Nigg, E. A. (2004) Polo-like kinases and the orchestration of cell division. *Nat. Rev. Mol. Cell Biol.* **5**, 429–40.
2. Petronczki, M., Lénárt, P., and Peters, J. M. (2008) Polo on the Rise – from Mitotic Entry to Cytokinesis with Plk1. *Dev. Cell* **14**, 646–59.
3. Strebhardt, K., and Ullrich, A. (2006) Targeting polo-like kinase 1 for cancer therapy. *Nat. Rev. Cancer* **6**, 321–30.
4. Elia, A. E., Cantley, L. C., and Yaffe, M. B. (2003) Proteomic screen finds pSer/pThr-binding domain localizing Plk1 to mitotic substrates. *Science* **299**, 1228–31.
5. Elia, A. E., Rellos, P., Haire, L. F., Chao, J. W., Ivins, F. J., Hoepker, K., Mohammad, D., Cantley, L. C., Smerdon, S. J., and Yaffe, M. B. (2003) The molecular basis for phosphodependent substrate targeting and regulation of Plks by the Polo-box domain. *Cell* **115**, 83–95.

6. Reindl, W., Yuan, J., Kramer, A., Strebhardt, K., and Berg, T. (2008) Inhibition of Polo-like Kinase 1 by Blocking Polo-Box Domain-Dependent Protein-Protein Interactions. *Chem. Biol.* **15**, 459–66.
7. Watanabe, N., Sekine, T., Takagi, M., Iwasaki, J., Imamoto, N., Kawasaki, H., and Osada, H. (2009) Deficiency in chromosome congression by the inhibition of Plk1 polo box domain-dependent recognition. *J. Biol. Chem.* **284**, 2344–53.
8. Reindl, W., Yuan, J., Kramer, A., Strebhardt, K., and Berg, T. (2009) A Pan-Specific Inhibitor of the Polo-Box Domains of Polo-like Kinases Arrests Cancer Cells in Mitosis. *Chembiochem* **10**, 1145–48.
9. Reindl, W., Strebhardt, K., and Berg, T. (2008) A high-throughput assay based on fluorescence polarization for inhibitors of the polo-box domain of polo-like kinase 1. *Anal. Biochem.* **383**, 205–9.
10. Owicki, J. C. (2000) Fluorescence polarization and anisotropy in high throughput screening: perspectives and primer. *J. Biomol. Screen.* **5**, 297–306.

Chapter 6

Assessment of Hepatotoxicity Potential of Drug Candidate Molecules Including Kinase Inhibitors by Hepatocyte Imaging Assay Technology and Bile Flux Imaging Assay Technology

Jinghai J. Xu, Margaret C. Dunn, Arthur R. Smith, and Eric S. Tien

Abstract

Kinases are members of a major protein family targeted for drug discovery and development. Given the ubiquitous nature of many kinases as well as the broad range of pathways controlled by these enzymes, early safety assessments of small molecule inhibitors of kinases are crucial in identifying new molecules with sufficient therapeutic window for clinical development. Failure or attrition of drug candidates in late-stage pipelines due to hepatotoxicity is a significant challenge in the drug development field. Herein we provide detailed methods for the *h*epatocyte *i*maging *a*ssay *t*echnology (HIAT) and the *b*ile flux *i*maging *a*ssay *t*echnology (BIAT) to evaluate drug-induced liver injury (DILI) potentials for drug candidates. Optimized culturing methods for primary human hepatocytes, both freshly isolated and prequalified cryopreserved cells, are also presented. The applications of these high-content cellular imaging technologies in the evaluation of p38 and Her2 kinase inhibitors are highlighted to illustrate the usefulness of the research methodology in a compound screening as well as mechanistic investigative setting.

Key words: Mechanism-based drug profiling, Translational toxicology, Hepatocellular damage, High-content screening and analysis, Primary cell culture, Cellular imaging, Drug safety evaluation, Discovery toxicology, Toxicity test

1. Introduction

Kinases have long been targets for small molecule and biologic therapies due to their diverse functionality and central roles in signaling pathways. Therapeutics have been designed to inhibit kinases to treat inflammation, cancer, and a multitude of other diseases (1, 2). The p38 mitogen-activated protein kinase (MAPK) and human epidermal growth factor receptor 2 (Her2) are two examples of kinases that have been targeted to treat inflammation and cancer, respectively (3–6). The challenge with targeting such influential proteins is the potential for affecting nonspecific pathways that can lead to undesirable outcomes (i.e., side effects) (7–9).

Drug-induced liver injury (DILI) has been cited as the major impediment for drug development and the leading cause of drug withdrawal after approval for marketing by drug regulatory agencies around the world (10). While significant efforts and investments have been made to screen out drug molecules that have the propensity to form reactive metabolites that can covalently bind biomolecules, recent validation studies have shown that the correlation between such covalent binding studies and clinical manifestation of DILI is rather poor (11). On the one hand, it is well-known that some drugs can form covalent binding adducts in the liver without causing hepatotoxicity at therapeutically used doses. Good examples of these include acetaminophen (10) and paroxetine (12). On the other hand, it is known that other drugs can cause clinical hepatotoxicity without any evidence of reactive metabolite formation or covalent binding. Those examples include drugs that can induce steatohepatitis (e.g., perhexiline), cholestasis (e.g., erythromycin estolate), or other mixed hepatocellular and hepatobiliary injuries (e.g., telithromycin, ximelagatran). Hence, a renewed thinking in experimental testing paradigm to better predict human clinical DILI drugs is needed.

We have applied a combined design of employing more relevant human cellular systems (i.e., primary human hepatocytes), testing at physiologically relevant concentrations (i.e., liver-relevant multiples of therapeutic C_{max}), and measuring a panel of prelethal but highly toxicologically relevant endpoints (i.e., quantitative imaging measurements of major toxicity mechanisms), toward predicting clinical DILI (13). Since the combined testing strategy utilized primary human hepatocyte cultures and cellular imaging technology, we called it *h*epatocyte *i*maging *a*ssay *t*echnology (HIAT). In a comprehensive validation study of more than 300 drugs and chemicals, HIAT has been demonstrated to exhibit a true-positive rate of 50–60% for even the idiosyncratic human hepatotoxic drugs and an exceptionally low false-positive rate of 0–5% (13). As such, the overall concordance of HIAT (which is a rapid in vitro test) and human idiosyncratic DILI is on par with the traditional combined animal testing strategies employing rodents, dogs, and monkeys over a much longer period of time (14). If one further combines HIAT, which identifies many idiosyncratic human hepatotoxic drugs missed by the animal toxicological studies, with the more traditional preclinical safety studies, one can achieve a true-positive rate of over 75% while still maintaining a very low false-positive rate of 0–5% (assuming no false-positive DILI findings by animal testing). In addition, the drug-induced intrahepatic cholestasis mechanism was previously not covered by the HIAT method. Hence, we have extended the previous work to include *b*ile flux *i*maging *a*ssay *t*echnology (BIAT) to investigate cholestatic mechanisms and pathways. In this chapter, we describe the proper human hepatocyte culturing techniques, the combination of cellular imaging measurements one can apply on these cultures, and the applications of such methodologies on both p38 and Her2 small molecule kinase inhibitors. These applications span from identifying potential mechanisms of hepatotoxicity (p38 and Her2) to selecting better drug candidates devoid of such hepatotoxic potential (i.e., identifying best-in-class compound among all known p38 inhibitors).

The key to any toxicology and safety assessment in primary human hepatocytes is properly cultured cells. The main characteristics of properly cultured hepatocytes are: sandwich culture with extracellular matrices, confluent cell monolayer with few dead cells, three-dimensional morphology with tight cellular junctures that exhibit bile canaliculi, and hepatobiliary transport functions. Hepatocytes cultured in such a configuration exhibit their natural polarity (sinusoidal membrane vs. canalicular membrane) with both expression and function of a compendium of drug uptake and efflux transporters (15, 16). Fundamentally, it is the right balance of such uptake and efflux transporters that dictate how much drug cells "see" intracellularly, which ultimately dictate the correct and quantitative prediction of drug-induced effects, both pharmacologic and toxicological effects. Immortalized human hepatic cell lines or other hepatoma cell lines often lack such cellular polarity, or transporter balance which could lead to erroneous prediction (17, 18). Mastery of hepatocyte culture techniques opens up an impressive array of drug discovery opportunities centered on the human liver. Since it is long known that human livers differ from animal livers in drug uptake transporters, metabolizing and conjugating enzymes, efflux transporters, and a plethora of other hepatic metabolism and signaling pathways, it is our belief that by employing properly cultured human hepatocytes, better translational medicine predictions can be made toward the ultimate human outcome.

Proper evaluation of hepatotoxic potential also requires a combined measure of multiple indicators of cellular health. This is analogous to a person taking a blood test where multiple biomarkers are simultaneously measured to predict human health and diagnose potential illness. The HIAT (13) is a multiplexed imaging assay designed to maximize the predictive value toward clinical DILI, including idiosyncratic DILI, from a single in vitro experiment. The BIAT, the second assay protocol described in this chapter, measures the activity of the bile salt export pump (BSEP) but the technique opens up the possibility of examining other hepatobiliary transporters depending on the specific fluorescent probes used.

A skilled person in the field can easily adapt these protocols toward other imaging (e.g., steatosis, phospholipidosis, cytoskeletal effects, mitochondrial stress, endoplasmic reticulum (ER) stress, apoptosis, immunofluorescence, protein trafficking, distribution, and concentration, cytomics, etc.), and biochemical measurements (e.g., protein production, biomarker discovery and validation, ELISA, enzyme leakage, genomics, proteomics, metabonomics, lipidomics, ribonomics, etc.), for both drug safety and drug efficacy evaluation purposes.

1.1. Application Notes of HIAT and BIAT for Small Molecule Kinase Inhibitors: Practical Experiences Post Assay Development and Validation

The MAPK p38 alpha represents a point of convergence for multiple signaling processes that are activated during inflammation, making it a key potential target for the modulation of cytokine production (7). However, despite many years of research and development by several biopharmaceutical companies, no p38 alpha inhibitor has become drug to date. Among the top reasons of attrition for these drug candidates are dose-limiting side effects, especially elevated liver enzymes and skin rash (9).

Since HIAT has been developed and validated with over 300 drugs and drug candidates (13), the selection of safer p38 MAPK inhibitors was among the first real-world applications of HIAT. Figure 1 shows a representative result of a panel of p38 alpha inhibitors and their imaging profile results in HIAT. As expected, perhexiline (positive control) showed several adverse signals as indicated by gray-colored cells. Fluoxetine and Famotidine (both negative controls) showed no adverse signals in any of the imaging measurement, as indicated by clear cells and recapitulated the findings by Xu et al. (13). The development of the first seven p38 alpha inhibitors was stopped in human clinical trials due to adverse liver signals (i.e., elevated liver enzymes in patients' serum). These compounds showed varying degrees of adverse HIAT signals as indicated by gray-colored cells in Fig. 1. Drugs #8 and 9 are second-generation p38 alpha inhibitors that are still in phase 2 clinical trials and have exhibited much better liver signals in the clinic so far. Essentially they performed like the two negative control drugs in HIAT. More interestingly, the last eight p38 alpha inhibitors are from two entirely different structural series (i.e., third-generation inhibitors). They also performed much "cleaner" than the first-generation p38 inhibitors, with series 1 (S1) displaying better profile than series 2 (S2). In this study, we tested drug #7 at 100 times of its human therapeutic single-dose C_{max}. For all the other drugs, since their clinical therapeutic C_{max} values have not been determined or reported, we compared their pharmacological IC50 potency values to drug #7 in the same predictive pharmacology assay which is the induction of TNF alpha from lipopolysaccharide or LPS-treated human monocytes (7). Their clinically required therapeutic C_{max} values were approximated based on linear proportionality of their pharmacological IC50 values vs. drug #7.

6 Assessment of Hepatotoxicity Potential of Drug Candidate Molecules...   87

(monocyte) —[TNFa]→ "Cmax projection"   (hepatocyte) —HIAT→ "DILI projection"

Drug	Nuclei Count	Nuclei Area	ROS Intensity	TMRM Intensity	Lipid Intensity	GSH Content	GSH Area	Lipid Count	Clinical Outcome / Comment
Perhexiline	1.4	1.5	0	0	3.6	0.08	0.3	23.11	Positive DILI
Fluoxetine	1.1	1.1	0.6	1.8	0.2	0.83	0.97	0.08	Negative Prozac®
Famotidine	1.2	1.1	0	1.6	0.1	0.78	0.92	0	Negative Pepcid®
1	1.3	0.8	0	0	1	0.08	0.28	0.1	Ph 2 DILI
2	1.2	1.2	0.5	0.3	3.8	0.37	0.09	23.23	Ph 2 DILI
3	1	1.3	1.5	0.2	5.8	0.36	0.38	77.28	Ph 2 DILI
4	0.9	1.1	38	1.9	2.5	2.75	0.56	15.96	Ph 2 DILI
5	1.2	1	0.2	0.8	0.2	0.53	0.71	0.05	Ph 1 DILI
6	1.1	1.2	0	1.7	2.6	0.72	0.8	5.15	Ph 1 DILI
7	1.1	1.1	0	0.7	2.5	0.87	0.96	20.15	Ph 1 DILI
8	1	1	0	0.8	0.2	0.93	0.97	0.02	Ph2 active
9	0.9	0.9	0.3	0.7	0.1	0.63	0.88	0	Ph2 active
10	1.2	1.1	0.0	0.6	0.0	0.9	0.9	0.0	3rd-Gen S1
11	1.1	1.0	0.0	0.8	0.2	1.0	0.9	0.1	3rd-Gen S1
12	1.0	1.0	0.0	0.8	0.0	0.9	1.0	0.1	3rd-Gen S1
13	1.0	1.0	0.0	0.8	0.1	0.8	1.0	0.2	3rd-Gen S1
14	1.0	0.9	0.0	0.9	0.0	0.9	1.0	0.0	3rd-Gen S1
15	1.0	1.0	0.0	1.0	0.0	0.9	1.0	0.0	3rd-Gen S1
16	1.0	1.0	0.0	0.4	0.0	1.3	1.0	0.1	3rd-Gen S2
17	1.0	0.9	0.0	0.5	1.4	1.0	0.9	2.8	3rd-Gen S2

Fig. 1. Application of HIAT (hepatocyte imaging assay technology) in identifying safer p38 alpha inhibitors. Clear cells indicate normal signals or signals indistinguishable from all the negative control drugs, including Fluoxetine and Famotidine. *Gray-shaded cells* indicate adverse signals in HIAT, which included increased ROS intensity, decreased TMRM intensity, decreased GSH content and area, and increased lipid count. For details on how the assay was trained, validated, and appropriate threshold selected by machine learning approaches, please refer to ref. 13.

Such a therapeutic window-based hepatotoxicity prediction schema is described on the top of Fig. 1, and justifications for using 100 times human therapeutic single-dose C_{max} were discussed in ref. 13. It is interesting to note that both drug efficacy (as measured in human monocytes) and toxicity prediction (as measured in human hepatocytes) are based on experimental data of human primary cells in this case.

In another case of small molecule kinase inhibitors, CP-724,714 is a potent, selective, and orally active inhibitor of human epidermal growth factor receptor-2 (erbB2/Her2/neu) kinase. It showed initial promise in treating patients bearing advanced Her2 positive tumors (19). However, subsequent clinical development of this drug was discontinued due to serious hepatotoxicities including jaundice and cholestatic liver damage. BIAT was applied to better understand and characterize the cholestatic property of this drug. CP-724,714 induced dose-dependent inhibition of the rate-limiting

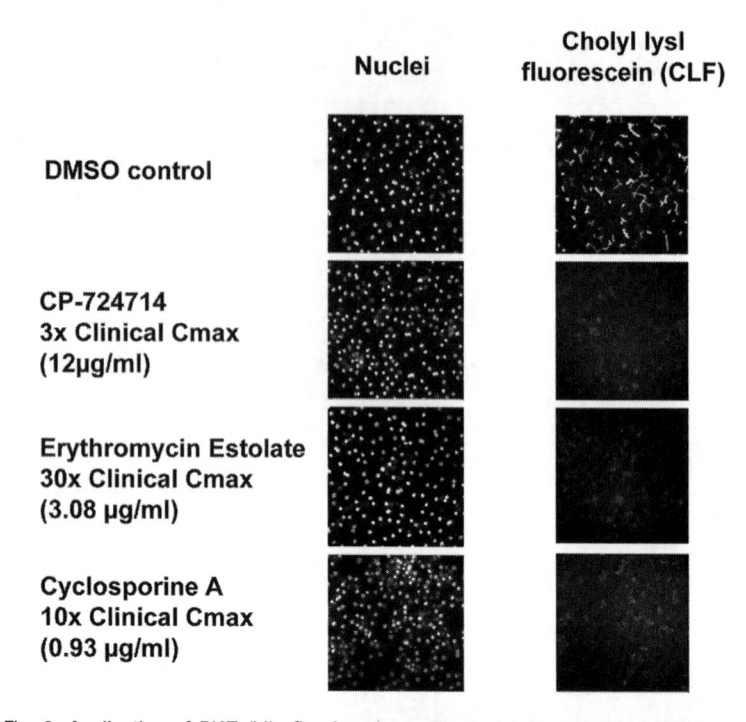

Fig. 2. Application of BIAT (bile flux imaging assay technology) in understanding and characterizing drug-induced cholestasis effect by the orally available small molecule Her2 inhibitor, CP-724,714. Erythromycin estolate and cyclosporine A were used as positive control drugs for the BIAT. The primary human hepatocytes cultured in the sandwiched configuration were treated with CP-724,714 or control drugs of interest for 15 min in the presence of a fluorescent bile acid probe, CLF. For more information about this Her2 inhibitor and its detailed mechanistic hepatotoxicity studies, please refer to ref. 20.

step of bile flow, the BSEP. As shown in Fig. 2, erythromycin estolate and cyclosporine A are two positive control drugs for the BIAT. They abolished cholyl lysyl fluorescein (CLF) transport or "flux" into the bile canaliculi at 30× and 10× of their clinical therapeutic C_{max} values, respectively. On the other hand, CP-724,714 abolished CLF transport into the bile canaliculi at 3× of its therapeutic C_{max}. Therefore, CP-724,714 is a much more potent inducer of intrahepatic cholestasis than either erythromycin estolate or cyclosporine A. In addition, CP-724,714 has the propensity to be taken up to hepatocyte by hepatic uptake transporters at a higher rate than efflux transporters, and affect the mitochondrial health of hepatocytes (20). These combined properties of CP-724,714 may have led to clinical manifestations of DILI in susceptible patients in the clinic (19). Going forward, it is these kinds of costly late-stage drug attritions due to DILI that our HIAT and BIAT methodologies, and further improvements or derivative works thereof, are aiming to avoid.

The protocols in this section are written for the plating of cryopreserved hepatocytes but can be easily adapted to the plating of fresh cells (as explained in Subheading 4, Note 2, they are actually easier than plating cryopreserved cells). Proper evaluation of cryopreserved cell lots is critical before making a quality purchase of a large number of vials from this lot (see Subheading 2.2 below).

2. Materials

2.1. Media Preparation

1. Cryopreserved Hepatocyte Recovery Medium (CHRM): for successful implementation of this protocol, please use the commercially available and prepackaged material sold by CellzDirect (Durham, NC, USA, now part of Life Technologies, and Invitrogen).

2. Plating Media: Dulbecco's minimal essential medium (DMEM) without phenol red, supplemented with 5% fetal bovine serum (FBS), 50 U/ml penicillin, 50 µg/ml streptomycin, 4 µg/ml bovine insulin, 1 µM trichostatin A, 1 µM dexamethasone, 2 mM L-glutamine.

3. Culturing and Imaging Media: William's E Medium (WEM) without phenol red, supplemented with 15 mM HEPES buffer, 1× ITS+ [6.25 µg/ml transferrin, 6.25 µg/ml selenous acid, 5.35 µg/ml linoleic acid, and 1.25 µg/ml bovine serum albumin (BSA)], 50 U/ml penicillin, 50 µg/ml streptomycin, 1 µM trichostatin A, 0.1 µM dexamethasone, 2 mM L-glutamine.

4. Drugging Media: WEM with phenol red, 15 mM HEPES buffer, 5% FBS, 50 U/ml penicillin, 50 µg/ml streptomycin, 4 µg/ml bovine insulin, 1 µM trichostatin A, 0.1 µM dexamethasone, 2 mM L-glutamine.

2.2. Source of Human Hepatocytes

The quality of cells is crucial for the success of this protocol. Therefore, platable and culturable human hepatocytes (either fresh or cryopreserved) are purchased from CellzDirect (Durham, NC, USA). For cryopreserved cells, regular contacts with the technical staff at CellzDirect should be maintained to inform the availability of best-quality lots. Pictures of cells after plating should be exchanged, and the morphology of cells that are similar to those published by Bi et al. (please refer to figures and detailed protocols in ref. 21) is used as a pre-requisite for a usable lot in this hepatotoxicity testing protocol.

2.3. Other Reagents and Supplies

1. Dulbecco's phosphate-buffered saline (PBS, containing Ca^{2+} and Mg^{2+}), Hanks balanced salt solution (HBSS, containing Ca^{2+} and Mg^{2+}), Trypan Blue stock solution, and other regular

media components can be purchased from a number of suppliers.
2. Rat tail collagen I.
3. Phenol red free Matrigel.
4. Ultra pure dimethyl sulfoxide (DMSO).
5. Drug substances of interest (e.g., Famotidine, Fluoxetine, Perhexiline, Metformin, Erythromycin estolate, cyclosporine A).
6. Further standard laboratory chemicals.
7. Fluorescent dyes: tetramethyl rhodamine methyl ester (TMRM), CM-H$_2$DCFDA, mBCl, Hoechst 33342, CLF, DRAQ5.
8. Cell culture plates: 96-well tissue culture grade plates (clear, flat-bottom, and UV-transparent).
9. 96-Well sterile V bottom trough microtiter plates (MTP), 50 ml conical tubes.
10. Sterile hydrophobic plate seals (AeraSeal films) and film foller.
11. Sterile V-Groove 96-well reservoir and sterile 96-well V-bottom plates.

2.4. Image Instrumentation and Analysis

1. An automatable epifluorescence microscopic imager, including an environmental chamber and on-deck liquid transfer, was used in this study [Kinetic Scan Reader (KSR), made by Cellomics, now part of Thermo Scientific]. If only a few compounds are tested at a time, manual pipetting can replace on-deck liquid transfer.
2. Image analysis software: several suitable software packages are available for converting raw images to quantitative measurements in a semiautomated manner (e.g., ImagePro Plus by Media Cybernetics; image analysis software provided by microscope vendors including Cellomics).

2.5. General Cell Culture Instruments

1. A high-quality mammalian cell incubator that can maintain uniform saturating humidity and 37°C/5% CO$_2$/95% air-flow environment.
2. A sonicating heated water bath with temperature adjustment.
3. A centrifuge with g-force adjustment (for $100 \times g$ at room temperature).
4. A biosafety cabinet and other appropriate safety equipment to safely handle primary cell work.
5. A hemocytometer.
6. A microscope (to count cells and to check cell attachment and morphology).
7. P20, P200, P1000 pipettors and sterile tips.

8. P200 8-channel pipettor and sterile tips.
9. Two 96-channel Soken PP550 personal pipetting stations, with sterile P550 tips, tip loader/ejector, adjustable stage height and pipetting speed, were purchased from Apricot Designs (Covina, CA).
10. Refrigerator, freezer, and liquid nitrogen storage container.

3. Methods

3.1. Thawing and Plating Cryopreserved Human Hepatocytes

1. Prepare everything for the plating steps, including steps 1–5 below, before removing cryopreserved hepatocyte vials from liquid nitrogen Dewar tank (see Note 1). As with any proper human cell culture experiments, apply good laboratory safety practice and proper sterile techniques. Twenty-four hours prior to plating, freshly apply collagen coating to 96-well plates with rat tail collagen I at 50 µg/ml concentration (in a solution of Ca^{2+} and Mg^{2+} containing PBS with 0.02 N acetic acid) and incubate at 37°C overnight. For clear, flat, and UV-transparent imaging purposes, we coated 96-well tissue culture grade plates purchased from BD Biosciences. It is our experience that freshly coated plates provide the most reproducible results.

2. Wash plates three times with Dulbecco's PBS (PBS containing Ca^{2+} and Mg^{2+}) to remove residual collagen/acetic acid.

3. Aliquot 48 ml plating medium into a 50 ml conical tube and warm to 37°C.

4. Prefill collagen-coated 96-well plates with 55 µl/well of Plating Medium (seeding the cell suspension on top of media provides better cell distribution across the well). Plates are placed into 37°C/5% CO_2/95% air, saturating humidity incubator for warming.

5. In sterile Eppendorf tube, prepare 100 µl of 0.08% Trypan Blue in Dulbecco's PBS.

6. See Subheading 4, Note 2 for procedures of plating freshly isolated hepatocytes. Remove one vial of cryopreserved hepatocytes from liquid nitrogen Dewar and placed on ice. Briefly twist the cap to relieve the internal pressure and re-tighten. It is critical that the time on ice be kept as short as possible, and definitely less than 1 min.

7. Thaw hepatocytes in 37°C water bath by gently moving the vial through the water. Do not submerge the vial completely and do not remove the vial from the water during the thawing process. Just prior to complete thawing, a small amount of ice will be present. This takes usually ~ 80–95 s depending on the

volume in the vial. Watch the thawing process very closely as over thawing will result in decreased cell viability.

8. Once thawed, remove the vial from the water bath and spray with 70% alcohol, then wipe dry with clean paper towel before placing in the biosafety hood.
9. Quickly pour the contents of the vial to the 50 ml conical tube containing 48 ml of warmed Plating Medium. Rinse the cryo vial with 1 ml of fresh warm Plating Medium. Pour the contents of the vial into the 50 ml conical tube containing the thawed hepatocytes.
10. Gently invert the 50 ml tube three times for thorough mixing of the cells.
11. Place the 50 ml conical tube in centrifuge and spin at room temperature for 5 min at $100 \times g$.
12. Remove tube from centrifuge and without disturbing the cell pellet, spray with 70% alcohol, and then wipe dry before placing in biosafety hood. Avoid re-inverting the tube or any other motions that may disrupt the cell pellet.
13. Uncap the tube and in a single motion, gently pour off the supernatant into a disposable waste container.
14. Gently tap the bottom of the tube to loosen the pellet and re-suspend in 5 ml of warm Plating Medium.
15. Gently rock the tube back and forth being careful not to invert the cell mixture onto the cap of the tube. Continue the gentle rocking motion until the pellet is completely suspended.
16. In sterile Eppendorf tube, combine 100 µl of 0.08% Trypan Blue (in Dulbecco's PBS) with 100 µl of your cell suspension (final concentration of Trypan Blue is 0.04%). Incubate cells with Trypan Blue for 1 min at room temperature, inverting the tube several times before transferring a 10 µl volume to each side (chamber) of a hemocytometer. Avoid using pipette tips with fine (small) openings as that may shear and damage hepatocytes. Quickly count the number of viable cells (i.e., clear cytoplasm) and dead cells (i.e., blue cytoplasm). Good quality lot and good thawing technique should yield fewer than 10% dead cells. Do not use automated cell counters (see Note 3).
17. Dilute the cell suspension to 0.75×10^6 viable cell/ml in pre-warmed Plating Medium. By default, dead cells are not counted toward viable cells.
18. Prior to seeding, be sure to invert the 50 ml conical tube of plating suspension several times as hepatocytes tend to settle and clump quickly.
19. Pour cell suspension into a sterile V bottom trough and seed cells to 96-well collagen-coated plates using an 8-channel pipettor and sterile tips.

20. Mix the hepatocyte suspension by rocking the V bottom trough back and forth 5–6 times before adding 80 µl/well to the first column of the MTP, repeat the mix step for each column. See Note 4 for adjusting seeding volume of cells that may come in different size.
21. Place plate in a 37°C/5% CO_2/95% air incubator with saturating humidity and incubate for 4–6 h. Cell attachment should be confirmed visually for each plate using an inverted light microscope before proceeding to the next step.
22. After confirming cell attachment, remove the plate from the incubator and place in biosafety hood. Remove the plastic plate lid and place a sterile hydrophobic plate seal over the entire 96-well plate. Use a roller to seal the sterile plate seal. Holding each plate firmly in one hand, shake the plate back and forth vigorously for ~5 s, then turn the plate 90° and repeat the vigorous shaking. This will help remove any dead cells which have loosely attached to the plates.
23. Set up sterile drape in biosafety hood. Remove plate seal, aspirate the existing media using a 96-channel pipettor with stage height set such that there will be ~30 µl of medium left in each well. This is important because at no aspiration step should any pipette tips touch the cell layer directly to cause any cell dislodgement from the bottom of the plate. The remaining medium in the wells will be flicked onto the sterile drape material by inverting the plate and then firmly blotting the plate on the drape. This procedure will ensure that the remaining loose dead cells from the previous shake step will be removed, without causing any dislodgement of healthy cells.
24. Working quickly after the remaining media has been removed (i.e., do not let cells sit dry). Pipette 125 µl/well prewarmed Culturing Medium using the 96-well pipettor, at slow speed, in 25 µl increment, and then incubate plate for 20–24 h in a 37°C/5% CO_2/95% air, saturating humidity incubator. See Notes 5 and 6 for tips on liquid transfer using the Soken.

3.2. Matrigel Overlay

1. Place sterile "V-Groove" 96-well reservoir, a box of sterile P1000 pipettor tips, a 50-ml sterile conical tube, and a sealed rack of plastic tips for the 96-well Apricot PP550 Soken in −20°C freezer the night before. Keeping all materials that get into contact with Matrigel cold will prevent the Matrigel from gelling prematurely during the overlay step.
2. Take one vial of phenol red free Matrigel from −20°C freezer (see Note 7). Place the vial in a bucket filled with ice. The vial should be nearly submerged in the ice. Place bucket in a 4°C refrigerator so that the Matrigel will thaw slowly overnight.

3. Place an appropriate amount of Culturing Medium into the sterile 50 ml conical tube and place on ice in a 4°C refrigerator. The exact amount depends on the number of plates to overlay. The hepatocyte medium used throughout the protocol has been selected to aid in maintaining hepatocyte differentiation, including the use of trichostatin A (see Note 8).

4. Retrieve cold P1000 tip box from −20°C freezer, pipette Matrigel solution into 50 ml conical tube, add back ~1 ml cold media to the Matrigel aliquot tube with the same tip (slowly around sides of tube) and then transfer this liquid back to working Matrigel solution. The final Matrigel concentration in Culturing Medium should be 0.25 mg/ml (see Note 9). Invert the 50 ml conical tube to mix content well. Place on ice.

5. Retrieve cold "V-groove" reservoir from −20°C freezer, pour Matrigel mixture into cold reservoir, and place on ice.

6. Retrieve cold 96-well pipettor tips and load cold pipettor tips to the 96-well pipettor. Prefill sufficient Matrigel media into the cold tips to do two cell plates.

7. In concert with the previous step, one should aspirate the cell culture medium from one cell plate using the 96 channel pipettor. The remaining medium in the wells is flicked onto a sterile drape material by inverting the plate and then firmly blotting the plate on the drape.

8. Quickly add back 125 µl of chilled Matrigel using the 96 channel pipettor, set at slow dispensing speed, and dispense 25 µl increments (see Note 10).

9. Repeat the above step for the second cell plate.

10. Incubate cell plates for 20–24 h at 37°C/5% CO_2/95% air, saturating humidity in an incubator. If this overlay step is performed correctly, within 24 h the healthy human hepatocyte morphology should emerge (i.e., confluent cell monolayer, three-dimensional morphology, and tight cellular junctures that exhibit bile canaliculi formation) (see Fig. 3).

3.3. Drug Treatment for HIAT

A number of controls are required in HIAT measurements. DMSO is used as the drug vehicle control. Negative compound controls are provided by Famotidine (human average single-dose therapeutic C_{max} is 0.104 µg/ml so final test concentration is 10.4 µg/ml; 100× C_{max}) and Fluoxetine (human average single-dose therapeutic C_{max} is 0.014 µg/ml so final test concentration is 1.4 µg/ml; 100× C_{max}). A positive compound control is the use of Perhexiline (human average single-dose therapeutic C_{max} is 0.6 µg/ml so final test concentration is 60 µg/ml, 100× C_{max}). For the rationale behind the use of 100× human average single-dose therapeutic C_{max}, please refer to the validation study by Xu et al. (13).

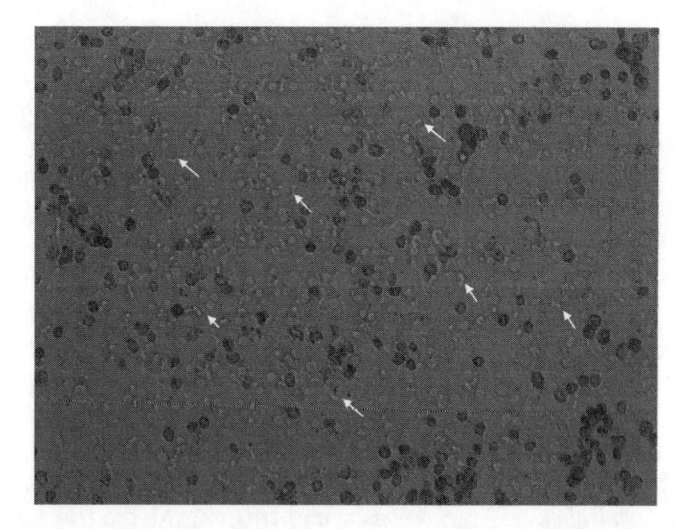

6 Assessment of Hepatotoxicity Potential of Drug Candidate Molecules...

Fig. 3. Images of healthy human hepatocyte cultures showing a confluent cell monolayer, three-dimensional morphology, and tight cellular junctures that exhibit bile canaliculi structures (indicated by *white arrows*). Cryopreserved human hepatocytes were thawed, plated, and Matrigel overlaid as described in this protocol. This picture was taken on day 5 (day 1 designated as the day of cell thawing and plating).

1. Vehicle controls: Fill all wells in column 1 and column 7 with 125 µl Drugging Medium containing 0.4% v/v DMSO.

2. Compound controls: prepare a 10.4 µg/ml Famotidine solution in Drugging Medium. Prepare a 1.4 µg/ml Fluoxetine solution in Drugging Medium. Prepare a 60 µg/ml Perhexiline solution in Drugging Medium.

3. Test compound solubilization: initially dissolve all test compounds in ultra pure DMSO. Then dilute with warm phenol red Drugging Media containing 5% serum to the desired test compound concentration (containing 0.4% DMSO). Start with a concentration of 100× human single-dose therapeutic C_{max}, either measured clinically or projected preclinically. Recommended dose response titrations are 100×, 30×, 10×, 3×, 1× C_{max}. Since Drugging Medium contains 5% serum, which also facilitates drug solubilization, total human C_{max} values are used.

4. To ensure complete compound solubilization, sonicate compound solutions in a heated water bath for 30 min at ~ 40°C. Visually inspect all diluted compounds for any pH-associated color changes in phenol red media and compound insolubility. Incubate all diluted compound solutions at 37°C for a minimum of 30 min to enhance solubility. Re-inspect compounds for solubility and pH-associated color effect. Compounds that remain insoluble in media and change in media color should be noted as such.

5. Transfer 125 µl of the warm diluted compounds to a 96-well "V-bottom" intermediate plate.

6. Dosing cells: Use one Apricot PP550 Soken to remove existing cell culture medium while the second Apricot PP550 Soken is used to add drug/media. Again, a coordinated sequence of media removal and drug addition to the cells can be done by using two pipetting instruments sequentially. First mix diluted compounds up and down three times. Then aspirate old media from each well, taking care not to disrupt Matrigel layer nor touching the cells. Then add 125 µl of Drugging Mixture to each well, at slow speed, in 25 µl increments. Place cell plate back into cell culture incubator for 24 h.

3.4. Staining and Image Acquisition for HIAT

1. Prewarm an appropriate volume of Drugging Media (for 1× wash) and Imaging Media (no serum, no phenol red) to 37°C in water bath (see Note 11 about precautions regarding single use of fluorescent probes and light sensitivities).

2. Turn the KSR and its environmental chamber on ~2 h before starting the image acquisition step in order to equilibrate the environmental chamber and lamp to steady states. The environmental chamber, the liquid handling arm, and the waste line should be cleaned or flushed regularly according to the manufacturer's instructions to minimize microbial growth or contamination.

3. Mitochondrial membrane potential: 3× TMRM – add 15 µl of stock (0.2 mM) to 50 ml Imaging Media (3× concentration is 0.06 µM, final concentration at the cells is 0.02 µM); 1× TMRM – add 5 µl of stock to 50 ml Imaging Media (final concentration at the cells is 0.02 µM); 0.5× TMRM – add 2.5 µl of stock to 50 ml Imaging Media (final concentration at the cells is 0.01 µM). TMRM stock should be aliquoted to single use and stored at −20°C (see Note 11).

4. Wash once to remove residual drugs. Remove existing media from cell plate using one Apricot PP550 Soken and add 200 µl Drugging Medium with second Apricot PP550 Soken in 25 µl increments, at slow speed, pipette tips to the side, and not touching Matrigel layer.

5. Remove existing media from cell plate at slow speed, using one Apricot PP550 Soken and add 125 µl 1× TMRM with second Apricot PP550 Soken in 25 µl increments, at slow speed, tips to the side, and not touching Matrigel layer. Incubate plate at 37°C for 1 h for the mitochondrial stain. Prepare the next three steps during this hour.

6. Nuclei: 3× DRAQ5 – add 135 µl of stock (5 mM) to 5 ml Imaging Media (3× concentration is 135 µM, final concentration on the cells is 0.045 µM). DRAQ5 stock should be aliquoted to single use and stored at 4°C.

7. Reactive oxygen species (ROS): 3× CM-H$_2$DCFDA – add 30 µl of stock (5 mM) to 5 ml Imaging Media (3× concentration is 30 µM, final concentration at the cells is 10 µM). CM-H$_2$DCFDA stock is stored at –20°C. Routinely, two vials (each containing 50 µg probe) are pulled from cold storage if staining one plate of cells. Solubilize by adding 17.2 µl ultra pure DMSO to each tube. Vortexed both tubes, then transfer the contents of one tube to the second. Vortex this second tube again before transferring 30 µl to the Imaging Media.

8. Combine 5 ml volumes of 3× DRAQ5, 3× CM-H$_2$DCFDA, and 3× TMRM in a 50 ml conical tube to make a 1× probe mix. Mix thoroughly by inverting the tube and place back into a 37°C water bath for warming.

9. Remove existing media from cell plate slow speed, using one Apricot PP550 Soken and add 125 µl probe mix with a second Apricot PP550 Soken in 25 µl increments, at slow speed, tips to the side, and not touching Matrigel layer. Then incubate plates at 37°C for 45 min.

10. Remove probe mix using one Apricot PP550 Soken and add 200 µl of Imaging Media (25 µl increments, at slow speed, tips to side, and not touching Matrigel layer) to wash away excess probes.

11. Next, remove wash media with one Apricot PP550 Soken and add 100 µl of 0.5× TMRM with the second Apricot PP550 Soken (25 µl increments, slow speed, tips to side, and not touching Matrigel layer). Leave probe mixture on cells during the image acquisition step.

12. Load the plate into the Cellomics KSR with the lid off. The environmental chamber on the KSR will keep the cells alive during the image acquisition.

13. Glutathione content: prepare 2× monochlorobimane (mBCl) – add 15 µl of stock (160 mM) to 15 ml Imaging Media (2× concentration is 160 µM, final concentration at the cells is 80 µM). Weigh out 2 mg of mBCl and prepare a 160 mM stock solution in ultra pure DMSO on the day of staining.

14. Transfer 15 ml prewarmed mBCl mixture to Cellomics KSR reagent reservoir (located on the KSR deck and kept at 37°C). Use the on-line pipettor of the KSR to add 100 µl of the 2× mBCl to each column of a 96-well plate, incubate on deck for 1 min, then acquire the images for that column as below. Repeat for the next column.

15. Fluorescence is measured for four different dyes (each in a separate channel). The 20× objective is used to collect images for all four fluorescence channels with an appropriate filter set (XF 93). Dyes are excited and their fluorescence are monitored at excitation and emission wavelengths of: 655 ± 15 and

730 ± 25 nm for DRAQ5 (channel 1 – nuclei/lipids); 475 ± 20 and 515 ± 10 nm for CM-H$_2$DCFDA (channel 2 – ROS); 549 ± 4 and 600 ± 12.5 nm for TMRM (channel 3 – mitochondrial membrane potential); 365 ± 25 and 515 ± 10 nm for mBCl (channel 4 – glutathione content).

16. Capture six images per well (six fields per well) using the "Acquire Only" protocol of the instrument. Use fixed exposures that are predetermined using control wells at about mid-linear range of the camera.

17. Proceed with image analysis.

3.5. Image Analysis for HIAT

The images from all wells are quantitatively analyzed using the image analysis macro in Image Pro Plus v4.5 (Media Cybernetics, Silver Spring, MD). See Note 12 for the use of other image analysis softwares.

The nuclei images (from the Draq5 channel 1) are segmented according to the intensity differences between nuclei and background pixels. The segmented nuclei are then gated by area, perimeter, and intensity to set aside brightly condensed dead cells, cell clumps, and/or cellular debris. A binary mask and a dilated binary mask (kernel size 5×5 octagon, seven iterations) are created from the segmented nuclei as in a nuclear outline. The dilated binary mask is Boolean "AND" with a Voronoi diagram to create a "zone of influence" for each cell. The Voronoi diagram is created by inverting the nuclear mask to highlight the background as the objects of interest. Thinning the image of the object backgrounds by thinning the filter results in the intermediate edges between objects, i.e., the Voronoi diagram. Invert the Voronoi diagram. This creates the "regions of influence" for each object. The nuclear masks and "zone of influence" are saved in the Count/Size dialog box in Image Pro Plus and are used in later processing steps. The resulting valid nuclei are counted by the "count object" function in ImagePro and exported to Excel as "Total Nuclei Count," "Nuclei Average Intensity," "Nuclei Area," and "Nuclei Area per Cell."

In order to measure ROS fluorescence intensity (from the CM-H$_2$DCFDA channel 2), a fixed intensity threshold value is chosen to identify true ROS positive cells. The segmented objects and resulting binary mask is Boolean "AND" with the raw grayscale ROS image to create an intensity mask. The previously saved "zone of influence" is overlaid by Boolean "AND" with the intensity mask. Total intensity is measured and exported to Excel as "ROS Total Intensity" and "ROS Intensity per Cell."

Mitochondria are stained by TMRM (channel 3), a mitochondrial membrane potential indicator. A fixed intensity threshold value is chosen from the 0.4% DMSO control wells. TMRM total intensity is measured and exported to Excel as "TMRM Total Intensity" and "TMRM Intensity per Cell," using the same steps as ROS measurements.

A duplicate Draq5 grayscale nuclear image is used to determine lipid count and lipid intensity. The gray level histogram is used to calculate the minimum intensity value on the duplicate grayscale image. This background value is subtracted from the duplicate grayscale image. The subtracted image is further processed by employing a top hat filter (kernel size 5 × 5) to detect lipid particles that are brighter than background. The previously saved nuclear mask is subtracted from the Draq5 grayscale nuclear image to subtract the nuclei from the image (hence the remaining spots are "lipid spots"). A fixed intensity threshold value is chosen from the Perhexiline positive control wells such that only the bright lipid particles would be included. The lipid particles are further gated by area and roundness. Valid lipid particles are segmented and the resulting binary mask is Boolean "AND" with the original Draq5 grayscale image to get true intensity values for the masked particles. The previously saved "zone of influence" mask is loaded to the masked intensity image. Total intensity is measured and exported to Excel as "Lipid Intensity" and "Lipid Intensity per Cell." The resulting valid lipid particles are counted by the "count object" function in Image Pro Plus and exported to Excel as "Lipid Count" using the "Population Density" measurement.

The Glutathione (GSH) content is quantified by the amount of cellular uptake of the cell permeant monochlorobimane (mBCL channel 4) probe. The images are segmented according to the intensity differences between GSH and background pixels. GSH total intensity, average intensity (mean density), and area is measured and exported to Excel as "GSH Total Intensity," "GSH Total Intensity per Cell," "GSH Total Area," "GSH Area per Cell," and "GSH Average Intensity," using the same steps as described above.

The image analysis routine is automated on a plate-by-plate basis. The entire HIAT procedure can be trained on a relatively small training set of drugs. Table 1 gives an example list of such a drug training set and their expected HIAT results. Once all images are saved, more sophisticated image analysis algorithms can be envisioned and statistical and computational analysis can be applied to HIAT. However, the areas of automated image analysis technologies and extraction of numerical data from cohorts of images for training, testing, and prediction are beyond the scope of this chapter.

3.6. Hepatocyte Culture for the BIAT

Cryopreserved or fresh human hepatocytes are cultured as described above. For the purpose of BIAT, the human hepatocytes are typically plated on day 1, Matrigel overlay applied on day 2, media changed on day 3 and 4, and drug dosed on day 5. The extra day will ensure good bile canaliculi formation (and hence transporter functions) prior to evaluating functional bile flux imaging by the fluorescent bile acid CLF.

Table 1
Example data of the hepatocyte imaging assay technology (HIAT)

Drug name	Literature DILI in vivo classification	Therapeutic C_{max} (µg/ml)	In vitro score	Positive DILI tags
Famotidine	Negative	0.104	Negative	
Fluoxetine	Negative	0.014	Negative	
Nefazadone	Positive	0.4349	Positive	ROS, mito, lipid
Perhexiline	Positive	0.6	Positive	Mito, lipid, GSH
Cimetidine	Positive	3.89	Negative	
Levofloxacin	Negative	5.7	Negative	
Troglitazone	Positive	2.82	Positive	Mito, lipid, GSH
Rosiglitizone	Negative	0.373	Negative	
Asprin	Negative	0.995	Negative	
Nimesulide	Positive	6.5	Positive	Mito, lipid, GSH
Diclofenac	Positive	2.367	Positive	ROS, mito, lipid, GSH
Flufenamic acid	Negative	13	Negative	
Zomepirac	Negative	2.4	Negative	
Sulindac	Positive	11.4	Positive	ROS, lipid
Diflunisal	Positive	124	Positive	Lipid, GSH
Acetaminophen	Negative when used at normal dose	21	Negative	
Erythromycin	Negative	1.33	Negative	
Telithromycin	Positive	2.25	Positive	Lipid

Published reference compounds were assessed with HIAT and compared to literature classifications of drug-induced liver injury (DILI) in humans. For orally dosed drugs (all drugs listed here), 100× human therapeutic single-dose C_{max} was used as a relevant concentration for testing in this short-term (24 h) in vitro hepatotoxicity assay (13). *Clear cells*: true negative drugs. *Gray-shaded cells*: true-positive drugs. *Black-shaded cells*: false-negative drug. Positive DILI tags were those imaging channels that were found to be significantly different from all the DILI negative drugs in this table

3.7. Drug Treatment for BIAT

1. Vehicle controls: all wells in rows 1 and 2 are filled with 125 µl per well phenol red free, 5% serum containing Drugging Medium containing 0.4% DMSO. See Table 2 for an example plate layout. Negative controls: Fluoxetine, $C_{max} = 0.014$ µg/ml, negative at 30× C_{max}; Metformin, $C_{max} = 3.1$ µg/ml, negative at 30× C_{max}. Positive controls: Erythromycin estolate, $C_{max} = 3.08$ µg/ml, positive at 30× C_{max}; cyclosporine A, $C_{max} = 0.93$ µg/ml, positive at 10× C_{max}.

Table 2
Typical plate layout for the bile flux imaging assay technology (BIAT) using a single 30× C_{max} concentration and duplicate treatment (C & D, E & F, G & H)

	1	2	3	4	5	6
A	DMSO	DMSO	DMSO	DMSO	DMSO	DMSO
B	DMSO	DMSO	DMSO	DMSO	DMSO	DMSO
C	Compound 1	Compound 4	Compound 7	Compound 10	Compound 13	Compound 16
D	30×	30×	30×	30×	30×	30×
E	Compound 2	Compound 5	Compound 8	Compound 11	Compound 14	Compound 17
F	30×	30×	30×	30×	30×	30×
G	Compound 3	Compound 6	Compound 9	Compound 12	Compound 15	Compound 18
H	30×	30×	30×	30×	30×	30×

Other dose titration schema can be envisioned based on this experimental design (e.g., 100×, 30×, 10×, 3×, and 1× C_{max}). The speed of the current live-cell image acquisition instrument is still relatively slow (compared to a low-resolution but fast plate reader). To minimize any fluorescent signal degradation over time, only the left half of a 96-well plate is used within one processing batch

2. Prepare a 10 µM solution of CLF in phenol red free, serum-free Imaging Medium by adding an appropriate amount of the 10 mM stock (stock is aliquoted and stored at −20 °C) to pre-warmed Imaging Medium (1:1,000 dilution). See Note 11 regarding precautions about single use of fluorescent probes and light sensitivities.

3. Prepare working stock of drugs to test at 2× final concentration and 0.8% DMSO, in Drugging Medium, in sterile tubes.

4. Invert and vortex working stocks in tubes. Sonicate if necessary. Transfer a 300 µl volume to its appropriate position on a sterile 96-well polypropylene V bottom intermediate plate. This constitutes the master 2× drug plate to dose the hepatocytes.

5. Using the Apricot PP550 Soken pipettor, mix the master 2× drug intermediate plate and dispense 65 µl of 2× drug into a fresh polypropylene V bottom plate. Drugs that change the color of phenol red should be noted at this step.

6. Next, using an 8-channel hand pipettor, add 65 µl/well of 10 µM CLF solution (changing tips after each column) to the intermediate plate containing 65 µl of 2× drug solutions (final volume is 130 µl of 2× drugs + 2× CLF to make a mixture that contains 1× drug + 1× CLF).

7. Fast inhibition method: this method is used to detect fast binders and disrupters of transporter function. One Apricot PP550 Soken is used to remove existing media while a second Apricot

PP550 Soken is used to add drug/probe. Existing media is removed from cell plate at slow speed, with tips to side, and tips set at a height that do not contact or disrupt the Matrigel. Ideally, ~30 μl of liquid is left behind in each well during the medium removal step. Anything less than that will leave a dry island in the well. For this assay to work appropriately, the Matrigel must not be disturbed or any portion of the well left dry at any time. The 2× drug/probe solutions are mixed prior to adding to the cells. Then, add 125 μl of drug/probe to each well, at slow speed, in 25 μl increments, with tips to side. After adding drug/probe, the plate is placed back in the incubator for 15 min. At the 15 min time point, proceed to Trypan Blue Quench step described below.

8. Slow inhibition method: this method is used to detect slow binders and/or disrupters of transporter trafficking. Incubated plate with 1× drugs only without CLF for 60 min. To create a 1× drug plate, transfer 70 μl from the master 2× drug plate prepared above to a fresh polypropylene V bottom plate that has been prefilled with 70 μl of prewarmed phenol red free, 5% serum containing Drugging Media. Dose cells as described above and incubate for 60 min. During this incubation, re-mix a master 2× drug intermediate plate and dispense 65 μl (2× drug) into a fresh polypropylene V bottom intermediate plate and proceed with the CLF addition steps outlined above, adding 65 μl of 10 μM CLF to the 65 μl of 2× drugs (final volume in the intermediate plate will be 130 μl of 2× drugs + 2× CLF to make 1× drug + 1× CLF). At the 60 min time point, remove the 1× drugs from the cell plate with an Apricot PP550 Soken (as above) and then add back the 2× drug/probe solutions. Add a total of 125 μl of drug/probe to each well, at slow speed, in 25 μl increments, with tips to side. Incubate for 15 min and then proceed with Trypan Blue Quench step described below.

9. Trypan Blue Quench: the purpose of this step is to use a diluted Trypan Blue solution to quench extracellular residual CLF signal or CLF signals that have been taken up nonspecifically by dead cells. Trypan Blue enters the dead cells with compromised membrane, quenches CLF fluorescence associated with such dead cell clumps, and significantly enhances the signal-to-noise ratio of truly transported CLF signal in bile canaliculi. In advance of this step, prepare a 0.025 mg/ml solution of Trypan Blue in HBSS (containing Ca^{2+} and Mg^{2+}) by diluting 0.4% Trypan Blue stock solution 1:16 in HBSS. At the end of the drug/CLF incubation, remove cell plate from the incubator and use an Apricot PP550 Soken to remove the drug/CLF. Using the Apricot PP550 Soken, add 100 μl/well of the 0.25 mg/ml Trypan Blue solution and incubate at room

temperature exactly for 1 min. The next steps need to be done quickly to stay within the 1 min timeframe. At the end of the 1 min Trypan Blue Quench, remove Trypan Blue using one Apricot PP550 Soken and add 200 µl warmed HBSS (slow speed, 25 increments) to the cell plate using a second Apricot PP550 Soken. Set the Apricot PP550 to mix the 200 µl HBSS wash buffer on slow speed with "volume fill" set to 100 µl. Do not lower the tips to the bottom of the well for the mix cycle as it runs the risk of disrupting the Matrigel overlay which might compromise the integrity of the bile canalicular structures and function (CLF signal would drop considerably upon imaging). Repeat the above wash once. After the final wash, remove the HBSS using the same Apricot PP550 Soken, then transfer plate to the second Apricot PP550 and add 100 µl to each well prewarmed phenol red free Imaging Medium.

3.8. Image Acquisition for BIAT

1. Load plate onto the Array Scan KSR. Again, the environmental chamber and the lamp of the KSR should be already equilibrated for about 2 h ahead of the measurement. The lid should be kept on as there is no liquid transfer steps needed in this image acquisition protocol.

2. CLF and nuclei image acquisition: fluorescence is measured for two different dyes (each in a separate scan over the same area). This is because the CLF probe and the Hoechst nuclear dye are not compatible if multiplexed together. The CLF signals are acquired first, before the Hoechst staining and image acquisition at the next step below. The 20× objective is used to collect images for both fluorescence channels with the XF100 GFP filter set used for CLF-stained bile canaliculi signal and the XF93 Hoechst filter set used for Hoechst-stained nuclei signal. Dyes are excited and their fluorescence monitored at their excitation and emission wavelengths of: 475 ± 20 and 515 ± 10 nm for CLF (channel 1 – bile canaliculi) and 365 ± 25 and 515 ± 10 nm for Hoechst 33342 (channel 1 – nuclei). Exposure for all channels are fixed and predetermined using control wells to be around mid-linear ranges for the camera. Six images are captured per well (six fields per well) using the "Acquire Only" protocol of the instrument.

3. At the conclusion of the CLF scan, the plate is re-stained with Hoechst 33342. Add 15 µl of 10 mg/ml stock (stored at 4°C) to 15 ml prewarmed phenol red free Imaging Medium (1:1,000 dilution). Remove existing Imaging Medium from cell plate using Apricot PP550 Soken (slow speed, tips to side), add 100 µl Hoechst 33342 using a second Apricot PP550 Soken. The plate is incubated at 37°C for 10 min. Remove Hoechst 33342 using one Apricot PP550 Soken and add 100 µl prewarmed phenol red free Imaging Medium to each well using

the second Apricot PP550. Put a lid on the plate and load into the ArrayScan KSR and scan initiated for nuclei channel as described above.

3.9. Image Analysis of BIAT

Images are analyzed using automated image analysis macros using Image Pro Plus v4.5 (Media Cybernetics, Bethesda, MD, USA). The total intensity of CLF accumulated in the bile canalicular space (from the FITC channel) is quantified by first applying an edge detection filter followed by a fixed threshold for background subtraction. CLF total intensity is measured and exported to Excel as "CLF Total Intensity." The nuclei images are acquired in a separate scan (from the Hoechst channel) and are processed as previously described for HIAT. The CLF fluorescent intensity values are normalized by the total nuclei count from the same image fields (i.e., the sum of CLF fluorescent intensity values divided by the sum of nuclei count from a total of six image fields from the same well). The numerical mean of such normalized values from the DMSO vehicle control wells is set at 100%, hence all the drug-treated wells are calculated as a relative percentage to the vehicle control wells. See Note 12 for the use of other image analysis softwares.

4. Notes

1. Prior to thawing cryopreserved hepatocytes, ensure that all required reagents are prepared ahead of time, all items that will come in contact with cells must be in sterile condition, and all required equipment and instrument must be calibrated, cleaned, and ready to go (see Subheading 3.1, step 1).

2. Freshly isolated hepatocytes typically do not need the CHRM media and can be spun down at $100 \times g$ for 5 min and then re-suspended with the same protocol as the cryopreserved cells. They can then processed exactly like the cyropreserved hepatocytes described above (see Subheading 3.1, steps 6–10, which can be skipped for freshly isolated hepatocytes).

3. Do not use automated cell counters to count primary human hepatocytes, as hepatocytes tend to clump in automated cell counters leading to inaccurate count. Count both live and dead cells using hemocytometer. If the percentage of dead cells exceeds 10%, the use of a low-speed, iso-density Percoll centrifugation method may be used to get rid of dead cells (22) (see Subheading 3.1, step 16).

4. Since different lots of primary hepatocytes may vary in size, it is recommended that different volumes of cells (e.g., 50, 60,

70, 80, 90, 100, 110 µl) be seeded for the first few columns of a separate test plate to determine the best seeding volume (i.e., best seeding number of cells per well) for all subsequent plates. Visual inspection under a microscope provides the best guide for this step: cells should be 80–90% confluent right after seeding, such that after cell attachment (and some spreading), the culture is essentially a 100% confluent monolayer (see Subheading 3.1, step 20).

5. Ideally, two automated personal pipetting stations are set up in a biosafety hood for working with primary hepatocyte cultures. One station is dedicated to adding medium while the second station removes medium. This ensures that cells will not experience "dry wells" during the medium change. It is equally important that the stage height on the pipetting stations is set such that the tips do not disrupt the cell or Matrigel layer during any medium removal step. Other pipetting instruments (or even manual pipetting solutions) can certainly be used here, so long as: (a) the tips of pipettes do not touch the cell nor Matrigel layer, (b) the speed the liquid transfer can be set to low, and the position of liquid transfer can be set to one side of the well, and (c) the orifice of tips is wide enough to transfer viscous primary cell suspension without shearing or damaging cells, or Matrigel solution without causing gelling inside the tips (see Subheading 3.1, step 24).

6. Even loading of the 96-well Apricot PP550 Soken tips is critical to avoid disruption of Matrigel overlay. Load tips as normal, remove head from loader, and observe the ends of the tips to ensure that they are evenly loaded. If an older loader is used, a pad made of clean paper towels plated in between the loader block and pipette head may help to ensure even compression and loading of tips (see Subheading 3.1, step 24).

7. Aliquot Matrigel ahead of time in single use vials such that one can overlay two 96-well plates with the same set of chilled tips. Store aliquots in −20°C freezer (see Subheading 3.2, step 1).

8. Trichostatin A is an HDAC inhibitor and has been found at low concentrations to aid in maintaining hepatocyte differentiation (23, 24) (see Subheading 3.2, step 3).

9. Matrigel stock concentrations vary between lots. For example, if the current Matrigel stock is 10 mg/ml, one would aliquot Matrigel into 1.25 ml single aliquot tubes and store in −20°C freezer and each aliquot would be enough to make 50 ml of media for overlay on cells, at a final Matrigel concentration of 0.25 mg/ml. Once a lot of Matrigel has been qualified to work for the described assays, it is highly recommended that sufficient quantity of this lot be procured to minimize lot-to-lot variability (see Subheading 3.2, step 4).

10. Matrigel will start to solidify as it warms, so move swiftly to prepare and add to cells once all materials have been removed from cold storage. In particular, Culturing Medium should be kept on ice, along with Matrigel, just prior to combining. The Matrigel/media solution in the cold reservoir should also be kept on ice (after swirling and rocking several times to mix the content), just prior to adding to the cell plates. Consistent and even Matrigel overlay is critical to ensure consistency in cell morphology (see Subheading 3.2, step 8).

11. It is highly recommended that all fluorescent probes be solubilized in ultra pure solvent such as 100% DMSO, then aliquoted to single-use size to minimize freeze–thaw cycles and light exposure. For example, we routinely solubilize 1 mg dry CLF in 108 µl of 100% DMSO to achieve a 10 mM solution. This solution is then aliquoted in 5 µl increments for frozen storage and for single use. Wrap all fluorescent probes in foils to protect them from light. Avoid bright light when working with fluorescent probes. We typically keep the lamps inside and around the biosafety hood off, and curtains or shades down. The ceiling light in the ArrayScan KSR room should also be turned off during image acquisition (see Subheading 3.4, step 3).

12. In addition to using Image Pro Plus v4.5 for automated image analysis, other image analysis softwares can also be used, so long as each fluorescence channel can be independently calculated, selections of objects of interest can be independently verified, and the entire image analysis routine can be automated across an entire plate or sets of 96-well plates (see Subheadings 3.5 and 3.9).

Acknowledgments

The authors would like to thank Drs. David de Graaf, Jeffery Chabot, Peter Henstock, Michael Aleo, Denise Robinson-Gravatt, and other research program team members for their support in the development and validation of HIAT and BIAT protocols.

References

1. Duan, W., and Wong, W. S. (2006) Targeting mitogen-activated protein kinases for asthma. *Curr. Drug Targets* 7, 691–698.
2. Wong, K. K. (2009) Recent Developments in Anti-Cancer Agents Targeting the Ras/Raf/MEK/ERK Pathway. *Recent Patents Anticancer Drug Discov.* 4, 28–35.
3. Schindler, J. F., Monahan, J. B., and Smith, W. G. (2007) p38 pathway kinases as anti-inflammatory drug targets. *J. Dent. Res.* 86, 800–811.
4. Hendriks, B. S., Hua, F., and Chabot, J. R. (2008) Analysis of mechanistic pathway models in drug discovery: p38 pathway. *Biotechnol. Prog.* 24, 96–109.
5. Konecny, G. E., Pegram, M. D., Venkatesan, N., Finn, R., Yang, G., Rahmeh, M., Untch, M., Rusnak, D. W., Spehar, G., Mullin, R. J.,

Keith, B. R., Gilmer, T. M., Berger, M., Podratz, K. C., and Slamon, D. J. (2006) Activity of the dual kinase inhibitor lapatinib (GW572016) against HER-2-overexpressing and trastuzumab-treated breast cancer cells. *Cancer Res.* **66**, 1630–1639.

6. Moulder, S. L., Yakes, F. M., Muthuswamy, S. K., Bianco, R., Simpson, J. F., and Arteaga, C. L. (2001) Epidermal growth factor receptor (HER1) tyrosine kinase inhibitor ZD1839 (Iressa) inhibits HER2/neu (erbB2)-overexpressing breast cancer cells in vitro and in vivo. *Cancer Res.* **61**, 8887–8895.

7. Dominguez, C., Powers, D. A., and Tamayo, N. (2005) p38 MAP kinase inhibitors: many are made, but few are chosen. *Curr. Opin. Drug Discov. Devel.* **8**, 421–430.

8. Guo, F., Letrent, S. P., Munster, P. N., Britten, C. D., Gelmon, K., Tolcher, A. W., and Sharma, A. (2008) Pharmacokinetics of a HER2 tyrosine kinase inhibitor CP-724,714 in patients with advanced malignant HER2 positive solid tumors: correlations with clinical characteristics and safety. *Cancer Chemother. Pharmacol.* **62**, 97–109.

9. Xu, J. J., Hendriks, B. S., Zhao, J., and de Graaf, D. (2008) Multiple effects of acetaminophen and p38 inhibitors: towards pathway toxicology. *FEBS Lett.* **582**, 1276–1282.

10. Antoine, D. J., Williams, D. P., and Park, B. K. (2008) Understanding the role of reactive metabolites in drug-induced hepatotoxicity: state of the science. *Expert Opin. Drug Metab. Toxicol.* **4**, 1415–1427.

11. Obach, R. S., Kalgutkar, A. S., Soglia, J. R., and Zhao, S. X. (2008) Can in vitro metabolism-dependent covalent binding data in liver microsomes distinguish hepatotoxic from nonhepatotoxic drugs? An analysis of 18 drugs with consideration of intrinsic clearance and daily dose. *Chem. Res. Toxicol.* **21**, 1814–1822.

12. Zhao, S. X., Dalvie, D. K., Kelly, J. M., Soglia, J. R., Frederick, K. S., Smith, E. B., Obach, R. S., and Kalgutkar, A. S. (2007) NADPH-dependent covalent binding of [3H]paroxetine to human liver microsomes and S-9 fractions: identification of an electrophilic quinone metabolite of paroxetine. *Chem. Res. Toxicol.* **20**, 1649–1657.

13. Xu, J. J., Henstock, P. V., Dunn, M. C., Smith, A. R., Chabot, J. R., and de Graaf, D. (2008) Cellular imaging predictions of clinical drug-induced liver injury. *Toxicol. Sci.* **105**, 97–105.

14. Olson, H., Betton, G., Robinson, D., Thomas, K., Monro, A., Kolaja, G., Lilly, P., Sanders, J., Sipes, G., Bracken, W., Dorato, M., Van Deun, K., Smith, P., Berger, B., and Heller, A. (2000) Concordance of the toxicity of pharmaceuticals in humans and in animals. *Regul. Toxicol. Pharmacol.* **32**, 56–67.

15. LeCluyse, E. L., Audus, K. L., and Hochman, J. H. (1994) Formation of extensive canalicular networks by rat hepatocytes cultured in collagen-sandwich configuration. *Am. J. Physiol.* **266**, C1764–1774.

16. Liu, X., LeCluyse, E. L., Brouwer, K. R., Gan, L. S., Lemasters, J. J., Stieger, B., Meier, P. J., and Brouwer, K. L. (1999) Biliary excretion in primary rat hepatocytes cultured in a collagen-sandwich configuration. *Am. J. Physiol.* **277**, G12–21.

17. Hariparsad, N., Carr, B. A., Evers, R., and Chu, X. (2008) Comparison of immortalized Fa2N-4 cells and human hepatocytes as in vitro models for cytochrome P450 induction. *Drug Metab. Dispos.* **36**, 1046–1055.

18. Le Vee, M., Jigorel, E., Glaise, D., Gripon, P., Guguen-Guillouzo, C., and Fardel, O. (2006) Functional expression of sinusoidal and canalicular hepatic drug transporters in the differentiated human hepatoma HepaRG cell line. *Eur. J. Pharm. Sci.* **28**, 109–117.

19. Munster, P. N., Britten, C. D., Mita, M., Gelmon, K., Minton, S. E., Moulder, S., Slamon, D. J., Guo, F., Letrent, S. P., Denis, L., and Tolcher, A. W. (2007) First study of the safety, tolerability, and pharmacokinetics of CP-724,714 in patients with advanced malignant solid HER2-expressing tumors. *Clin. Cancer Res.* **13**, 1238–1245.

20. Feng, B., Xu, J. J., Bi, Y. A., Mireles, R., Davidson, R., Duignan, D. B., Campbell, S., Kostrubsky, V. E., Dunn, M. C., Smith, A. R., and Wang, H. F. (2009) Role of hepatic transporters in the disposition and hepatotoxicity of a HER2 tyrosine kinase inhibitor CP-724,714. *Toxicol. Sci.* **108**, 492–500.

21. Bi, Y. A., Kazolias, D., and Duignan, D. B. (2006) Use of cryopreserved human hepatocytes in sandwich culture to measure hepatobiliary transport. *Drug Metab. Dispos.* **34**, 1658–1665.

22. Kreamer, B. L., Staecker, J. L., Sawada, N., Sattler, G. L., Hsia, M. T., and Pitot, H. C. (1986) Use of a low-speed, iso-density percoll centrifugation method to increase the viability of isolated rat hepatocyte preparations. *In Vitro Cell Dev. Biol.* **22**, 201–211.

23. Vinken, M., Henkens, T., Vanhaecke, T., Papeleu, P., Geerts, A., Van Rossen, E., Chipman, J. K., Meda, P., and Rogiers, V. (2006) Trichostatin a enhances gap junctional intercellular communication in primary cultures of adult rat hepatocytes. *Toxicol. Sci.* **91**, 484–492.

24. Papeleu, P., Vanhaecke, T., and Rogiers, V. (2006) Histone deacetylase inhibition: A differentiation therapy for cultured primary hepatocytes? *Curr. Enz. Inhib.* **2**, 91–104.

Chapter 7

Kinase Inhibitor Selectivity Profiling Using Differential Scanning Fluorimetry

Oleg Fedorov, Frank H. Niesen, and Stefan Knapp

Abstract

Fast, robust, and inexpensive screening methods are the heart of drug discovery processes. Moreover, it is useful to have access to several established assay formats, for validation purposes. If a targeted protein is an enzyme, the logical and widely used approach is the direct measurement of the effect of the added ligands on its activity. A variety of enzymatic assay formats have been successfully applied for inhibitor screening of protein kinases. However, enzymatic assays require an active enzyme with a known substrate and often time-consuming assay optimization. Several alternative approaches have been recently developed that detect binding of ligands to proteins. This chapter overviews and provides the experimental protocol of the successful application of differential scanning fluorimetry (DSF) in our laboratory for fast and robust screening of medium-sized (<10,000) inhibitor libraries. DSF monitors the thermal stabilization of the native protein structure upon ligand binding. It allows selectivity profiling of any protein kinase without prior knowledge of either substrate or activity of the kinase under investigation. Comparative studies revealed that generated data is highly reproducible and correlates well with the results from other ligand binding methodologies, direct binding constants as well as enzymatic assays.

Key words: Kinase, Protein stability, Inhibitor selectivity, Compound screening, Differential scanning fluorimetry

1. Introduction

Protein kinases play central roles in all cellular processes. Not surprisingly, the deregulation of kinase activity results in a variety of disorders. The list of kinases implicated in human diseases is ever increasing and suggests that a significant proportion of the members of the kinome represent potential drug targets. To fully utilize the enormous potential for the development of inhibitors against a large number of kinases as chemical probes or lead compounds for drug discovery, their selectivity against the 518 human kinases will have to be individually assessed. In order to achieve this, inhibition data must be collected for representative kinase panels (1–3). Traditionally, kinase screening relies on assays that utilize direct measurements of enzymatic activities (4). However, for a successful generation of large data arrays, appropriate substrates need to be identified. In addition, many kinases need to be activated by an upstream signaling partner which, in many cases, is unknown. Moreover, the enzymatic assays need to be individually optimized with respect to the substrate, concentration of ATP, as well as the buffer composition, in order to yield a satisfactory signal-to-noise ratio These requirements may not always be possible to meet, for example, if the target is a novel and less well-studied kinase, or if multiple forms are involved in their mechanism of activation (5). Furthermore, when selectivity data against a sizable kinase panel is required for the assessment, the traditional screening approach may become costly and time consuming. To address these limitations, alternative approaches have been developed, based on competition binding assays (6, 7). However, these methods are difficult to establish and are therefore usually outsourced to a specialized company. A generic method, based on the effect of thermal stabilization of the protein structure upon ligand binding, proved to be especially useful for screening of kinase inhibitors (8). The general protocol for this assay, called differential scanning fluorimetry (DSF), has been published previously (9). Here, we present its adaptation for kinase screening.

The stability of a protein is related to its Gibbs free energy of unfolding, ΔG_u, which is temperature dependent. The stability of proteins decreases with temperature; as the temperature increases, the ΔG_u decreases and becomes zero under reversible unfolding conditions where the concentrations of folded and unfolded protein are equal. The temperature at this point, the melting temperature (T_m) of the protein, increases upon ligand binding if differences in heat capacity of the unfolding reaction can be neglected. This stability increase is a direct consequence of the increase in ΔG_u as a result of the free energy contribution of ligand binding (Fig. 1a). Due to the small differences in surface exposure between the folded and the unfolded state upon binding of a low molecular weight ligand, its influence on the heat capacity can usually be neglected, and a linear correlation between ligand binding affinity and melting temperature is observed. Even though the above consideration is only true for two-state reversible unfolding events, the resulting ΔT_m data, in particular for kinases, correlate well with experimentally determined K_D and IC_{50} values (10); it has been shown that the stabilizing effect of compounds upon binding is proportional to the concentration and affinity of the ligands (11, 12). However, caution should be taken when comparing screening data of different family members based on their ΔT_m values, for protein kinase screening this assay proved to be very predictive and stable (8, 13). For example, we correlated binding data generated in our laboratory

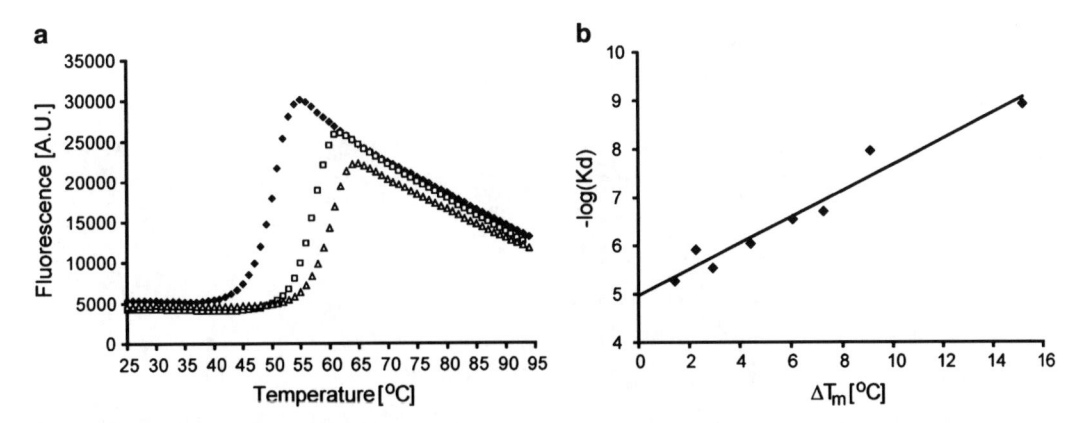

Fig. 1. (a) Unfolding of AAK1, reference (kinase in the presence of DMSO); (*filled diamond*) kinase in the presence of 10 μM of JNJ-7706621, (*open triangle*) kinase in the presence of 10 μM of Sunitinib. (b) Correlation between ΔT_m and the logarithm of the binding constant. Values are taken from Table 1, $R^2 = 0.949$.

with data generated using an in vitro competition binding assay developed at AMBIT (3) (Table 1) and showed that the data correlated very well ($R^2 = 0.949$), as demonstrated in the table and in Fig. 1b.

DSF monitors thermal unfolding of proteins in the presence of a fluorescent dye and is typically performed using a real-time PCR instrument (9). The fluorescent dyes that can be used for DSF are highly fluorescent in nonpolar environment, such as the hydrophobic sites on unfolded proteins, compared to aqueous solution where the fluorescence is quenched. To date, the dye with the most favorable properties for DSF is SYPRO orange, due to its high signal-to-noise ratio and relatively high wavelength for excitation, nearly 500 nm. This excitation wavelength decreases the likelihood that small molecules would interfere with dye and distort the unfolding curve. For T_m determination, the fluorescence intensity is plotted as a function of the temperature generating a sigmoidal curve that can be described by a two-state transition (Fig. 1a). The inflection point of the transition curve (T_m) is then calculated using simple equations such as the Boltzmann equation,

$$y = \mathrm{LL} + \frac{(\mathrm{UL} - \mathrm{LL})}{1 + \exp\left((T_m - x)/a\right)}, \quad (1)$$

where "LL" and "UL" are the values of minimum and maximum intensities, respectively, and "a" denotes the slope of the curve within T_m. A correlation between the thermal scan rates and the measured T_m is observed, resulting in apparently higher melting temperatures at higher scan rates. This correlation is, however, not linear and decreases at higher scan rates, so that experiments can be run faster and the throughput of the assay be increased, while the overall ranking of inhibitor potency remains similar (Fig. 2). Compared to screens at the traditionally applied scan rate of 1°C/min

Table 1
Comparison between measured ΔT_m and K_D values

Inhibitor	K_D (nM)[a]	ΔT_m(°C)
SB-202190	>10,000	0.7
SB-203580	>10,000	0.2
Staurosporine	1.2	15.2
Gefitinib	>10,000	1.4
Erlotinib	1,200	2.3
Imatinib	>10,000	−0.2
LY-333531	900	4.4
Sunitinib	11	9.1
JNJ-7706621	200	7.2
Dasatinib	>10,000	0.6
PTK-787	>10,000	−0.4
VX-680/MK-0457	290	6.1
BIRB-796	>10,000	−0.7
Lapatinib	>10,000	−0.4
ZD-6474	>10,000	0.1
Flavopiridol	5,300	1.4
GW-786034	2,900	2.9
SB-431542	>10,000	0.0

[a]Data are from ref. 3

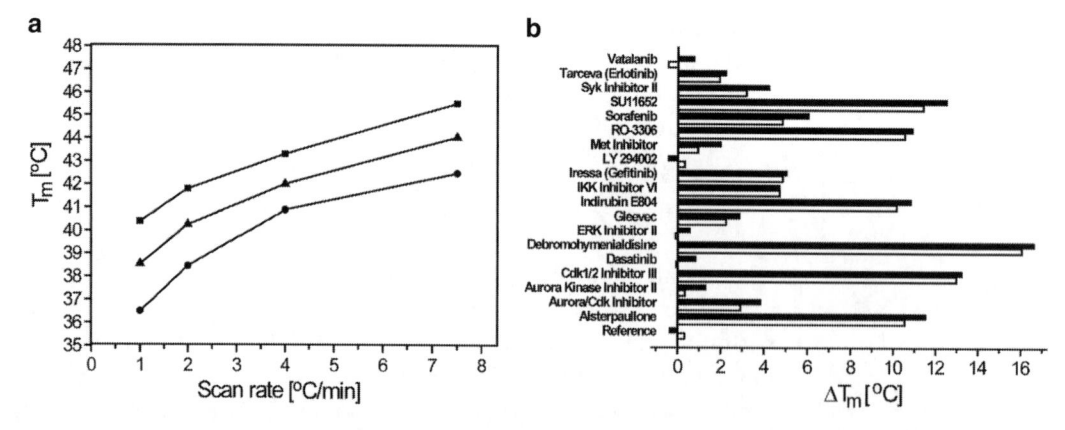

Fig. 2. Influence of the scan rate on the measurement of stability in STK17. (a) Dependence of the transition midpoint, T_m, on the scan rate and NaCl concentration. 50 mM NaCl (*spheres*), 150 mM NaCl (*triangles*), and 500 mM NaCl (*squares*). (b) Change in stability, ΔT_m, in the presence of selected kinase inhibitors measured at scan rates of 1 C/min (*white bars*) and of 7.5°C/min (*black bars*).

7 Kinase Inhibitor Selectivity Profiling Using Differential Scanning Fluorimetry   113

(resulting in a measurement time of 1 h and 11 min per screened plate), screening of several thousand compounds per day is feasible using a fast temperature ramp and a single RT-PCR machine without compromising the results.

2. Materials

2.1. Reagents

1. Assay buffer: 10 mM HEPES–NaOH, pH 7.5, 500 mM NaCl.
2. Kinase inhibitors: 0.5 mM in DMSO (see Note 1).
3. Kinase of interest: 2 µM in assay buffer.
4. Dimethyl sulfoxide (DMSO).
5. SYPRO orange: 5,000× stock in DMSO.

2.2. Consumables

1. 10 ml Plastic tubes.
2. DMSO-resistant 96-well plates.
3. Adhesive aluminum seals.
4. Standard U-bottom 96-well microplates.
5. White QPCR low-profile plates (see Note 2).
6. Optical PCR seals.

2.3. Tools and Instruments

1. 10 and 50 µl Multichannel pipettes.
2. Smooth rubber roller for aluminum plate foil (from any DIY store).
3. Hand applicator for plate foil.
4. Real-time PCR instrument, such as the Mx3005p (Agilent) because of its broad range of excitation and emission wavelengths. SYPRO orange can be monitored using filters commonly provided with the machines (for the Mx3005p, combine FAMex, 492 nm and ROXem, 610 nm).

2.4. Software

1. Excel-based Worksheet "DSF Analysis" available from: ftp://ftp.sgc.ox.ac.uk/pub/biophysics.
2. Data analysis and fitting software, e.g., Prism 5.

3. Methods

3.1. Preparation of Compound Storage Plates

1. Design the layout of the screening plate. Include reference positions (DMSO only, without compound) as well as controls (water only; DMSO often causes destabilization of proteins).

2. Thaw all compound stock solutions needed to setup the plate, by placing all compound vials for ~5 min into a trough filled to ~1 cm depth with room temperature water.

3. Fill the reference and the control wells of the 96-well storage plate with 100% DMSO and distilled water, respectively.

4. Place a sufficient volume of each compound stock solution (in DMSO) into the wells of the compound plate (DMSO-resistant standard microplate) to yield a final concentration of 0.5 mM of each compound in 200 µl volumes. It may be necessary to vortex the compound stock solution in order to ensure that it is completely dissolved after thawing. Use a pipette to mix the well solutions.

5. Prepare copies of the master plate (20–50 µl per well) to avoid unnecessary rounds of thawing and freezing for all material.

6. Attach aluminum foil seals to plates and store at −20°C or below.

7. Important: ensure the plates are sealed well (using the rubber roller) in order to prevent evaporation and cross contamination.

3.2. Setting Up the Plate

3.2.1. Experimental Setup

When setting up a compound screen, distribute the buffered protein solution including the dye into the wells of the plate, and then transfer the compound solution (in a small volume to limit the DMSO concentration) from each well of the source plate into the PCR plate (see Note 3). The SYPRO orange dye is delivered as a 5,000× solution in 100% DMSO. Compound stocks are also in 100% DMSO and need to be diluted in the final screening conditions by at least 50× to avoid DMSO concentrations of more than 2%. As a result of these limitations, the smallest volume that can be dispensed determines the final volume per well in the PCR plate. Manual 10 µl multichannel pipettes allow accurate pipetting of 0.5 µl volumes. As a result, the total reaction volume will typically be 20 µl. A protein concentration of 75 µg/ml (i.e., 2 µM for a kinase domain of a molecular mass of 35 kDa) is normally sufficient to accurately measure the T_m. Try to maintain a ratio between protein and compound of at least 1:5. For compounds that have an expected affinity (K_D) below 1 µM, it is most practical to screen the compounds at 10 µM concentrations because most compounds are soluble in aqueous solution at this concentration (see Note 4).

3.2.2. Equipment Preparation

1. Warm up the Xenon lamp in the PCR instrument for the time recommended by the manufacturer.

2. Thaw the compound or buffer/additive plate during the lamp warm up time by placing it in a shallow trough of room temperature water.

3. Measure the protein concentration, preferably by its absorbance at 280 nm (14).

4. Calculate the volume of protein stock solution necessary to prepare 2.1 ml of a 2 μM solution.

5. Prepare 2.1 ml of assay buffer, supplemented with 5× SYPRO orange (1:1,000 dilution of the stock solution) in a plastic tube.

6. Add the protein to this buffer solution and mix carefully using a 1 ml pipette.

7. Aliquot protein solution into wells (170 μl each) of one row of the standard U-bottom-shaped microplate.

8. Using a 50 μl multichannel pipette, aliquot 19.5 μl of the protein solution into each of the wells of the PCR plate. To avoid creating bubbles, mix gently and empty the pipette on the side of the well.

9. Spin the compound plate briefly (200×g, 1 min) to collect the solution in the bottom of the wells and then remove the aluminum sealing foil.

10. Using a 10 μl pipette, transfer 0.5 μl of each compound into the PCR plate containing the protein solution.

11. Reseal the compound plate with a new aluminum sealing foil. Ensure that the plate is well-sealed by using a smooth rubber roller.

3.3. Experiment Procedure

Place the PCR plate into the PCR instrument and run the temperature scan from 25 to 95°C at a rate of 3°C/min. Depending on the PCR instrument used, the rate may be selected by adjusting the cycle duration, such that, e.g., a duration of 0.15 min corresponds to a scan rate of 4°C/min. Our recommendation for the cycle duration is a time of 0.23 min, which is the shortest time increment that allows three readings per cycle and results in an experiment length of approximately 25 min.

3.4. Data Analysis

The Excel-based tool "DSF Analysis" is available for free download from our FTP site (ftp://ftp.sgc.ox.ac.uk/pub/biophysics) facilitates most of the data processing, analysis, and visualization. Most of its functions are explained in an accompanying instruction manual, also available from this site (see Note 5). Please note that this tool has been designed specifically for data analysis of the Mx3005p PCR instrument.

1. Export the data to Excel. In the MxPro software, choose the "Analysis" tab, then click on the "Analysis Selection/Setup" tab and select all wells by mouse click in the upper left corner of the displayed plate layout. Click on the tab "Results," tick "Amplification plots" from the options given on the upper right corner, and select "R (Multicomponent view)." From the main menu, select "File\Export Chart Data\Export Chart Data

to Excel\Format 2 – Horizontally Grouped by Plot." Excel will open, and the file can then be processed further (see below).

2. Open the "DSF Analysis" Excel tool, as well as the Excel file containing the thermal denaturation plots (called "amplification plots"). Mark the entire data table by clicking the upper left corner. Drag (Ctrl+C) and drop (Ctrl+V) data into the worksheet "Chart Data Horizontal."

3. To enable fitting for T_m values using a standard fitting software such as Prism 5 (GraphPad), the curves are reduced to the actual transition by the "DSF analysis" worksheet. If necessary, the temperatures denoting the intensity minimum before the transition and the maximum amplitude can be corrected manually, within the worksheet "All Graphs."

4. Transfer the results of the curve processing into the fitting software (a template for use with Prism 5 can be found on our FTP site) from the table within the worksheet "Processed Data."

5. Transfer the fitting results (i.e., the T_m values) back into the "DSF Analysis" tool, into the designated space within "Processed Data."

4. Notes

1. The stability of compounds at −20°C may vary, and the integrity of the compounds should be checked frequently with Mass Spectrometry or NMR. It is advisable to prepare and store all compound stock solutions that are needed for a certain plate before starting with the setup. DMSO is very hygroscopic and should be protected from exposure to moisture as much as possible. Such exposure can cause precipitation of compound during the storage at high concentrations in DMSO if the absorption is high. In addition, exposure of the compounds to warm temperatures should be avoided whenever possible (see Subheading 2.1).

2. Compared to frosted PCR plates, white plates have more consistent optical properties and decreased refraction, thus enhancing the signal and should be preferred (see Subheading 2.2).

3. For pipetting, stack the flexible PCR plates into standard microplates (see Subheading 3.2.1).

4. Compound profiling using DSF is most appropriate for compounds with values for K_D below 1 µM, because shifts in T_m are very pronounced and allow a clear ranking of compounds depending on the affinity (Fig. 1, see Subheading 3.2.1)

5. If IC_{50} or K_D values are available for several benchmark compounds, the relationship between T_m and affinity can be

visualized by plotting T_m values vs. the logarithm of the affinity, as illustrated in Table 1 and Fig. 2b for AAK1, for which published K_D values were used (3) (see Subheading 3.4).

Acknowledgments

The Structural Genomics Consortium is a registered charity (number 1097737) that receives funds from the Canadian Institutes for Health Research, the Canadian Foundation for Innovation, Genome Canada through the Ontario Genomics Institute, GlaxoSmithKline, Karolinska Institutet, the Knut and Alice Wallenberg Foundation, the Ontario Innovation Trust, the Ontario Ministry for Research and Innovation, Merck & Co., Inc., the Novartis Research Foundation, the Swedish Agency for Innovation Systems, the Swedish Foundation for Strategic Research and the Wellcome Trust.

References

1. Goldstein, D. M., Gray, N. S., and Zarrinkar, P. P. (2008) High-throughput kinase profiling as a platform for drug discovery. *Nat. Rev. Drug Discov.* 7, 391–397.
2. Bamborough, P., Drewry, D., Harper, G., Smith, G. K., and Schneider, K. (2008) Assessment of chemical coverage of kinome space and its implications for kinase drug discovery. *J. Med. Chem.* 51, 7898–7914.
3. Karaman, M. W., Herrgard, S., Treiber, D. K., Gallant, P., Atteridge, C. E., Campbell, B. T., Chan, K. W., Ciceri, P., Davis, M. I., Edeen, P. T., Faraoni, R., Floyd, M., Hunt, J. P., Lockhart, D. J., Milanov, Z. V., Morrison, M. J., Pallares, G., Patel, H. K., Pritchard, S., Wodicka, L. M., and Zarrinkar, P. P. (2008) A quantitative analysis of kinase inhibitor selectivity. *Nat. Biotechnol.* 26, 127–132.
4. Bain, J., Plater, L., Elliott, M., Shpiro, N., Hastie, C. J., McLauchlan, H., Klevernic, I., Arthur, J. S., Alessi, D. R., and Cohen, P. (2007) The selectivity of protein kinase inhibitors: a further update. *Biochem J.* 408, 297–315.
5. Chene, P. (2008) Challenges in design of biochemical assays for the identification of small molecules to target multiple conformations of protein kinases. *Drug. Discov. Today* 13, 522–529.
6. Fabian, M. A., Biggs, W. H., 3rd, Treiber, D. K., Atteridge, C. E., Azimioara, M. D., Benedetti, M. G., Carter, T. A., Ciceri, P., Edeen, P. T., Floyd, M., Ford, J. M., Galvin, M., Gerlach, J. L., Grotzfeld, R. M., Herrgard, S., Insko, D. E., Insko, M. A., Lai, A. G., Lelias, J. M., Mehta, S. A., Milanov, Z. V., Velasco, A. M., Wodicka, L. M., Patel, H. K., Zarrinkar, P. P., and Lockhart, D. J. (2005) A small molecule-kinase interaction map for clinical kinase inhibitors. *Nat. Biotechnol.* 23, 329–336.
7. Bantscheff, M., Eberhard, D., Abraham, Y., Bastuck, S., Boesche, M., Hobson, S., Mathieson, T., Perrin, J., Raida, M., Rau, C., Reader, V., Sweetman, G., Bauer, A., Bouwmeester, T., Hopf, C., Kruse, U., Neubauer, G., Ramsden, N., Rick, J., Kuster, B., and Drewes, G. (2007) Quantitative chemical proteomics reveals mechanisms of action of clinical ABL kinase inhibitors. *Nat. Biotechnol.* 25, 1035–1044.
8. Fedorov, O., Marsden, B., Pogacic, V., Rellos, P., Muller, S., Bullock, A. N., Schwaller, J., Sundstrom, M., and Knapp, S. (2007) A systematic interaction map of validated kinase inhibitors with Ser/Thr kinases. *Proc. Natl. Acad. Sci. USA* 104, 20523–20528.
9. Niesen, F. H., Berglund, H., and Vedadi, M. (2007) The use of differential scanning fluorimetry to detect ligand interactions that promote protein stability. *Nat. Protoc.* 2, 2212–2221.
10. Bullock, A. N., Debreczeni, J. E., Fedorov, O. Y., Nelson, A., Marsden, B. D., and Knapp, S. (2005) Structural basis of inhibitor specificity

of the human protooncogene proviral insertion site in moloney murine leukemia virus (PIM-1) kinase. *J. Med. Chem.* **48**, 7604–7614.

11. Matulis, D., Kranz, J. K., Salemme, F. R., and Todd, M. J. (2005) Thermodynamic stability of carbonic anhydrase: measurements of binding affinity and stoichiometry using ThermoFluor. *Biochemistry* **44**, 5258–5266.

12. Pantoliano, M. W., Petrella, E. C., Kwasnoski, J. D., Lobanov, V. S., Myslik, J., Graf, E., Carver, T., Asel, E., Springer, B. A., Lane, P., and Salemme, F. R. (2001) High-density miniaturized thermal shift assays as a general strategy for drug discovery. *J. Biomol. Screen.* **6**, 429–440.

13. Pogacic, V., Bullock, A. N., Fedorov, O., Filippakopoulos, P., Gasser, C., Biondi, A., Meyer-Monard, S., Knapp, S., and Schwaller, J. (2007) Structural analysis identifies imidazo[1,2-b]pyridazines as PIM kinase inhibitors with in vitro antileukemic activity. *Cancer Res.* **67**, 6916–6924.

14. Pace, C. N., Vajdos, F., Fee, L., Grimsley, G., and Gray, T. (1995) How to measure and predict the molar absorption coefficient of a protein. *Protein Sci.* **4**, 2411–2423.

Chapter 8

Chemoproteomic Characterization of Protein Kinase Inhibitors Using Immobilized ATP

James S. Duncan, Timothy A.J. Haystead, and David W. Litchfield

Abstract

Protein kinase inhibitors have emerged as indispensable tools for the elucidation of the biological functions of specific signal transduction pathways and as promising candidates for molecular-targeted therapy. However, because many protein kinase inhibitors are ATP-competitive inhibitors targeting the catalytic site of specific protein kinases, the large number of protein kinases that are encoded within eukaryotic genomes and the existence of many other cellular proteins that bind ATP result in the prospect of off-target effects for many of these compounds. Many of the potential off-target effects remain unrecognized because protein kinase inhibitors are often developed and tested primarily on the basis of in vitro assays using purified components. To overcome this limitation, we describe a systematic approach to characterize ATP-competitive protein kinase inhibitors employing ATP-sepharose to capture the purine-binding proteome from cell extracts. Protein kinase inhibitors can be used in competition experiments to prevent binding of specific cellular proteins to ATP-sepharose or to elute bound proteins from ATP-sepharose. Collectively, these strategies can enable validation of interactions between a specific protein kinase and an inhibitor in complex mixtures and can yield the identification of inhibitor targets.

Key words: Protein kinase inhibitors, Chemoproteomics, ATP-sepharose, Protein kinase CK2, Mass spectrometry, 2D Gel electrophoresis

1. Introduction

Protein kinase inhibitors have emerged as attractive candidates for molecular-targeted therapy and as useful tools for investigating the functions of specific protein kinases and protein kinase-mediated signaling pathways in different biological responses (1–4). While effective active site and allosteric site inhibitors have been described, a large proportion of protein kinase inhibitors that are currently available represent compounds that target the

ATP binding site of protein kinases. Since there are more than 500 protein kinases sharing a similar architecture encoded within the human genome (5), it has proven difficult to design inhibitors specific for individual protein kinases. The challenge of achieving specificity is illustrated by the observation that many protein kinase inhibitors, initially described as specific, turn out to be effective inhibitors of other protein kinases (6–9). This problem arises in part because characterization of protein kinase inhibitors has traditionally relied on in vitro studies involving binding or enzyme assays performed with a limited number of purified protein kinases. Compounding the likelihood that kinase inhibitors may have additional cellular targets (i.e., off-targets) is the fact that, in addition to protein kinases, a broad variety of other cellular proteins bind to or utilize ATP as a substrate. Off-target interactions may not necessarily negate the utility of protein kinase inhibitors for investigation of protein kinase function in experimental systems or as therapeutic agents. Nevertheless, it is important that unbiased strategies be employed to systematically profile the cellular targets of protein kinases.

In order to perform a systematic evaluation of ATP-competitive protein kinase inhibitors, we employed ATP-sepharose to capture the purine-binding proteome from cell extracts (10, 11). Two variations of this strategy were employed to characterize inhibitors of protein kinase CK2 (12), an enzyme that has emerged as a potential therapeutic target because it is elevated in a number of tumors and displays oncogenic activity in mice (13–16). The complementary approaches that we devised for evaluating CK2 inhibitors are: (1) elution experiments where CK2 inhibitors were used to release proteins from ATP-sepharose and (2) competition experiments where CK2 inhibitors were included in incubations of cell extracts with ATP-sepharose. We subsequently performed immunoblot analysis to verify inhibitor interactions with CK2 as well as mass spectrometry following electrophoresis on 1D or 2D gels to identify other inhibitor targets. Using these strategies, we verified that the CK2 inhibitors do indeed bind to CK2 in complex mixtures. At the same time, we identified a number of other cellular targets for the CK2 inhibitors, potentially providing at least a partial explanation for the failure of inhibitor-resistant CK2 mutants to rescue cells from all of the effects of treatment with the CK2 inhibitors (12). This chapter describes the use of ATP-sepharose employing both the elution with inhibitors and inhibitor competition strategies together with immunoblotting or 2D gels and mass spectrometry to characterize cellular targets of the inhibitors (Fig. 1). While these approaches were illustrated using CK2 inhibitors, it is expected that they can be readily adapted for the evaluation of inhibitors for other protein kinases or ATP-utilizing enzymes.

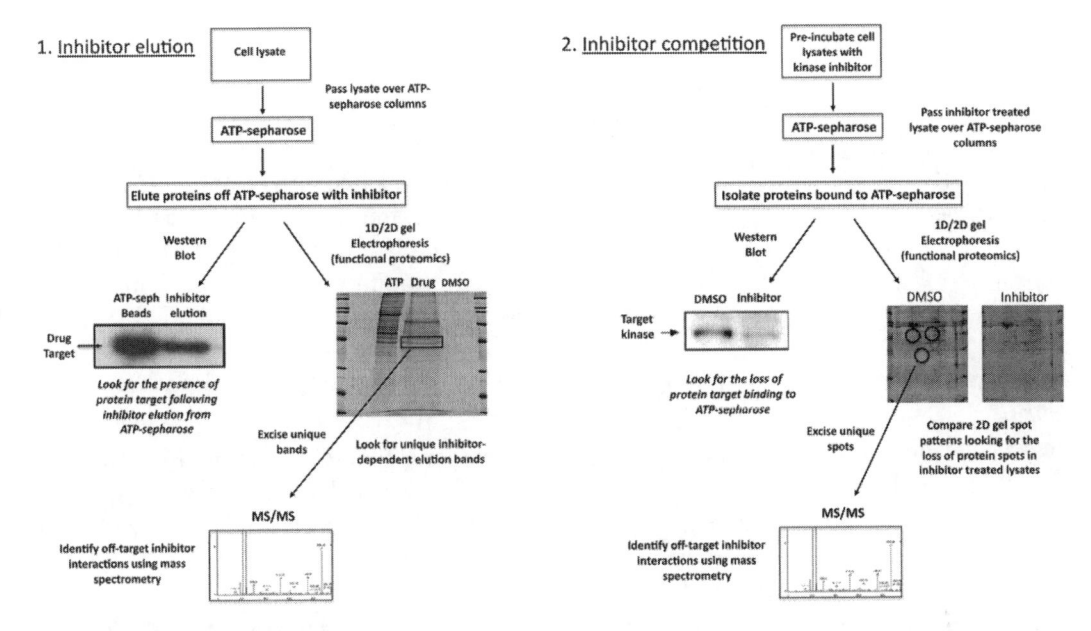

Fig. 1. Protein kinase affinity purification and unbiased identification of inhibitor targets using γ-linked ATP-sepharose. (1) In the inhibitor elution strategy, a specific protein kinase inhibitor is selected to elute bound protein kinases from ATP-sepharose. Briefly, cell lysates are incubated with ATP-sepharose beads and washed extensively to remove nonspecific bound proteins. Elution of inhibitor targets from ATP-sepharose is carried out via the incubation of ATP-sepharose beads with increasing inhibitor concentration. Inhibitor–target interactions are evaluated via Western blot analysis using specific antibodies, and/or by 2D gel electrophoresis in conjunction with mass spectrometry. Proteins eluted from ATP-sepharose with kinase inhibitor compared to the drug carrier elution profiles represent potential inhibitor targets. (2) The inhibitor competition assay provides a complementary strategy for the unbiased evaluation of protein kinase inhibitor targets that involves the preincubation of cell lysates with the kinase inhibitor of interest, followed by incubation with ATP-sepharose. Binding of the kinase inhibitor to target protein prevents interaction with ATP-sepharose, which can be determined via Western blot using specific antibodies and/or 2D gel electrophoresis in combination with mass spectrometry.

2. Materials

2.1. Cell Culture and Lysis

1. Cell lines: human cervical carcinoma (HeLa) S3 cells are grown in 1 l spinner flasks. Human osteosarcoma U2-OS cells are grown on 10- or 15-cm tissue culture plates. All cells are grown at 37°C in an atmosphere of 5% CO_2 (see Note 1).

2. Dulbecco's modified Eagle's medium (DMEM) containing 10% fetal bovine serum, penicillin (100 U/ml), and streptomycin (100 μg/ml) on 10- or 15-cm tissue culture plates.

3. N-terminal HA epitope-tagged CK2α′ or CK2α′$^{V67/I175/A}$ is available from the authors on request.

4. Cells lysis buffer: 20 mM Tris–HCl (pH 7.5), 150 mM NaCl, 1 mM EDTA, 1 mM EGTA, 1.0% Triton X-100, 0.5% NP-40, 2.5 mM sodium pyrophosphate, 1 mM Na_3VO_4, 1 μg/ml leupeptin, and 1 mM PMSF.

5. Cell lifters.
6. Sonicator (e.g., Fisher Scientific, Sonic Dismembrator Model 100).

2.2. Protein Kinase CK2 Inhibitors

1. TBB (4,5,6,7-Tetrabromo-1H-benzotriazole) (17), TBBz (4,5,6,7-tetrabromo-1H-benzimidazole) (18), and DMAT (2-dimethylamino-4,5,6,7-tetrabromo-1H-benzimidazole) (19) (see Note 2). All CK2 inhibitors are dissolved in DMSO at a concentration of 10 mM.

2.3. ATP-Sepharose Affinity Chromatography

1. γ-Phosphate ATP-sepharose: synthesized as described previously (20).
2. ATP-sepharose columns: Poly-Prep Chromatography columns packed with 100 μL ATP-sepharose. Micro Bio-Spin columns packed with 30 μl ATP-sepharose. ATP-sepharose affinity columns and ATP-sepharose beads are stored in Buffer A at 4°C.
3. Equilibration buffer (Buffer A): 50 mM NaCl, 50 mM HEPES, pH 7.4, 10 mM $MgCl_2$, 1% NP40, 1 μg/ml leupeptin, 1 μg/ml aprotinin, 1 mM dithiothreitol.
4. High-salt wash buffer (Buffer B): 1 M NaCl, 50 mM HEPES, pH 7.4, 10 mM $MgCl_2$, 1% NP40, 1 μg/ml leupeptin, 1 μg/ml aprotinin, 1 mM dithiothreitol.
5. Amicon Ultra 10K centrifuge tubes.

2.4. SDS-Polyacrylamide Gel Electrophoresis

1. For our studies, gel electrophoresis was performed using a Mini-Protein 3 system (BioRad). There are a number of other comparable systems for electrophoresis available.
2. Lower separating buffer (4×): 1.5 M Tris–HCl, pH 8.8, 0.4% SDS. Stored at room temperature.
3. Upper stacking buffer (4×): 0.5 M Tris–HCl, pH 6.8, 0.4% SDS. Stored at room temperature.
4. 30% Acrylamide/Bis solution (29:1 with 3.3%C) stored at 4°C.
5. *N,N,N,N'*-Tetramethyl-ethylenediamine (TEMED).
6. Ammonium persulfate: 10% (w/v) solution in water prepared fresh prior to gel preparation.
7. SDS-PAGE running buffer (10×): 0.25 M Tris base, 1.9 M glycine, 1% (v/v) SDS in water.
8. Protein molecular weight markers: any broad range prestained or unstained standards may be used.

2.5. Western Blotting

1. For our studies, electrophoretic transfer was performed using a Transblot Semi-Dry Cell (BioRad). There are a number of other comparable systems available.

2. Transfer Buffer: 25 mM Tris base, 192 mM glycine, 20% (v/v) methanol in water.
3. PVDF membranes, 3 MM chromatography paper.
4. Tris-buffered saline (TBS): 20 mM Tris–HCl, pH 7.5, 500 mM NaCl.
5. Tris-buffered saline with Tween (TBST): 0.05% (v/v) Tween 20 in TBS.
6. Phosphate-buffered saline (PBS): 137 mM NaCl, 2.7 mM g KCl, 10 mM Na_2HPO_4, 1.76 mM KH_2PO_4, pH 7.2.
7. Phosphate-buffered saline with Tween (PBST): 0.05% (v/v) in PBS.
8. Bovine serum albumin (BSA).
9. Blocking Buffer: 5% BSA in PBST, 5% BSA in TBST, or 5% nonfat milk in TBST. Selection of blocking solutions is determined by the primary antibodies to be used for immunoblotting. For our studies, blocking in preparation for the use of rabbit anti-CK2 antibodies is performed using 5% BSA/TBST while blocking for the use of anti-HA 3F10 antibodies is performed using 5% BSA/PBST. Blocking in preparation for the use of anti-HSP90 antibodies is performed using 5% nonfat milk/TBST.
10. Primary antibody dilution buffer: 5% BSA in TBST or 5% nonfat milk in TBST.
11. Primary antibodies: anti-CK2α polyclonal rabbit antiserum directed against the C-terminal synthetic peptide $\alpha^{376-391}$ and anti-CK2α' polyclonal rabbit antiserum directed against the C-terminal synthetic peptide $\alpha'^{333-350}$ were previously described (21). Anti-HSP90 antibodies are polyclonal rabbit antibodies and anti-HA 3F10 antibodies are rat monoclonal antibodies conjugated to biotin. Anti-CK2α and anti-CK2α' are used at dilutions of 1:5,000 in 5% BSA/TBST. Biotinylated anti-HA 3F10 antibodies are used at a dilution of 1:100 in 5% BSA/PBST. HSP90 antibodies are used at a dilution of 1:1,000 in 5% nonfat milk/TBST.
12. Secondary antibodies: horseradish peroxidase (HRP)-conjugated goat anti-rabbit and HRP-conjugated anti-biotin antibodies.
13. Western blot detection: ECL Plus Western Blotting Detection System, BioMax XAR X-ray film, flat bed scanner, image processing software.

2.6. 2D-Gel Electrophoresis

1. IPG buffer pH 4–7 and IPG buffer pH 3–10.
2. 2D lysis buffer: 7 M urea, 2 M thiourea, 4% (w/v) CHAPS, 1 mM benzamidine, 2.5 μg/ml leupeptin, 20 μg/ml pepstatin, 10 μg/ml aprotinin, 1 mM DTT, 200 mM Na_3VO_4,

100 µM microcystin, and 0.5% (v/v) IPG, pH 4–7, or IPG pH 3–10 buffer.

3. Rehydration buffer: 7 M urea, 2 M thiourea, 4% CHAPS, 50 mM DTT, 0.5% IPG buffer, and bromophenol blue (trace). This buffer can be stored in 50 ml aliquots at –20°C.

4. Immobiline dry strips: 7 cm pH 4–7 or 13 cm pH 3–10.

5. The first dimension (isoelectric focusing) equipment: the IPGphor II system with ceramic strip holders was used in this study but alternative systems are available.

6. Equilibration buffer for second dimension: 50 mM Tris–HCl, pH 8.8, 6 M urea, 30% glycerol, 20% w/v, bromophenol blue (trace). This buffer can be stored at –20°C. For first equilibration, add fresh DTT to 10 mg/ml. For second equilibration, add fresh iodoacetamide to 25 mg/ml.

7. Second dimension (SDS-PAGE) equipment: the two systems used in this study are a Bio-Rad Mini-Protein 3 Dodeca Cell (7-cm IPG strips), or a Hoefer SE 600 vertical gel apparatus (13-cm IPG strips). Alternative systems are available.

8. Agarose sealing solution: SDS-PAGE running buffer (1×) with 0.5% agarose and bromophenol blue (trace). This reagent can be made in 100 ml batch sizes in an Erlenmeyer flask by heating in a microwave followed by dispensing 10 ml aliquots. The reagent can be stored at room temperature in screw-capped tubes.

9. Fixing solution: 50% methanol (v/v), 7% (v/v) acetic acid in water.

10. 2D gel stain: Sypro Ruby.

11. Wash solution: 10% methanol (v/v), 7% (v/v) acetic acid in water.

2.7. 2D Gel Electrophoresis Quantification/ Analysis and Mass Spectrometry

1. Gel imaging: the ProXPRESS 2D Proteomic imaging system was used in this study. Alternatives software tools are available.

2. 2D spot recognition software: the Phoretix 2D evolution software was used in this study. Alternatives software tools are available.

3. Spot excision from gel: the Ettan Spot Picker was used in this study. Alternatives software tools are available.

4. Re-suspension buffer for excised gel spots: 50% methanol and 5% acetic acid in water.

5. Trypsin digestion: the MassPREP automated digestor was used in this study. Alternatives software tools are available.

6. Peptide re-suspension buffer following lyophilization: 30% acetonitrile, 0.1% trifluoro acetic acid (TFA).

7. MALDI Matrix: 10 mg/ml α-cyano-4-hydroxycinnamic acid (CHCA) in 50% acetonitrile, 25 mM ammonium citrate, 0.1% TFA.

8. Mass spectrometer: The 4700 Proteomics Analyzer MALDI TOF/TOF Mass Spectrometer was used in this study. Alternatives software tools are available.

9. Protein Identification: The GPS Explorer Workstation version 3.0 series was used in this study. Alternatives software tools are available.

3. Methods

Previous studies have demonstrated that ATP that is immobilized through its γ phosphate can be effectively utilized to bind protein kinases and other ATP-utilizing enzymes (10–12, 20). To investigate the cellular targets for ATP-competitive protein kinase inhibitors, we have employed two complementary strategies. The first of these strategies involves the use of the protein kinase inhibitors to elute bound proteins from ATP-sepharose. When antibodies are available to detect specific protein kinases, this approach can be employed to validate that the kinase inhibitor can effectively compete with ATP for binding to its intended target. Since immunoblots offer high sensitivity, these experiments can be performed with relatively small amounts of cellular protein (<10 mg). In the example described here, we have evaluated the ability of inhibitors for protein kinase CK2 to elute one of the CK2 isoforms (CK2α′) from ATP-sepharose. To further characterize interactions between CK2 and its inhibitors, parallel studies were performed using mutants of CK2α′ where two hydrophobic residues (V67 and I175) shown to be responsible for close contacts between its ATP binding site and the inhibitors were substituted with alanine (12, 22, 23). Notably, CK2 inhibitors are much less effective at the elution of this form of CK2 than with wild-type forms of the enzyme. These studies were performed using adherent human osteosarcoma U2-OS cells that were transfected with wild-type and mutant forms of CK2. The second approach that we have described involves the identification of proteins that fail to bind to ATP-sepharose when the protein kinase inhibitors are included during binding reactions. Although immunoblots could again be employed to evaluate specific protein kinases, one of the strengths of this approach is the prospect of performing an unbiased analysis of inhibitor targets. Accordingly, in the example that we have described using this approach, our objective was to identify proteins by mass spectrometry. Since larger amounts of cellular protein are required to enable isolation of sufficient quantities for identification by mass spectrometry, these studies were performed using human cervical carcinoma HeLa cells that can be readily grown in suspension to obtain large quantities of cellular protein.

3.1. Inhibitor Validation: Inhibitor Elution of Targets from ATP-Sepharose

1. Grow adherent cells in 15-cm tissue culture dishes. For the example illustrated, human osteosarcoma U2-OS cells were used that transiently express CK2α′ or CK2α′$^{V67/I175/A}$ with N-terminal HA epitope tags (designated HA-CK2α′ and HA-CK2α′R) to enable detection (24). Grow five plates for each sample (see Note 3).

2. Wash cells twice with PBS (10 ml) and then scrape from the 15 cm plates using 0.5 ml lysis buffer and a cell lifter.

3. Sonicate lysates for 2 × 10 s on ice.

4. Clear samples by centrifugation at 4°C for 15 min at 80,000 × g and determine protein concentration by, e.g., the BCA assay (25).

5. Before proceeding, remove a small aliquot of cell lysate and store at −80°C. This sample can later be used for western blot analysis of the levels of the protein of interest.

6. Pack ATP-sepharose into Poly-Prep Chromatography columns (100 μL) or into micro Bio-Spin columns (30 μL) and equilibrate with Buffer A (five column volumes).

7. Adjust lysates (10^8 cell equivalents) in Buffer A to 1 M NaCl and pass over a 100 μL ATP-sepharose packed into a Poly-Prep Chromatography column. For 30 μL of ATP-sepharose packed into micro Bio-Spin columns, use 10 mg of cell extract (see Note 4).

8. Collect the flow-through of the lysates passed over the ATP-sepharose.

9. Wash ATP-sepharose beads extensively with Buffer A (100 column volumes), followed by washing with Buffer B (5 column volumes) and finally re-equilibrate beads with Buffer A.

10. Elute inhibitor-interacting proteins is performed by step-wise addition of 0.5 ml of increasing concentration of protein kinase inhibitor in Buffer A (e.g., 1 μM, 40 μM, 400 μM, and 1 mM). Buffer A may contain up to 10% DMSO to facilitate solubility of the kinase inhibitor. However, increasing concentrations of DMSO result in increased nonspecific elutions. The elution step is carried out 3× to ensure complete dissociation of protein bound to ATP. Perform one control experiment without inhibitor but with DMSO at the same concentration as used for the inhibitor elutions (see Note 5).

11. Collect inhibitor elutions in 1.5-ml Eppendorf centrifuge tubes and keep on ice for immediate analysis or put at −80°C for long-term storage.

12. Spin concentrate elution fractions (0.5 ml each) to approximately 50–100 μL volume using Amicon Ultra 10K centrifuge tubes.

13. Determine protein concentration by, e.g., the Bradford assay (26). It is convenient to use a 96-well plate for this purpose and UV absorbance is monitored at A_{595nm}.

Inhibitor: DMAT
Blot: anti-HA

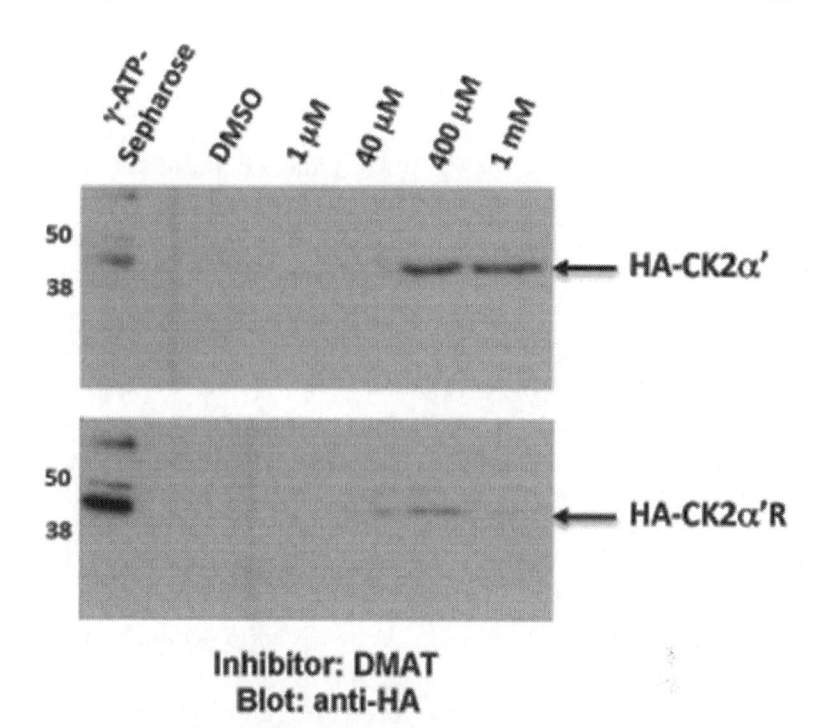

Fig. 2. Validation of kinase inhibitor interactions with CK2α' using γ-linked ATP-sepharose. (a) Elution of CK2α' from ATP-sepharose using CK2 inhibitor DMAT and demonstration of reduced interaction of DMAT with an inhibitor-resistant CK2α' mutant. U2-OS cells expressing HA-CK2α' or HA-CK2α'R (V67A/I175A) were harvested in Buffer A adjusted to 1 M NaCl and incubated with ATP-sepharose conjugated beads. Following an extensive bead wash, HA-CK2α' or HA-CK2α'R were eluted from ATP-sepharose with increasing concentrations of CK2 kinase inhibitor DMAT (1 μM, 40 μM, 400 μM, and 1 mM). Elution with the drug carrier (DMSO) was used as a control. Elution of HA-CK2α' and/or CK2α'R from ATP-sepharose was detected via Western blot analysis using anti-HA 3F10 antibodies. (b) Preincubation of cell lysates with CK2 inhibitors greatly reduced binding of endogenous CK2α' to ATP-sepharose in inhibitor competition assays. HeLa S3 cell lysates were preincubated with 100 μM of CK2 inhibitors (TBBz, TBB, or DMAT) or the control drug carrier DMSO and passed over ATP-sepharose columns. Beads were washed extensively, isolated, and bound proteins captured via incubation with 2D lysis buffer. Detection of bound CK2α' to ATP-sepharose was carried out via Western blot analysis using anti-CK2α' antibodies. Binding of HSP90 to ATP-sepharose was used as a loading control, detected with anti-HSP90 antibodies.

14. For subsequent analysis by Western blotting (27), re-suspend samples in 2× laemmli buffer (28) and boil for 4 min in preparation for SDS-PAGE (Fig. 2a). Use prestained protein markers as standards (see Note 6).

3.2. Identification of Protein Kinase Inhibitor Targets: Inhibitor Competition

1. Grow suspension cells in spinner flasks. To follow the example illustrated here, maintain human cervical carcinoma HeLa cells at densities between 1×10^5 and 5×10^5 cells/ml. Approximately 10^8 cell equivalents are required for each sample. To enable later statistical analysis of 2D gels, perform four replicates for each sample.

2. Pellet cells by centrifugation at $5,000 \times g$ at 4°C. Wash cell pellets 2× with PBS.

3. After removal of all liquid, weigh cell pellets and subsequently lyse in 1.5 volumes of Buffer A (dilute by cell volume "weight") and store on ice for 10 min.

4. Sonicate lysates for 2×10 s on ice and then subject lysates to centrifugation at $80,000 \times g$ for 30 min at 4°C.

5. Before proceeding further, remove a small aliquot of the cell lysates for later analysis of the levels of the protein of interest by western blotting. Store lysates at –80°C.

6. For inhibitor competition, incubate equal volumes of lysates with DMSO (inhibitor carrier control) and either of 100 μM TBB, TBBz, or DMAT for 2 h with gentle rocking at 4°C to allow inhibitor–protein interactions to occur (see Note 7).

7. During the incubation of inhibitors with cell lysates, equilibrate ATP-sepharose beads (100 μL per 10^8 cell equivalents) in Buffer A in 1.5 ml Eppendorf plastic centrifuge tubes.

8. Using a 200 μL pipette tip with the end cut off (using a razor blade or scalpel), transfer 100 μL of equilibrated ATP-sepharose beads to each tube containing the inhibitor-treated cell lysates.

9. Incubate at 4°C for 15 min with gentle rocking to enable binding. Then collect the ATP-sepharose beads by centrifugation and transfer beads into a Poly-Prep Chromatography column using a cut 200 μL pipette tip.

10. Wash ATP-sepharose columns extensively with 100 column volumes of Buffer A, and then with Buffer B (5 column volumes) before final re-equilibration with Buffer A.

11. Transfer ATP-sepharose beads in Buffer A to a 1.5-ml microcentrifuge tube using a cut 200 μL tip and incubate in 150 μL of 2D lysis buffer for 15 min with gentle rocking at 4°C to remove bound proteins from the ATP-sepharose beads (see Note 8).

12. Determine protein concentration by, e.g., the Bradford assay (26). It is convenient to use 96-well plates for this purpose and UV absorbance is monitored at A_{595nm}. The samples are now ready for Western blot analysis and/or isoelectric focusing (Fig. 2b).

3.3. Western Blot

1. Separate proteins by SDS-PAGE followed by transfer to PVDF membranes.

2. Following transfer, rinse membranes briefly with TBS and then block for 60 min.

3. After blocking, incubate membranes with the appropriate primary antibodies overnight at 4°C.

4. Following overnight incubation, remove the primary antibody solution i. Wash membranes with PBST or TBST and then incubate with the appropriate secondary antibodies including: HRP-GAR diluted 1:25,000 for anti-CK2α and anti-CK2α′ antibodies and 1:5,000 for anti-HSP90 antibodies or HRP-conjugated anti-Biotin antibodies diluted 1:10,000 for anti-HA 3F10 antibodies.

5. Following secondary antibody incubation, wash membranes with PBST or TBST and visualize by enhanced chemiluminescence (ECL) using an X-ray film.

6. Convert X-ray film images to digital images using a flatbed scanner.

3.4. 2D Gel Electrophoresis: Isoelectric Focusing

1. Mix protein samples (150 μg for 7 cm IPG strips and 250 μg for 13 cm IPG strips) with rehydration buffer. Apply the samples to the immobiline dry strips (7 cm pH 4–7 or 13 cm pH 3–10) in ceramic strip holders (29, 30).

2. Distribute the sample (0.125 ml for 7 cm strips, 0.25 ml for 13 cm strips) into the ceramic holder and use tweezers to carefully place the IPG strip, gel side down, over the sample. It is important to avoid bubbles when placing the strip over the sample.

3. Overlay the IPG strip with mineral oil (~0.5 ml for 7 cm strips, ~1 ml for 13 cm strips) to prevent evaporation and minimize crystallization of the urea.

4. Run the isoelectric focusing step using the IPGphor II system and using the following programs (all steps at 20°C). For the 7 cm IPG strips: Step 1, 20 V for 12 h; Step 2, 100 V for 100 V-h; Step 3, 500 V for 500 V-h; Step 4, 1,000 V for 1,000 V-h; Step 5, 2,000 V for 2,000 V-h; Step 6, 4,000 V for 4,000 V-h; and Step 7, 8,000 V for 16,000 V-h. For the 13-cm IPG strips, the program is as follows: Step 1, 20 V for 12 h; Step 2, 100 V for 2 h; Step 3, 500 V for 500 V-h; Step 4, 1,000 V for 1,000 V-h; Step 5, 2,000 V for 4,000 V-h; Step 6, 4,000 V for 8,000 V-h; Step 7, 6,000 V for 12,000 V-h; and Step 8, 8,000 V for 64,000 V-h.

5. Following completion of isoelectric focusing, remove the IPG strips from the ceramic strip holders with forceps. Incubate the strips with equilibration buffer containing freshly added DTT (10 mg/ml) with gentle rocking for 15 min at room temperature to reduce the proteins.

6. Incubate IPG strips with equilibration buffer containing freshly added iodoacetamide (25 mg/ml) with gentle rocking for 15 min at room temperature to alkylate cystein side chains.

7. Apply the equilibrated IPG strips to SDS-PAGE gel electrophoresis.

3.5. 2D Gel Electrophoresis: SDS-PAGE

1. These instructions are for the use of a Bio-Rad Mini-Protean 3 Dodeca Cell gel system (for 7-cm IPG strips) or a Hoefer SE 600 vertical gel apparatus (for 13-cm IPG strips) but can be readily adapted to other electrophoresis systems.
2. Wash glass plates extensively with detergent, followed by 95% ethanol, followed by distilled water. Then dry glass plates in an oven.
3. Prepare a 1.5 mm, 10% gel by mixing 12.2 ml of distilled water, 7.5 ml of 1.5 M Tris–HCl, pH 8.8, 10.0 ml of acrylamide/bis solution, 0.15 ml 20% (w/v) SDS, 0.15 ml 10% (w/v) ammonium persulfate (APS), and 0.02 ml of TEMED. Pour the gel leaving sufficient room for the 2D gel IPG strip (approximately 1.5 cm) and overlay with distilled water.
4. Utilizing tweezers, carefully place the equilibrated IPG strip on the top of the solidified gel ensuring that the plastic backing adheres to one of the glass plates.
5. If desired, a protein size marker can be applied to pre-cut filter paper (3 mm × 3 mm). Insert the filter paper directly adjacent to the IPG strip.
6. Apply 0.5% agarose sealing solution uniformly to the top of gel using a Pasteur pipette.
7. Prepare SDS-PAGE running buffer by diluting 100 ml of the 10× stock into 900 ml of distilled water and mix thoroughly.
8. Once the agarose sealing solution has completely solidified, fill upper and lower chambers of electrophoresis unit with the appropriate buffers.
9. Complete the assembly of electrophoresis unit and connect to power supply. Gels are run until the dye fronts reach the bottom of the gel (~1 h at 180 V for Bio-Rad Mini-Protean 3 Dodeca Cell gel system with 7 cm IPG strips or 4 h at 200 V for Hoefer SE 600 vertical gel system with 13 cm IPG strips).

3.6. 2D-Gel Electrophoresis Staining and Imaging

1. Following separation of proteins on SDS-PAGE gel electrophoresis, transfer gels to a large plastic dish and fix for 30 min at room temperature (twice) using 100 ml of fixing solution.
2. Remove fixing solution and add 150 ml of fresh SYPRO Ruby stain to each gel (13 cm gels). Stain overnight at room temperature in the dark. Aluminum foil should be wrapped around the plastic container to ensure light protection. Staining more than 1 gel at time with the same dye solution or reusing the dye should be avoided as it reduces staining efficiency. This is particularly relevant for subsequent quantitative image analysis.
3. Following staining, wash the gels with 100 ml of wash solution for 30 min.

4. Image-stained gels using, e.g., the ProXPRESS 2D Proteomic imaging system. Gels are imaged with top illumination using 460/80 nm excitation and 650/150 nm emission at a resolution of 100 μm.

3.7. 2D Gel Electrophoresis: Quantification and Analysis

Several image analysis packages are available. In this study, the Phoretix 2D evolution software is used as an example.

1. Analyse gels for differences in protein spots between 2D gels utilizing the Phoretix 2D evolution software.
2. Import at least four gel images derived from different gels run for each treatment into the Phoretix software and align spots using the SameSpot tool.
3. Import the aligned images into the Progenesis PG220 software for analysis of spot differences and spot intensity.
4. Apply spot filtering to all aligned gels to normalize for pixel intensity and area with a normalized volume value of >0.005. Statistical analysis of spot changes is performed using ANOVA and the mean values are compared using a t-test.
5. For subsequent spot excision, generate a pick list and export to the Spot Picker.

3.8. Sample Preparation for Mass Spectrometry

1. Incubate gels in 50% (v/v) methanol, 5% (v/v) acetic acid.
2. Excise spots that are present in the DMSO control gels but absent in gels derived from samples where kinase inhibitors are incubated during the binding of cell extracts to ATP-sepharose. Spots can be excised manually using a sterile 1 ml pipette tip or using an automated Spot Picker (see Note 9).
3. Digest proteins in excised gel spots using trypsin inside the MassPREP automated digestor or a similar device. Resulting peptides are collected in conical PCR tubes.
4. Freeze peptides in liquid nitrogen for 30 s and lyophilize overnight. Following lyophilization, re-suspend peptides in 30% acetonitrile, 0.1% TFA.

3.9. Mass Spectrometry: Peptide Mass Fingerprinting

1. Mix equal volumes of peptide (0.7 μL) and MALDI matrix and spot on a MALDI plate.
2. After samples are spotted on plates, perform MALDI MS and/or MS/MS analysis on the MALDI mass spectrometer (see Note 10).
3. Calibrate the mass spectrometer using a standard recommended by the vendor.
4. Generate peptide mass fingerprints over the m/z range of 800–4,000 Da. The resulting spectra are evaluated using the GPS Explorer Workstation (version 3.0 series). Peaks are

picked using a minimal S/N threshold of 20. Exclude signals corresponding to trypsin autolysis products (842.5099, 870.509, and 2,211.1096).

5. Peptides are searched against the human Swiss-Prot database using the search engine MASCOT with oxidation set as a variable modification (M) and a peptide mass tolerance of 50 ppm. Accept protein identification if a minimum of five peptides match with a maximum mass error of 15 ppm and with no more than one missed cleavage site.

4. Notes

1. Our studies were performed using both suspension cells (HeLa S3) and adherent cells (U2-OS). Procedures can be readily adapted to other cell types (see Subheading 2.1).

2. The illustrated examples were performed with inhibitors of protein kinase CK2 that are commercially available. The procedures can be readily adapted to other protein kinase inhibitors (see Subheading 2.2).

3. The number of cells to be utilized for the validation of inhibitor interactions is dependent on the abundance of the protein kinase and the sensitivity of detection. In our example, we utilized epitope-tagged CK2 to enable detection of mutant forms of CK2 (see Subheading 3.1).

4. The sample should be adjusted to 1 M NaCl prior to ATP-sepharose incubation to minimize nonspecific interaction of protein with ATP-sepharose. Increasing salt concentration reduces protein–protein interactions minimizing identification of proteins bound to ATP binding proteins (see Subheading 3.1).

5. The concentrations of inhibitors employed for elution of proteins from ATP-sepharose may be dramatically higher than the Ki for the respective inhibitors. This is a consequence of the high local concentrations of immobilized ATP (see Subheading 3.1).

6. For the validation of interactions between CK2 and inhibitors, immunoblot analysis was employed to detect CK2. Immunoblot analysis was possible because of the availability of antibodies for the detection of CK2. In the absence of antibodies, this protocol can be adapted to enable the identification of proteins that are eluted from ATP-sepharose using other analytical strategies such as those described in Subheading 3.2 (see Subheading 3.1).

7. The concentrations of inhibitors employed to compete for protein binding to ATP-sepharose may be dramatically higher than the Ki for the respective inhibitors. This is a consequence

of the high local concentrations of immobilized ATP (see Subheading 3.2).

8. Although 2D gels were employed for our studies to examine the profiles of proteins that bind to ATP-sepharose in the presence or absence of CK2 inhibitors, it is envisaged that this strategy could be adapted to other methods for differential analysis of protein profiles (see Subheading 3.2).

9. The Ettan Spot Picker was employed for automated spot-picking from fluorescently labeled gels. Manual picking of spots can also be performed when gels are stained with visible dyes such as colloidal coomassie blue or silver stain (see Subheading 3.8).

10. Although we used the 4700 Proteomics Analyzer for protein identification, these methods can be readily adapted to the use of other mass spectrometers (see Subheading 3.9).

Acknowledgments

We are grateful to Laszlo Gyenis, John Lenehan, Maria Bretner, and Lee Graves for assistance and helpful discussions. We would also like to thank Cunjie Zhang and Christopher Ward in the Functional Proteomic Facility and Kristina Jurcic and Ken Yeung within the MALDI Mass Spectrometry Facility in the Schulich School of Medicine & Dentistry at the University of Western Ontario. Our work on the characterization of CK2 inhibitors and the development of functional proteomics strategies has been funded by the Canadian Cancer Society Research Institute and the Canadian Institutes of Health Research. James Duncan was supported by a Canada Graduate Scholarship from the Canadian Institutes of Health Research (CIHR) and by the CIHR-University of Western Ontario Strategic Training Initiative in Cancer Research and Technology Transfer.

References

1. Noble M.E., Endicott J.A., and Johnson L.N. (2004) Protein kinase inhibitors: insights into drug design from structure. *Science* **303**, 1800–1805.
2. Cohen P. (2002) Protein kinases--the major drug targets of the twenty-first century? *Nat. Rev. Drug Discov.* **1**, 309–315.
3. Sawyers C.L. (2003) Opportunities and challenges in the development of kinase inhibitor therapy for cancer. *Genes Dev.* **17**, 2998–3010.
4. Lydon N.B., and Druker B.J. (2004) Lessons learned from the development of imatinib. *Leuk. Res.* **28**, S29–38.
5. Manning G., Whyte D.B., Martinez R., Hunter T., and Sudarsanam S. (2002) The protein kinase complement of the human genome. *Science* **298**, 1912–1934.
6. Bain J., Plater L., Elliott M., Shpiro N., Hastie C.J., McLauchlan H., Klevernic I., Arthur J.S., Alessi D.R., and Cohen P. (2007) The selectivity of protein kinase inhibitors: a further update. *Biochem. J.* **408**, 297–315.
7. Bain J., McLauchlan H., Elliott M., and Cohen P. (2003) The specificities of protein kinase inhibitors: an update. *Biochem. J.* **371**, 199–204.

8. Davies S.P., Reddy H., Caivano M., and Cohen P. (2000) Specificity and mechanism of action of some commonly used protein kinase inhibitors. *Biochem. J.* **351**, 95–105.
9. Pagano M.A., Bain J., Kazimierczuk Z., Sarno S., Ruzzene M., Di Maira G., Elliott M., Orzeszko A., Cozza G., Meggio F., and Pinna L.A. (2008) The selectivity of inhibitors of protein kinase CK2: an update. *Biochem. J.* **415**, 353–365.
10. Graves P.R., Kwiek J.J., Fadden P., Ray R., Hardeman K., Coley A.M., Foley M., and Haystead T.A. (2002) Discovery of novel targets of quinoline drugs in the human purine binding proteome. *Mol. Pharmacol.* **62**, 1364–1372.
11. Haystead T.A. (2006) The purinome, a complex mix of drug and toxicity targets. *Curr. Top. Med. Chem.* **6**, 1117–1127.
12. Duncan J.S., Gyenis L., Lenehan J., Bretner M., Graves L.M., Haystead T.A., and Litchfield D.W. (2008) An unbiased evaluation of CK2 inhibitors by chemoproteomics: characterization of inhibitor effects on CK2 and identification of novel inhibitor targets. *Mol. Cell Proteomics* **7**, 1077–1088.
13. Landesman-Bollag E., Romieu-Mourez R., Song D.H., Sonenshein G.E., Cardiff R.D., and Seldin D.C. (2001) Protein kinase CK2 in mammary gland tumorigenesis. *Oncogene* **20**, 3247–3257.
14. Litchfield D.W. (2003) Protein kinase CK2: structure, regulation and role in cellular decisions of life and death. *Biochem. J.* **369**, 1–15.
15. Duncan J.S., and Litchfield D.W. (2008) Too much of a good thing: the role of protein kinase CK2 in tumorigenesis and prospects for therapeutic inhibition of CK2. *Biochim. Biophys. Acta* **1784**, 33–47.
16. Sarno S., and Pinna L.A. (2008) Protein kinase CK2 as a druggable target. *Mol. Biosyst.* **4**, 889–894.
17. Sarno S., Reddy H., Meggio F., Ruzzene M., Davies S.P., Donella-Deana A., Shugar D., and Pinna L.A. (2001) Selectivity of 4,5,6,7-tetrabromobenzotriazole, an ATP site-directed inhibitor of protein kinase CK2 ('casein kinase-2'). *FEBS Lett.* **496**, 44–48.
18. Zien P., Duncan J.S., Skierski J., Bretner M., Litchfield D.W., and Shugar D. (2005) Tetrabromobenzotriazole (TBBt) and tetrabromobenzimidazole (TBBz) as selective inhibitors of protein kinase CK2: evaluation of their effects on cells and different molecular forms of human CK2. *Biochim. Biophys. Acta* **1754**, 271–280.
19. Pagano M.A., Meggio F., Ruzzene M., Andrzejewska M., Kazimierczuk Z., Pinna L.A. (2004) 2-Dimethylamino-4,5,6,7-tetrabromo-1-H-benzimidazole: a novel powerful and selective inhibitor of protein kinase CK2. *Biochem. Biophys. Res. Commun.* **321**, 1040–1044.
20. Haystead C.M., Gregory P., Sturgill T.W., and Haystead T.A. (1993) Gamma-phosphate-linked ATP-sepharose for the affinity purification of protein kinases. Rapid purification to homogeneity of skeletal muscle mitogen-activated protein kinase kinase. *Eur. J. Biochem.* **214**, 459–467.
21. Gietz R.D., Graham K.C., and Litchfield D.W. (1995) Interactions between the subunits of casein kinase II. *J. Biol. Chem.* **270**, 13017–13021.
22. Battistutta R., De Moliner E., Sarno S., Zanotti G., and Pinna L.A. (2001) Structural features underlying selective inhibition of protein kinase CK2 by ATP site-directed tetrabromo-2-benzotriazole. *Protein Sci.* **10**, 2200–2206.
23. Sarno S., de Moliner E., Ruzzene M., Pagano M.A, Battistutta R., Bain J., Fabbro D., Schoepfer J., Elliott M., Furet P., Meggio F., Zanotti G., Pinna L.A. (2003) Biochemical and three-dimensional-structural study of the specific inhibition of protein kinase CK2 by [5-oxo-5,6-dihydroindolo-(1,2-a)quinazolin-7-yl] acetic acid (IQA). *Biochem. J.* **374**, 639–646.
24. Graham K.C., and Litchfield D.W. (2000) The regulatory beta subunit of protein kinase CK2 mediates formation of tetrameric CK2 complexes. *J. Biol. Chem.* **275**, 5003–5010.
25. Smith P.K., Krohn R.I., Hermanson G.T., Mallia A.K., Gartner F.H., Provenzano M.D., Fujimoto E.K., Goeke N.M., Olson B.J., and Klenk D.C. (1985) Measurement of protein using bicinchoninic acid. *Anal. Biochem.* **150**, 76–85.
26. Bradford M.M. (1976) A rapid and sensitive method for the quantitation of microgram quantities of protein utilizing the principle of protein-dye binding. *Anal. Biochem.* **72**, 248–254.
27. Towbin H., Staehelin T., and Gordon J. (1979) Electrophoretic transfer of proteins from polyacrylamide gels to nitrocellulose sheets: procedure and some applications. *Proc. Natl. Acad. Sci. USA.* **76**, 4350–4354.
28. Laemmli UK. (1970) Cleavage of structural proteins during the assembly of the head of bacteriophage T4. *Nature* **227**, 680–685.
29. Görg A., Obermaier C., Boguth G., Harder A., Scheibe B., Wildgruber R., and Weiss W. (2000) The current state of two-dimensional electrophoresis with immobilized pH gradients. *Electrophoresis* **21**, 1037–1053.
30. Görg A., Drews O., Lück C., Weiland F., and Weiss W. (2009) 2-DE with IPGs. *Electrophoresis* **30**, S122–132.

Chapter 9

Proteome-Wide Identification of Staurosporine-Binding Kinases Using Capture Compound Mass Spectrometry

Jenny J. Fischer, Olivia Y. Graebner (neé Baessler), and Mathias Dreger

Abstract

The enormous diversity of kinases and their pivotal role in cell signaling have set kinases in the focus of biomedical research. Profiling the kinome of tissues of different origin is essential for biomarker discovery. In drug research, it is necessary to comprehend the specificity profile of a given kinase inhibitor. Capture Compound Mass Spectrometry (CCMS) (Koster et al., Assay Drug. Dev. Technol. 5:381–390, 2007) addresses the need for a tool to physically isolate and reliably profile the binders of kinase inhibitors directly in biological samples. Capture Compounds™ are trifunctional probes: a selectivity function consisting of the kinase inhibitor interacts reversibly with the native target proteins in equilibrium, a photoactivatable reactivity function forms an irreversible covalent bond to the target protein upon irradiation, and a sorting function allows the captured protein(s) to be isolated and identified by mass spectrometric analysis in an affinity-driven manner. Capture Compounds™ with any kinase inhibitor as selectivity function can be synthesized. We here used staurosporine as the selectivity function because it targets and, therefore, allows profiling a broad range of kinases (Romano and Giordano, Cell Cycle 7:3364–3668, 2008). Furthermore, we give an example of the application of the staurosporine Capture Compound to isolate kinases from human liver-derived HepG2 cells.

Key words: Capture Compound Mass Spectrometry, Kinases, Kinase Profiling, Hepatocytes, HepG2, Tissue Profiling, Kinase inhibitors, Kinase profiling, Staurosporine

1. Introduction

The investigation of kinases is of outstanding interest, as they perform major roles in cell development (1), signaling, and metabolism (2). Mutations and dysregulation of kinases play causal roles in many human diseases. This affords the possibility of biomarker discovery and of developing agonists and antagonists of these enzymes for use in disease therapy (3). Kinases have become accessible to large scale profiling through chemical proteomics approaches, such as the use of kinase inhibitor beads, by which unprecedented numbers of kinases have been identified (4). At the same time, the selectivity profiling of different kinase inhibitors against large panels of kinases have provided a broad data basis for assessing the utility of certain inhibitors to address subsets of the kinome. As an example, staurosporine (Fig. 1) is a prototypical ATP-competitive kinase inhibitor that can target at least 253 kinases (5). On the contrary, with respect to protein families other than kinases, the use of multifunctional small-molecule probes has been demonstrated to provide for an outstanding analytical tool to profile, for the first time, even very low abundant proteins in biological samples (6). This approach circumvents typical drawbacks of small-molecule bead affinity-driven techniques, in which the solid support limits the accessibility of the immobilized ligand for protein interactions. Capture Compounds™ (Fig. 1a) are versatile multifunctional small-molecule probes to identify functionally selected protein families that at first interact in their native form reversibly with a common small molecule such as a nucleotide (7, 8), a methyltransferase inhibitor (9), or a kinase inhibitor (10) and are then isolated after freezing the equilibrium by photo-cross-linking to the Capture Compound. We here present the application of Capture Compound Mass Spectrometry (CCMS) (11) to address kinases from complex biological samples. We used staurosporine as selectivity function for the profiling of the mammalian kinome in the human hepatocyte cell line HepG2 (10).

The general design of Capture Compounds™ consists of three main functionalities (a) the small molecule or drug molecule to be investigated, (b) an adjacent photo-reactive functionality for photo-cross-linking and (c) a sorting function, e.g., biotin, for the isolation of captured proteins. The capture process is simple and easy to perform (Fig. 2). After incubation of the Capture Compound with

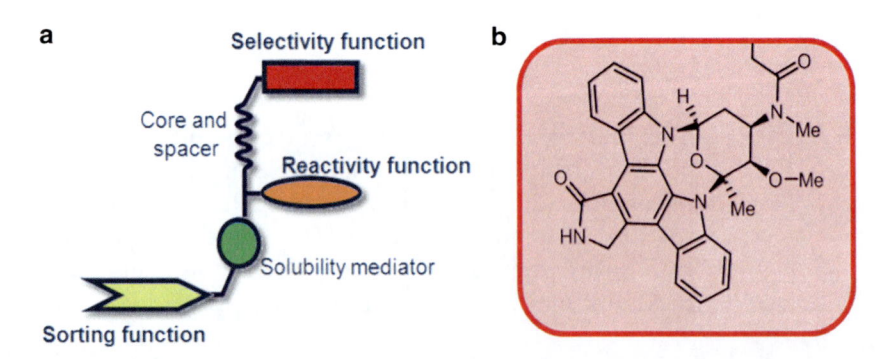

Fig. 1. Capture Compounds™ are trifunctional probes. Schematic depiction of Capture Compounds™ (a) and molecular structure of staurosporine with part of the linker leading to the scaffold (b). Capture Compounds™ are trifunctional probes: based on affinity, a selectivity function (staurosporine, *red*) interacts with the proteins in a biological sample at equilibrium, a reactivity function (*orange*) irreversibly forms a covalent bond, and a sorting function (*yellow*) allows the captured protein(s) to be isolated for mass spectrometric analysis.

Step 1. Capture Compound is added to the biological sample

Step 2. The Capture Compound binds the target protein(s) in an affinitiy driven manner.

Step 3. Induced by irradiation a covalent bond between the Capture Compound and the target protein(s) is formed.

Step 4. Magnetic beads bind the biotin of the Capture Compound, the Capture Compound is covalently attached to the protein.

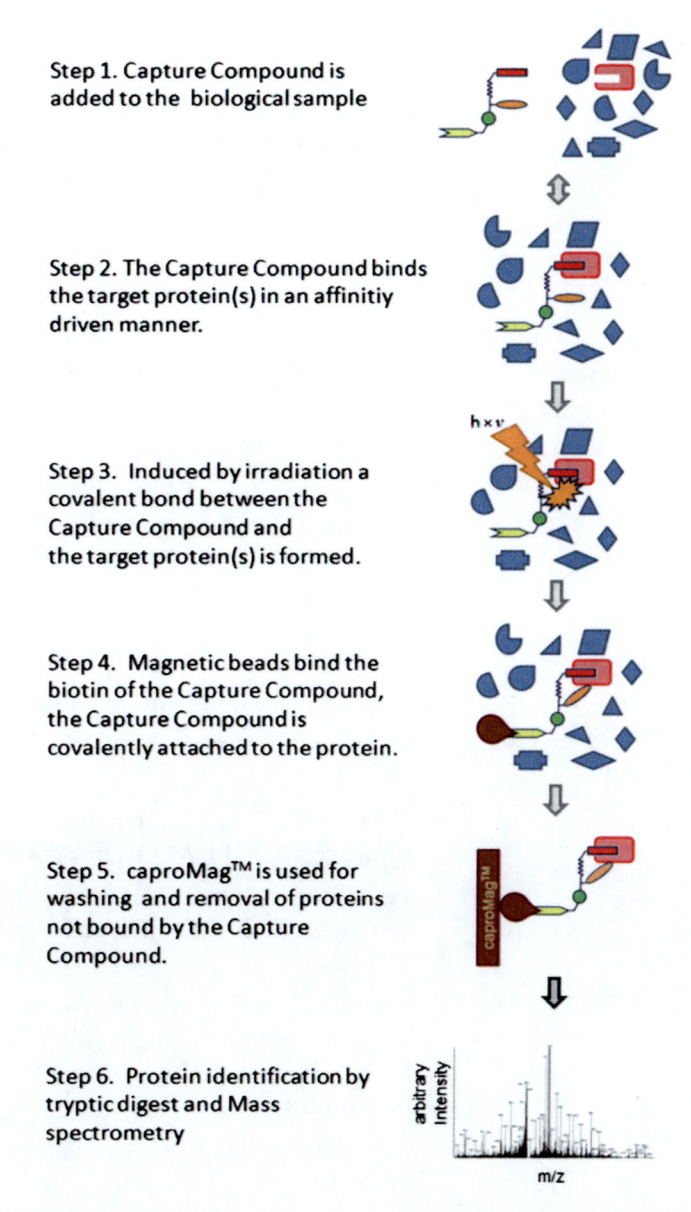

Step 5. caproMag™ is used for washing and removal of proteins not bound by the Capture Compound.

Step 6. Protein identification by tryptic digest and Mass spectrometry

Fig. 2. Schematic depiction of the Capture Compound Mass Spectrometry (CCMS) process.

the cell lysate and equilibrium binding of the target proteins by the selectivity group, photolysis leads to the generation of a photo-activated species such as a nitrene within the reactivity function. This leads to a covalent cross-link between the Capture Compound and the target proteins. Employing the sorting function biotin and strepta-vidin-coated magnetic beads, the Capture Compound–protein conjugates can be isolated, and unbound proteins are removed by stringent washing. The technology exclusively probes those proteins which interact with the small molecule that is part of the Capture Compound. The complexity of a biological sample is reduced to the interaction partners of the small molecule, resulting in an enrichment of the functionally selected proteins and, therefore, also allows identification of low abundant proteins. The captured proteins are trypsinized and subsequently identified by high resolution and high accuracy mass spectrometry.

2. Materials

2.1. Preparation of HepG2 Cell Lysate

1. HepG2 cell line: available from e.g., the German collection of microorganisms and cell lines (DSMZ).
2. Phosphate-buffered saline (PBS): ice-cold, sterile.
3. Cell lysis buffer: 6.7 mM MES, 6.7 mM sodium acetate, 6.7 mM HEPES, 1 mM EDTA, 10 mM ß-mercaptoethanol, 200 mM NaCl, pH 7.5, 1 tablet Complete Protease Inhibitor EDTA free.

2.2. Capture Experiment and Competition Control

1. Staurosporine Capture Compound: 50 µM in water.
2. Staurosporine competitor: 1 mM in water.
3. Streptavidin-coated magnetic beads: 1 µm diameter (see Note 1).
4. Capture Buffer (5×, CB): 100 mM HEPES, 250 mM potassium acetate, 50 mM magnesium acetate, 50% glycerol.
5. Wash Buffer (5×, WB): 250 mM Tris–HCl, pH 7.5, 5 mM EDTA, 5 M NaCl, 42.5 µM octyl-ß-d-glucopyranoside (see Note 2).
6. caproBox™ with filter: The caproBox™ is a device for irradiating samples with UV light (filter 330–380 nm) and simultaneously cooling, thereby avoiding denaturation of proteins during photo-cross-linking.
7. A magnet suitable for the handling of magnetic beads (see Note 3).
8. HepG2 cell lysate (see above and Notes 4 and 5).
9. 200 µL PCR tubes, ideally in 12-well stripe format.
10. Acetonitrile: LC-MS-grade.
11. Water: LC-MS-grade; the same quality is used in Subheadings 2.3 and 2.4.

2.3. Tryptic Digest and Preparation of Peptides for LC-MS/MS

1. Digestion buffer: 50 mM ammonium bicarbonate, 5 mM calcium chloride in LC-MS grade water. Store in aliquots at −20°C; thaw only once.
2. Trypsin: 1 µg/µl in 1 mM HCl, Enzyme must be of sequencing grade.
3. Formic acid: LC-MS grade.

2.4. Measurement of Peptides by LC-ESI-MS/MS

1. HPLC system: any state-of-the-art HPLC system capable of delivering flow rates below 1 μm/min.
2. Mass Spectrometer: any state-of-the-art tandem mass spectrometer capable of peptide fragmentation (see Note 6).
3. LC-MS/MS buffer A: LC-MS grade water with 0.1% (v/v) formic acid (FA).
4. LC-MS/MS buffer B: LC-MS grade acetonitrile (ACN) with 0.1% (v/v) FA.

2.5. Protein Identification by Sequence Database Searching

1. Protein sequence database: Download the latest UniProtKB/Swiss-Prot database release from www.expasy.org.
2. Protein identification software: Any software capable of identifying proteins from mass spectrometric data. Common examples include SEQUEST, Mascot, and XTandem. Most vendors of mass spectrometers supply this software along with the instrument.

3. Methods

In order to determine the kinases interacting with staurosporine in a given biological sample, incubation of the capture compound with a lysate leads to an equilibrium binding based on the affinity between the Capture Compound and the proteins. This equilibrium is then frozen by a photochemical reaction leading to the formation of a covalent bond between the Capture Compound and the interacting proteins. The proteins selectively bound by the selectivity function of the capture compound (the kinase inhibitor) have to be determined. To determine binding of any non-specific proteins, it is essential to perform the capture experiment and a competition experiment in parallel. In the competition experiment, the binding of the Capture Compound is competed for by preincubation of the lysate with an excess of the corresponding free (unmodified) small molecule. The results can be visualized by e.g., SDS-PAGE electrophoresis (an example is shown in Fig. 3a, b). Experiments carried out in parallel without irradiation (pull down) show lower amounts of isolated protein compared to capture experiments (Fig. 3a, c). After LC-MS/MS analysis, the specifically captured proteins can be determined by subtraction of the two data sets. A typical result of a capture experiment and a pull-down experiment from 400 μg HepG2 cell lysate as well as shot gun measurement from 5 μg cell lysate is shown in Fig. 3c. The method is also compatible with any state-of-the art stable isotope labeling technology, or assessment of the capture sample by 2D gel electrophoresis.

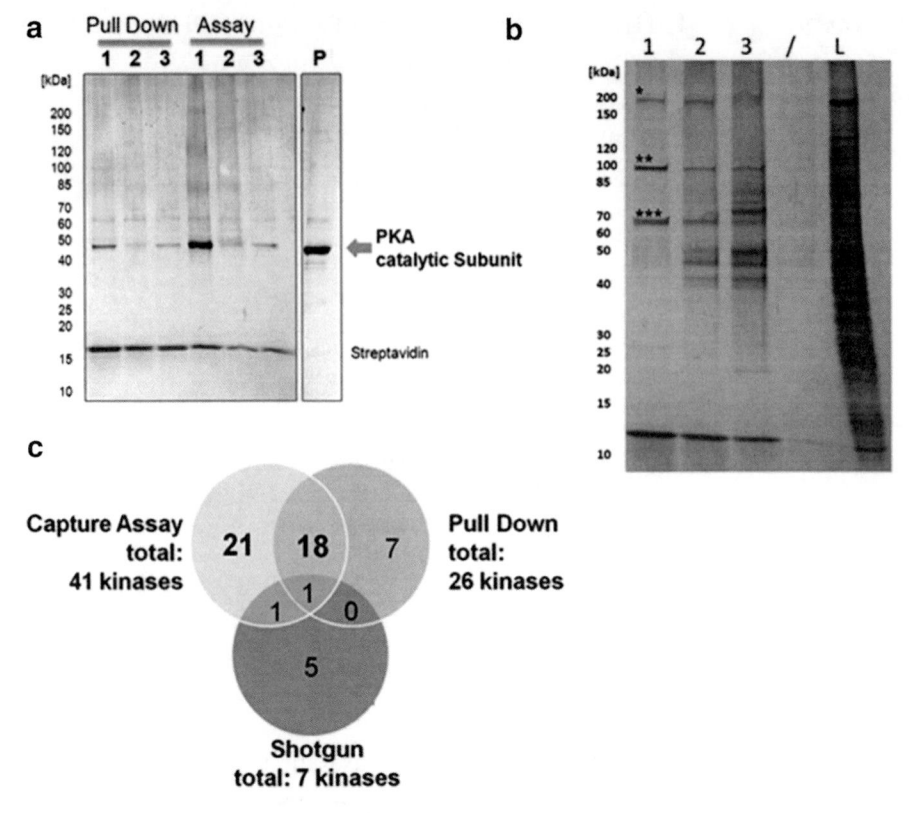

Fig. 3. Results of capturing kinases with staurosporine Capture Compound and comparison to pull-down assays. (**a**) Capturing of the purified catalytic subunit of PKA visualizes the superiority of the CCMS technology compared to a pull-down assay (without cross-linking). *Lane 1*: Capture assay, *lane 2*: competition control using free staurosporine, *lane 3*: control using a Capture Compound without selectivity function. (**b**) Silver stained SDS-PAGE visualizing the results of capturing proteins from a HepG2 cell lysate. *Lane 1*: control using a Capture Compound without selectivity function. Only naturally biotinylated proteins are isolated, *lane 2*: competition control using free staurosporine, *lane 3*: capture assay, *lane L*: HepG2 lysate corresponding to 0.5% of the amount of protein used for the capturing reaction. Naturally biotinylated proteins are also isolated by streptavidin beads and marked by *stars*: *Acetyl-CoA carboxylase 1, **Pyruvate carboxylase, ***Propionyl-CoA carboxylase beta chain. (**c**) Comparison of the number of kinases identified from a typical capture experiment, pull-down assay (only the strong binders are isolated) and shotgun analysis of the same lysate.

3.1. Preparation of HepG2 Cell Lysate

1. Grow cells in a 2 L spinner flask to a density of 3.7×10^5 cells/mL and a vitality of at least 90%.
2. Collect cells by gentle centrifugation and wash pellet three times with ice-cold phosphate-buffered saline.
3. Resuspended cells in 10 mL cell lysis buffer and homogenize three times in a French press at a pressure between 50,000 and 150,000 kPa.
4. Remove cell debris by ultracentrifugation at $30,000 \times g$ for 60 min at 4°C.
5. Filter lysate with a 0.22-μm filter.
6. Dialyze lysate using a molecular weight cutoff of 6–8 kDa overnight against the cell lysis buffer.

7. Remove proteins precipitated overnight by centrifugation at 4,000 × g for 10 min at 4°C.

8. Determine protein concentration by measuring UV absorbance at 280 nm (A_{280}) or according to Bradford (12).

9. Aliquot the lysates and snap-freeze in liquid nitrogen: store at below −60°C.

3.2. Capture Experiment and Competition Control

1. For several parallel experiments, it is recommended to prepare sufficient quantities of water, capture buffer, and cell lysate and to perform reactions within different wells of one 200-µLPCR strip. Here quantities for one reaction well are given. Mix gently by inversion after each addition (see Note 7).

2. Supplement a volume of ultra pure water for a final reaction mix volume of 100 µL with 20 µL 5× Capture Buffer (see Note 8). Mix and add HepG2 cell lysate corresponding to 0.4 mg total protein (see Notes 4 and 5). To the competition reaction, add 20 µL competitor and add an equivalent amount of water to the capture reaction.

3. If you suspect that the biological material contains high amounts of biotinylated proteins, pipette 50 µL of streptavidin-coated beads into fresh PCR-tubes. Hold magnet to the side of the tubes and remove liquid. Transfer the reaction mixtures into the bead-containing tubes and resuspend (see Note 2).

4. Mix (shaker or rotation wheel) the reaction and competition control at 4°C for 30 min to allow binding of the competitor to target proteins (and binding of naturally biotinylated proteins to the magnetic beads).

5. If streptavidin-coated beads were used to clear lysates of biotinylated proteins: Hold magnet against the tube walls and transfer the supernatants (reaction mixes) to fresh PCR-tubes. Discard the streptavidin-coated beads.

6. Add staurosporine Capture Compound in equal amounts to the capture reaction and competition control to a final concentration of 5 µM. The reaction volume should now be 100 µL. From this step onward, take care to protect the reactions from light (see Note 9).

7. Incubate reactions for 2 h at 4°C in the dark (shaker or radiation wheel).

8. Irradiate reactions in the caproBox™ for 10 min using the provided filter. Although the photoreactivity groups should now have completely reacted it is recommended that the reactions are not exposed to direct light until the digestion step.

9. Add 25 µL of 5× WB to each reaction and mix gently.

10. Add 50 µL of streptavidin-coated beads and incubate at 4°C for 1 h with mixing.

11. Insert the 200 µL PCR-reaction-tube-strip into the caproMag™ according to the manufacturer's instructions and collect the magnetic beads in the tube strip lids. Discard the reaction mix and replace by 200 µL 1× wash buffer (see Note 10). Resuspend the beads and again collect in the lids. Repeat washing with 1× WB another five times.
12. Wash the beads three times with 80% acetonitrile.
13. Wash the beads once with ultrapure water and collect the beads in lids (see Note 11). Avoid collecting water in the lids or remove manually. Alternatively, store the beads at this point in ultrapure water at 4°C until further use (see Note 12).

3.3. Tryptic Digest and Preparation of Peptides for LC-MS/MS

1. Fill 10 µL digestion buffer and 1 µL trypsin solution (or the equivalent of 1:100 enzyme:substrate w/w) into a new tube strip. Place lids with beads onto the new strip and resuspend by vigorously vortexing.
2. Digest proteins at 37°C with vigorous mixing overnight.
3. Centrifuge briefly and collect the beads by holding a magnet against the tube wall. Transfer supernatant containing the tryptic peptides to new tube (see Note 13).
4. Dry peptides in a vacuum centrifuge (~15 min).
5. Dissolve peptide pellet in 5.5 µL 5% formic acid, vortex, briefly incubate in an ultrasonic bath, and vortex again.
6. Transfer 5 µL of the dissolved peptides to a HPLC sample plate.

3.4. Nano LC System

1. Place sample plate into the autosampler of the LC system.
2. Inject the entire sample and separate peptides on a C18 reversed phase column. In this method, the following columns were used: Biosphere C_{18} precolumn (5 µm, 120 Å, 20 × 0.1 mm) and a Biosphere C_{18} analytical column (3 µm, 120 Å, 150 × 0.075 mm). Use a linear gradient of 5–40% LC-MS/MS buffer B in 80 min and a controlled flow rate of 300 nL/min.

3.5. Analysis of Peptides Using ESI-LC-MS/MS

Any state of the art tandem mass spectrometer may be used for the analysis of tryptic peptides generated by the above procedures. Below, we describe the method optimized for an LTQ-Orbitrap instrument.

1. The mass spectrometric analysis is performed in the data-dependent mode which automatically switches between orbitrap-MS and LTQ-MS/MS (MS^2) modes of data acquisition (see Notes 14 and 15).
2. Acquire full scan MS spectra (from m/z 400 to 2,000) in the orbitrap with a resolution of $r = 60,000$ at m/z 400 following the accumulation of ions to a target value of 500.000 charges in the linear ion trap.

3. Set the system to sequentially isolate the five most intense ions for fragmentation in the linear ion trap using collision-induced dissociation (CID) at a target value of 10.000 charges. The resulting fragment ions are recorded in the LTQ.

4. Target ions already mass selected for CID are dynamically excluded for the duration of 60 s.

5. Further mass spectrometric settings are as follows: spray voltage 1.7 kV, temperature of the heated transfer capillary 200°C, and relative normalized collision energy 35% for MS². The minimal signal required for MS² is 500 counts. Set activation q to $q=0.25$ and the activation time to 30 ms.

6. Set the lock mass to 445.120025 m/z. This corresponds to the molecular formula $(Si(CH_3)_2O)_6H^+$.

7. To clean the LC system, perform one blank run between two consecutive capture experiment measurements.

3.6. Peptide Identification via Database Search

Any appropriate software may be used for the identification of peptides and proteins from the mass spectrometric data. Below, we describe the method the search algorithm SEQUEST and the data visualization tool Scaffold.

1. Analyze the mass spectrometer output file (file extension .raw) using SEQUEST implemented in Bioworks 3.3.1 SP1 (Thermo Fisher Scientific).

2. Set the specific search parameters in the SEQUEST analyses as follows: 5 ppm precursor tolerance, 1 amu fragment ions tolerance, full trypsin specificity allowing for up to two missed cleavages.

3. Set the following variable modifications: phosphorylation at serine, threonine, and tyrosine, oxidation of methionines, deamidation at asparagine and glutamine, acetylation at lysine and serine, formylation at lysine, and methylation at arginine, lysine, serine, threonine, and asparagine. No fixed modifications are used in the database search.

4. Choose an appropriate protein sequence database against which the mass spectrometric data will be searched. Download for example the latest UniProtKB/Swiss-Prot database release from www.expasy.org.

5. Set the SEQUEST peptide identifications parameter as follows: minimum XCorr values of 2, 2.5, and 3 for singly, doubly, and triply charged peptides, respectively, a minimum ΔC_n of 0.1, a minimum probability ≤0.001.

6. Load all SEQUEST output files you wish to compare (e.g., the results of the capture and the competition experiment) into the program Scaffold 2.0 for the direct comparison of experimental results in one file.

4. Notes

1. Most complex biological samples contain naturally biotinylated proteins such as carboxylases. These naturally biotinylated proteins will be isolated from the reaction mixtures together with the kinases that are biotinylated through covalent reaction with the biotin-containing Capture Compound. Depending on the sample, these interfering signals may be quite strong and mask signals from captured kinases in SDS-PAGE or LC-MS/MS runs. Results obtained from samples containing many naturally biotinylated proteins can be significantly improved by carrying out the described depletion step. The amount of the beads used in this step might have to be adjusted on a case-by-case basis (see Subheading 2.2).

2. Staurosporine caproKit™ (caprotec bioanalytics GmbH, Berlin, Germany) contains staurosporine Capture Compound and competitor, Dynabeads®, 5× Capture Buffer and 5× Wash Buffer. Capture Compounds™ containing other selectivity functions can be also be ordered from caprotec bioanalytics GmbH (http://www.caprotec.com) or commissioned as custom synthesis (see Subheading 2.2).

3. caproMag™ is a magnetic device for the handling of magnetic beads (caprotec bioanalytics GmbH, Berlin, Germany). caproMag™ reduces the number of pipetting steps and thereby generates higher yields of purified bead-bound proteins. It is possible to separate the beads from the reaction and wash solutions by holding a conventional magnet to the side of the tubes or using any other commercially available rack for magnetic beads. However, the caproMag™ is strongly recommended since only this system is adjusted to handle 200 µl-PCR tube strips and allows the collection of beads in the lids so that tubes can be emptied without any pipetting steps. The caproMag™ has been designed especially for capture experiments, saves time, and reduces the risk of contaminations (see subheading 2.2).

4. Here, capturing from commercially available HepG2 lysate is given as an example. Preparation of lysates from other cell lines may have to be optimized on a case-by-case basis for this protocol. Generally, it is recommended that the lysates should be free from intact DNA (e.g., via benzonase digestion) and be buffered in the described lysis buffer. If a buffer change is necessary, it is recommended to use Zeba Desalt Spin Columns from Pierce for this purpose. Dithiol compounds such as dithiothreitol (DTT) should not be used, as they may interfere with the photoreaction. Instead, the use of ß-mercaptoethanol is advised. Strong denaturing lysis conditions (e.g., sonication) or agents (e.g., urea) must be avoided (see Subheading 2.2).

5. Capturing from subcellular fractions of mammalian tissue. For lysis and fractionation of organs such as liver, we recommend a motor-driven glass-Teflon homogenizer and 10 volumes of homogenization buffer per gram of tissue wet weight (0.32 M sucrose, 5 mM HEPES/NaOH pH 7.4, Roche Complete Protease Inhibitor Cocktail™ EDTA-free. Cellular fractions may then be obtained by (ultra-) centrifugation with different sucrose–Tris–HCl pH 8.1 gradients (Emig et al. (13)). The buffer of soluble fractions (e.g., cytosol) should be exchanged for the lysis buffer (see Note 4). Membrane fractions (e.g., mitochondria, microsomes) are solubilized in the lysis buffer supplemented with 0.5% n-dodecyl-ß-d-maltoside for 1 h at room temperature and then directly used in the capture reactions (see Subheading 2.2).

6. We use a split-less Easy-nLC™ liquid chromatography system from Proxeon Biosystems A/S with a Biosphere C_{18} precolumn (5 µm, 120Å, 20×0.1 mm) and a Biosphere C_{18} analytical column (3 µm, 120Å, 150×0.075 mm) that is online connected to a LTQ Orbitrap XL mass spectrometer. Any other similar set up may also be used (see Subheading 2.4).

7. The biological samples from which kinases are isolated may contain proteins prone to denaturation. Consequently, it is mandatory to keep samples cold and avoid thawing at all times. Note that the caproBox™ cools the samples to 4°C; the lamps emitting the UV light, however, also emit heat. Therefore, it is necessary to briefly centrifuge the vials before irradiation so that proteins adhering to the vial walls do not form precipitation seeds (see Subheading 3.2).

8. Although the given protocol should give optimum results in most cases, changes may still be necessary for some lysates. If results are not in accordance with expectations, varying NaCl concentrations between 100 mM and 300 mM in the capture reaction are recommended as starting point (see Subheading 3.2).

9. A major advantage of Capture Compounds™ lies in the formation of a covalent bond between the Capture Compound and the kinase. This permits both unperturbed affinity based equilibrium binding and subsequent stringent washing conditions. The covalent cross-link is achieved by a photoreaction at 310 nm. Normal overhead light contains only a small fraction of UV light. Still, to obtain reliable and reproducible results it is mandatory to protect the staurosporine Capture Compounds™ from light up to the time of controlled and cooled irradiation in the caproBox™. As a reference, in our laboratory, approximately 20% of the staurosporine Capture Compound has reacted within 1 h after exposure to normal laboratory light (see Subheading 3.2).

10. In some cases, proteins may precipitate during the washing steps. This can be seen by the formation of a brown film on the

walls of the reaction vials. Formation of such a brown film immediately indicates that the reaction has failed and should be broken off. Partial denaturation and precipitation of the proteins can be due to (a) thawing or heating (see Note 7) and (b) incompatibility between the lysis buffer and the wash buffer. If the recommended lysis buffer (see Note 4) was not used, the wash buffer should be changed too to reflect the composition of the actual lysis buffer used for the experiment. (c) A high amount of hydrophobic proteins (e.g., membrane fractions) in the sample. Try addition of 0.1–0.5% n-dodecyl-ß-d-maltoside to the wash buffer (see Subheading 3.2).

11. The identification of captured proteins is carried out by LC-MS/MS. Mass spectrometry is a highly sensitive method with the advantage of allowing the detection of very low protein amounts. In some cases, the presence of a protein can be unambiguously proven by only one peptide. Consequently, it is absolutely necessary to use exclusively LC-MS grade reagents in the final steps (starting with the water for the final bead wash). Avoid contamination of the experiments by external protein sources, e.g., keratin originating from dust or from the experimenter. Particularly during the final digestion steps, it is recommended to pay attention to clean work space, to wear a lab coat and possibly a hair net or ideally perform the final steps under a clean bench (see Subheading 3.2).

12. Depending on the experimental question it may be interesting to analyze the result of the capture experiments by SDS-PAGE followed by silver staining or Western blot. Generally, kinases have expression levels which are too low to be discerned as differential bands on a silver stained gel. Consequently, capture and control lanes may appear identical on the gel. Nevertheless, LC-MS/MS analysis allows the identification of specific differences in capture and control experiment (i.e., kinase capturing). If you need to demonstrate that one particular kinase binds the inhibitor, silver stained SDS-gels may be conclusive if the protein is used in a purified form. If binding of one particular protein of interest from a lysate must be shown Western blots are recommended. Western blots using streptavidin-horseradish peroxidase can also be used to visualize successful cross-linking of the biotin containing Capture Compound to the proteins. Note that naturally biotinylated proteins will also be isolated by the magnetic beads and will be contained in the capture experiment and the competition control. To analyze the reactions by SDS-PAGE, remove the water from the washed beads, resuspend in Laemmli buffer, and boil for 5 min. The beads are collected by holding a magnet to the tube walls and then pipetting the clear solution into the gel wells (see Subheading 3.2).

13. Due to the small volume of the peptide digest it is not recommended to collect the beads in the lids. The beads are collected by holding a magnet to the tube walls followed by pipetting the clear solution into fresh tubes (see Subheading 3.3).

14. To obtain reliable mass spectra, it is essential to have a stable electrospray during ESI-MS/MS analysis (see Subheading 3.5).

15. For other LC-MS/MS systems, measurement parameters and peptide identification algorithms must be adjusted individually. The program Scaffold enables direct comparison of many different single experiments within one file and enables identification of specifically captured proteins at one glance as well as an assessment of the reproducibility. Although not absolutely required, we recommend the use of this program (see Subheading 3.5).

References

1. Romano, G., and Giordano, A. (2008) Role of the cyclin-dependent kinase 9-related pathway in mammalian gene expression and human diseases, *Cell Cycle* 7, 3664–3668.
2. Cohen, P. (2002) Protein kinases--the major drug targets of the twenty-first century?, *Nat. Rev. Drug Discov.* 1, 309–315.
3. von Mehren, M. (2006) Beyond imatinib: second generation c-KIT inhibitors for the management of gastrointestinal stromal tumors, *Clin. Colorectal Cancer* 6 Suppl 1, S30–34.
4. Bantscheff, M., Hopf, C., Kruse, U., and Drewes, G. (2007) Proteomics-based strategies in kinase drug discovery, *Ernst Schering Found. Symp. Proc.*, 1–28.
5. Karaman, M. W., Herrgard, S., Treiber, D. K., Gallant, P., Atteridge, C. E., Campbell, B. T., Chan, K. W., Ciceri, P., Davis, M. I., Edeen, P. T., Faraoni, R., Floyd, M., Hunt, J. P., Lockhart, D. J., Milanov, Z. V., Morrison, M. J., Pallares, G., Patel, H. K., Pritchard, S., Wodicka, L. M., and Zarrinkar, P. P. (2008) A quantitative analysis of kinase inhibitor selectivity, *Nat. Biotechnol.* 26, 127–132.
6. Barglow, K. T., and Cravatt, B. F. (2007) Activity-based protein profiling for the functional annotation of enzymes, *Nat. Methods* 4, 822–827.
7. Luo, Y., Blex, C., Baessler, O., Glinski, M., Dreger, M., Sefkow, M., and Koster, H. (2009) From PKA to HCN: The cAMP-capture compound mass spectrometry as a novel tool for targeting cAMP binding proteins, *Mol. Cell. Proteomics* 12, 2843–2856.
8. Luo, Y., Fischer, J. J., Graebner Nee Baessler, O. Y., Schrey, A. K., Ungewiss, J., Glinski, M., Sefkow, M., Dreger, M., and Koester, H. (2010) GDP-Capture Compound - A novel tool for the profiling of GTPases in pro- and eukaryotes by capture compound mass spectrometry (CCMS), *J. Proteomics* 73, 815–819.
9. Dalhoff, C., Huben, M., Lenz, T., Poot, P., Nordhoff, E., Koster, H., and Weinhold, E. (2010) Synthesis of S-Adenosyl-L-homocysteine Capture Compounds for Selective Photoinduced Isolation of Methyltransferases, *ChemBioChem.* 11, 256–265.
10. Fischer, J. J., Baessler, O., Dalhoff, C., Michaelis, S., Schrey, A., Ungewiss, J., Andrich, K., Jeske, D., Kroll, F., Glinski, M., Sefkow, M., Dreger, M., and Koester, H. (2010) Comprehensive Identification of Staurosporine-Binding Kinases in the Hepatocyte Cell Line HepG2 using Capture Compound Mass Spectrometry (CCMS), *J. Proteome Res.* 9, 806–817.
11. Koster, H., Little, D. P., Luan, P., Muller, R., Siddiqi, S. M., Marappan, S., and Yip, P. (2007) Capture compound mass spectrometry: a technology for the investigation of small molecule protein interactions, *Assay Drug. Dev. Technol.* 5, 381–390.
12. Bradford, M. M. (1976) A rapid and sensitive method for the quantitation of microgram quantities of protein utilizing the principle of protein-dye binding, *Anal. Biochem.* 72, 248–254.
13. Emig, S., Schmalz, D., Shakibaei, M., and Buchner, K. (1995) The Nuclear Pore Complex Protein p62 Is One of Several Sialic Acid-containing Proteins of the Nuclear Envelope, *J. Biol. Chem.* 270, 13787–13793.

Chapter 10

Affinity Purification of Proteins Binding to Kinase Inhibitors Immobilized on Self-Assembling Monolayers

Marcus Bantscheff, Scott Hobson, and Bernhard Kuster

Abstract

Kinase inhibitors represent a relatively new class of drugs that offer novel therapies targeting specific malfunctioning kinase-mediated signaling pathways in oncology and potentially inflammation. As the ATP binding sites of the ~500 human kinases are structurally conserved and because most current drugs target the ATP binding site, there is a need to profile all the kinases that a drug may bind and/or inhibit. We have developed a chemical proteomics method that affinity purifies kinases from cell or tissue lysates using kinase inhibitors immobilized on self-assembling monolayers. The method can be applied to assess the selectivity of a given kinase inhibitor and thus to guide its preclinical or clinical development.

Key words: Kinase inhibitor, Chemical proteomics, Self-assembling monolayers, Mass spectrometry

1. Introduction

Kinase inhibitors represent a relatively new class of drugs targeting malfunctioning kinase-mediated signaling pathways (1). There are currently eight small-molecule inhibitors that are approved by the FDA and/or EMEA for the treatment of a number of human cancers. Given that all these molecules target the ATP binding site of a kinase, it is of paramount importance to establish to which of the ~500 human kinases and the several thousand ATP binding proteins an inhibitor may bind and inhibit. Traditionally, panels of recombinant kinase assays have been used for this purpose (2), but these panels are not complete, often do not recapitulate the activity of a kinase in vivo, and cannot assess binding/inhibition of nonkinase targets. To this end, we and others have developed chemical proteomics and chemical genomics methods that enable the assessment of binding specificity of a small molecule more broadly. In particular, the purification of protein binders using immobilized inhibitors and their subsequent identification by mass spectrometry has established systematic binding profiles for several kinase drugs (3–7). In this chapter, we describe one of these methods that utilizes self-assembling monolayers (8, 9) for the purification of specific drug–target interactions at low background protein binding.

2. Materials

Unless otherwise stated, the suppliers of laboratory chemicals are not critical but reagent purity should be at least analytical grade. Likewise, the origin of the used plasticware is not considered to be critical. All glassware should be thoroughly cleaned, rinsed extensively to remove traces of detergent, and subsequently dried in an oven.

2.1. Cell Lysis

1. Phosphate buffered saline (PBS).
2. Lysis buffer: 50 mM Tris/HCl pH 7.5, 5% glycerol, 1.5 mM $MgCl_2$, 150 mM NaCl, 25 mM NaF, and 1 mM $NaVO_4$. Add detergent (e.g., Tween-20) to a concentration of 0.8%. Add one complete EDTA-free tablet (protease inhibitor cocktail, Roche Diagnostics) per 25 ml of lysis buffer. Filter lysis buffer through a 0.22-μm filter (Millipore, SLGV013SL).
3. A standard cell homogenizer is needed for cell lysis (e.g., Potter S from B. Braun, Biotech International).
4. Ultracentrifugation: any ultracentrifuge and rotor may be used provided it can process the appropriate volumes and delivers the required g-force (e.g., 20,000×g step: Sorvall SLA600; 100,000×g step: Ti50.2).
5. Bradford protein assay kit (e.g., BioRad).

2.2. SAM Preparation

1. Gold-coated glass slides: 22-mm square gold-coated coverslips are available from Platypus technologies. Larger slides may also be used (see Note 1).
2. Polyethyleneglycol linkered alkanethiols: amino-EG6-undecanethiol (548.22 g/mol), carboxy-EG6-undecanethiol (524.71 g/mol), hydroxy-EG6-undecanethiol (468.69 g/mol) are available from (Dojindo, Japan).
3. Absolute ethanol, Argon 4.6.
4. Piranha solution: Carefully mix 50 ml of concentrated H_2SO_4 with concentrated H_2O_2 (~30%) at a ratio of 7:3 (v/v) in a glass beaker and allow to cool to room temperature (see Note 2).

2.3. Immobilization of Kinase Inhibitors

1. 10 mM PyBroP ((Benzotriazol-1-yloxy)-tripyrrolidinphosphonium hexafluorophosphate), in absolute ethanol (4.66 mg/ml).

2. 20 mM Diisopropylethylamine (DIEA) in absolute ethanol (8.75 µL DIEA in 2.5 ml ethanol), 1-Ethyl-3-[3-dimethylaminopropyl]carbodiimide (EDC), 1,3-Dicyclohexylcarbodiimide (DCCD), N-hydroxy-succinimide (NHS), acetic acid, PBS, abs ethanol, 6-well cell-culture plate, triethylamine (TEA), 2-Aminoethanol, ethylenediamine.

3. Kinase inhibitors: for this method, a kinase inhibitor must contain a primary or secondary aliphatic amine or a carboxylic acid group (see Note 3). The examples used in this chapter are Bisindolylmaleimide VIII and Purvalanol B.

2.4. Affinity Purification

1. Lysis buffer (see above) without detergent.
2. 6-well cell-culture plate (see above).

2.5. Sample Preparation for Mass Spectrometry

1. Formic acid, porcine trypsin (sequencing grade), HPLC-grade water, NH_4HCO_3, 0.5 M HCl.

2. Humidity chamber: the digestion of proteins by trypsin must be carried out in a humid chamber to prevent the SAM from drying up during digestion. This is easily achieved by placing a wet tissue at the bottom of a 6-well cell-culture plate and by sealing the plate using parafilm.

3. Centrifugal force vacuum concentrator for concentration of protein digests.

2.6. Identification of Proteins by Mass Spectrometry

1. The available equipment for the identification of proteins by mass spectrometry may vary greatly between laboratories. There are no particular requirements for this method except that the MS platform must be an LC-MS/MS system with sufficient sensitivity to sequence peptides at the femtomol level.

2. For the experiments exemplified in this chapter, tryptic fragments were analyzed by nanocapillary reversed-phase liquid chromatography tandem mass spectrometry (RP-LC-MS/MS) using a nano-LC system (CapLC, Waters) coupled to a quadrupole time-of-flight (QTOF Micro, Waters) mass spectrometer. 75-µm ID columns were self-packed using 5 µM C-18 material (Reprosil, Dr. Maisch, Germany).

3. HPLC solvents: HPLC-grade water, HPLC-grade acetonitrile, and HPLC-grade formic acid (98–100%).

4. Several database search algorithms are available and may be used for the matching of tandem mass spectra against a protein sequence database. We have used the Mascot search engine (Matrix Science, London).

3. Methods

Several experimental aspects are important for the identification of proteins binding to an immobilized inhibitor. First of all, the choice of protein source (cell culture, tissue) determines the range of kinases that can be identified as not all cell types express all proteins encoded by the genome. Second, all protein kinases need to be solubilized from the cells and tissues. As kinases are present in membranes, the cytosol, and the nucleus, the choice of lysis conditions and detergent is critical and will have to be adjusted on a case-by-case basis. Third, the specificity of the affinity purification depends on the density with which compounds are coupled to the surface of the SAMs. Our experience suggests that compound immobilization is generally straightforward, but only a fraction of the coupling capacity of the SAMs should actually be used. Fourth, the sensitivity of identifying bound kinases and other interacting proteins depends on the sensitivity of the employed LC-MS/MS system. Best results are obtained when top-grade nano-HPLC and mass spectrometers are used. For further details, see also data figures and notes section.

3.1. Lysis of Cells

1. Harvest cells from tissue culture cells and pelleted at $2,000 \times g$. Subsequently, wash cell pellet twice with 20 ml of ice-cold PBS.
2. Add two volumes of ice-cold lysis buffer to one volume of cell pellet and transfer the suspension into a cooled dounce tissue grinder.
3. Dounce the suspension 10× (using, for example, a mechanized POTTER S at a speed setting of 300/min) and transfer the homogenate into a 50-ml plastic tube and incubate for 30 min on ice.
4. Spin the crude lysate for 10 min at $20,000 \times g$ at 4°C and transfer the supernatant to a polycarbonate ultracentrifuge tube.
5. Spin the lysate for 1 h at $100,000 \times g$ at 4°C and transfer the supernatant into a fresh 50-ml plastic tube.
6. Determine the protein concentration of the lysate using a standard Bradford test. Prepare 50 mg aliquots, freeze in liquid nitrogen, and store at −80°C until use.

3.2. Preparation of the SAM

1. Preparation of the glass surface: Remove the gold-coated glass slides from the shipping container and immerse briefly 2× in absolute EtOH in a glass beaker (see Note 1). Dry the slides under a stream of argon. Immerse the slides in a glass beaker containing Piranha solution for 30 min or until no visible reactions are taking place anymore. Remove the gold-coated glass slides from Piranha

solution and immerse 2× in water followed by 2× in absolute ethanol (see Note 2). Dry the surfaces quickly with a stream of argon and proceed immediately with the next step.

3.2.1. Preparation of SAM Surface Containing Amine End Groups

1. Dissolve 2.73 mg of amino-EG6-undecanethiol in 1 ml Ethanol in a glass vial.
2. Dissolve 46.9 mg of hydroxy-EG6-undecanethiol in 1 ml Ethanol in a glass vial.
3. Pour 98 ml of Ethanol into a 250-ml beaker using a graduated glass cylinder.
4. Add both alkanethiol-containing solutions and mix thoroughly. This yields a solution containing 50 µM amino-EG6-undecanethiol and 1 mM total thiol.
5. Place the gold-coated slides into a thoroughly cleaned and dried glass container, so that they are not in contact with each other.
6. Add thiol-containing solution so that all glass slides are nicely covered and close the container so that it is airtight (see Note 4).
7. Incubate the glass slides overnight at room temperature.
8. Remove the slides from the glass container using tweezers and gently dry in a stream of argon.

This protocol yields approximately 5% amine-terminated SAMs.

3.2.2. Preparation of SAM Surface Containing Carboxy End Groups

1. Dissolve 2.62 mg of carboxy-EG6-undecanethiol in 1 ml Ethanol in a glass vial.
2. Dissolve 46.9 mg of hydroxy-EG6-undecanethiol in 1 ml Ethanol in a glass vial.
3. Pour 98 ml of Ethanol into a 250 ml beaker using a graduated glass cylinder.
4. Add both alkanethiol-containing solutions and mix thoroughly. This yields a solution containing 50 µM carboxy-EG6-undecanethiol and 1 mM total thiol.
5. Proceed as described in Subheading 3.2.1.

3.3. Immobilization of Kinase Inhibitor on the SAM

3.3.1. Kinase Inhibitors Containing a Primary or Secondary Amino Group

1. Prior to inhibitor immobilization, the SAM surface as prepared in Subheading 3.2.2 needs to be chemically activated.
2. Allow EDC reagent vial to warm up to room temperature and prepare a 400 mM solution in pure water. In parallel, prepare a 200 mM solution of NHS in water. Mix equal volumes of the EDC and NHS solutions.
3. Transfer the SAM containing glass slide into a new plastic 6-well plate (see Fig. 1 and Note 5).

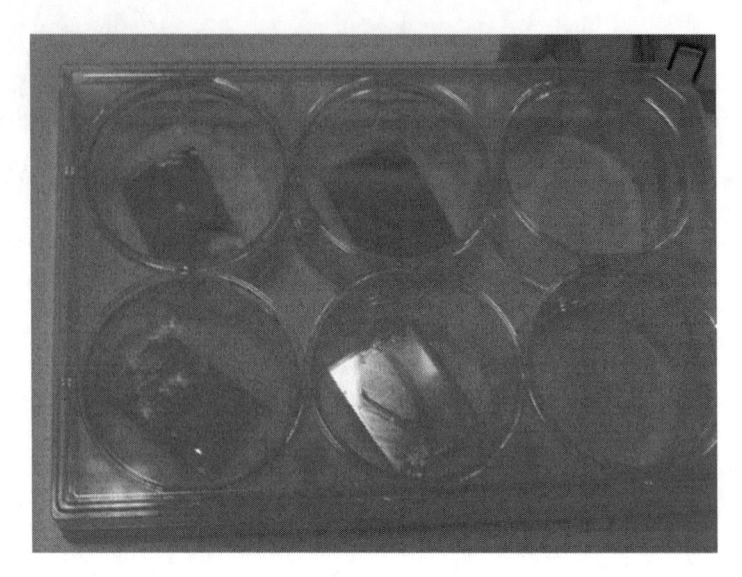

Fig. 1. Gold-coated glass slides in 6-well tissue culture plate.

4. Apply the mixed EDC/NHS reagent to the gold-coated side of the SAM. For SAMs prepared on coverslips use ~0.2 ml. Incubate for 15 min at room temperature. Remove surplus EDC/NHS reagent by two brief washings in PBS.

5. Prepare a 125 nmol/ml solution of the kinase inhibitor in PBS (see Note 6). Apply inhibitor to the activated SAM at 5 nmol/cm² and incubate overnight at room temperature (see Note 7).

6. In order to remove excess coupling reagents, wash the coupled SAM for 2× 10 s in a beaker filled with ethanol. Subsequently, wash coupled SAM for 2× 10 s in ~50 ml lysis buffer containing 0.4% detergent.

3.3.2. Kinase Inhibitors Containing a Carboxylic Acid Group

1. Prior to inhibitor immobilization on the SAM, the kinase inhibitor needs to be chemically activated.

2. Prepare a 10 mM solution of PyBroP in absolute ethanol. This solution is unstable and must be made fresh immediately prior to use. Prepare a 20 mM DIEA solution in absolute ethanol.

3. Mix 2.5 ml of each PyBroP and DIEA solutions and add 20 ml absolute ethanol. Add kinase inhibitor from an appropriate stock solution to the amount of 50 nmol/cm² of SAM surface.

4. Pour the above solution into a new plastic cell-culture 6-well plate and incubate the SAM at room temperature overnight.

5. Prepare NHS-activated acetic acid as blocking reagent by mixing equal volumes of 200 mM NHS and DCCD solutions in acetonitrile in a glass vial and by adding 11.4 µl of acetic acid

per ml solution. Mix thoroughly and after incubation at room temperature overnight, the solution is ready to use.

6. Unmodified amino groups on the SAM surface are blocked by adding 100 µl NHS-activated acetic acid solution and 100 µl 7.2 M TEA to the SAM. Incubate for at least 4 h at room temperature.

3.4. Affinity Purification

1. Keep SAM in lysis buffer until cell lysate is ready for use.
2. Thaw cell lysate quickly in a 37°C water bath and then keep on ice. Dilute lysate with lysis buffer (without detergent!) to 0.4% detergent and a protein concentration of 5–10 mg/ml (see Note 8). Transfer diluted lysate to a polycarbonate tube and spin for 20 min at $100,000 \times g$ at 4°C (see Note 9).
3. Incubate SAM with 1 ml of lysate in a 6-well plate overnight at 4°C on an orbital shaker (see Note 10).
4. Remove unbound proteins by three 10 s washes first using 50 ml lysis buffer with 0.4% detergent, second using 50 ml lysis buffer with 0.2% detergent, and third using 50 ml lysis buffer without any detergent. Blow off remaining liquid from the SAM by a stream of argon.

3.5. Identification of Interacting Proteins

1. Prior to mass spectrometric analysis, proteins purified on SAMs need to be digested into peptides.
2. Dissolve trypsin in 1 mM HCL to a concentration of 1 mg/ml and keep at −20°C until use. Dilute trypsin stock solution to 0.3 µg/ml in 50 mM NH_4HCO_3 pH 7.8. Add trypsin solution to SAM: 100–200 µl are needed for a coverslip. Incubate in a humid atmosphere for 3 h at 55°C without shaking. Collect the supernatant containing the peptides. Wash the SAM surface twice with 0.1% formic acid (100 µl for coverslips; 500 µl for microscope slides). Combine these three samples, freeze in liquid nitrogen, and dry in a centrifugal force vacuum concentrator.
3. For mass spectrometric analysis, reconstitute the sample in 20 µl 0.1% formic acid, vortex, incubate for 5 min in an ultrasonic bath and centrifuge the sample. Inject 5–20 µl of the sample into the LC-MS/MS system and separate tryptic peptides within 2 h on a 75 µm inner diameter C-18 reversed phase column using gradient elution (90 min linear gradient from 2 to 35% acetonitrile in 0.1% formic acid, followed by a 5 min wash step at 60% acetonitrile and 25 min reequilibration at 2% acetonitrile).
4. For protein identification, search the generated tandem mass spectra against an appropriate protein sequence data base (e.g., IPI, Swissprot, or other) with peptide and fragment mass tolerances set to values appropriate for the particular mass spectrometer used. Up to 3 missed cleavage sites should be

allowed and we recommend to use methionine oxidation as a variable modification (see Notes 11 and 12).

4. Notes

1. Never touch gold-coated glass slides with your hands. Use tweezers instead and hold the slides at the edges only. Make sure that you know which side of the SAM is gold coated (see Subheadings 2.2 and 3.2).

2. A Piranha solution is used to remove all organic matter from gold-coated substrates prior to functionalization of the substrate with the SAM. Please note that Piranha solution is extremely corrosive and thus should only be handled by a qualified person and following all appropriate safety precautions (lab coat, safety glasses, gloves, fume hood, waste disposal, etc, see Subheadings 2.2 and 3.2).

3. For this method to work, kinase inhibitors must contain a primary or secondary amine or a carboxylic acid group. Kinase inhibitors for which this is not the case, have to be chemically modified prior to immobilization (see Subheading 2.3).

4. Thiol groups are sensitive to oxidation by oxygen present in ambient air. Therefore, use thiol-containing solution immediately after preparation (see Subheading 3.2.1).

5. As an alternative to 6-well cell-culture plates, petri dishes may be used when experiments are scaled up to larger (or multiple) glass slides. All buffer volumes should be adjusted appropriately. BUT make sure that the amount of added kinase inhibitor is always calculated based on the surface area of the glass slides (see Subheading 3.3.1).

6. Kinase inhibitors tend to be poorly soluble in water. Therefore, 10–100 mM stock solutions should be prepared in DMSO or DMF (see Subheading 3.3.1).

7. Compound density on SAMS should be kept relatively low to ensure that putative binders have proper access to the immobilized small-molecule compound and to prevent unspecific interactions between bound proteins. The described density of 5% of the total surface should be considered as a rule of thumb. Lower densities might be required when purifying very large protein complexes. Coupling densities up to 20% may be used to increase kinase recovery. Please note that this may also increase unspecific protein binding (see Subheading 3.3.1).

8. We have tested several detergents. The procedure is compatible with most detergents. However, we note that results obtained

10 Affinity Purification of Proteins Binding to Kinase Inhibitors...

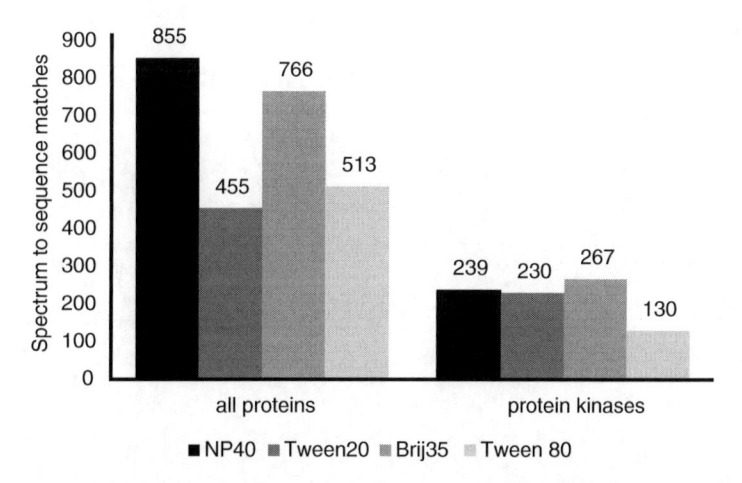

Fig. 2. Affinity enrichment on self-assembled monolayers is compatible with a variety of detergents. The immobilized CDK inhibitor purvalanol B purifies five to nine different protein kinases when using different detergents. While the amount of identified kinases is similar for Tween 20 and NP40 (judged by similar spectrum to sequence matches), significantly fewer nonkinase proteins were detected in the presence of 0.4% Tween 20, indicating a higher binding specificity.

with e.g., DDM were substantially worse than those performed with NP40 (see Subheading 3.4 and Fig. 2).

9. The described ultracentrifugation steps are absolutely required to remove any protein-containing particles from the protein preparation. Failure to do so will often result in high protein background binding presumably due to adsorption and precipitation of protein particles on the SAM surface (see Subheading 3.4).

10. High protein concentrations are desirable to achieve efficient binding (see Subheading 3.4).

11. The database search parameters that should be used for protein identification using Mascot depend on the instrument used (see Subheading 3.5).

12. The successful purification of kinases from lysates on SAMs is both a function of the affinity of a kinase to the immobilized ligand and the abundance of that protein in the lysate. It is, therefore, well possible that a low-affinity interaction of a very high abundant protein is more easily identified than a high-affinity interaction of a very low abundant protein (see Table 1). In order to increase binding selectivity and to confirm binding of the inhibitor to the ATP binding site, free ATP can be spiked into protein preparations during the binding step (see Fig. 3 and Subheading 3.5).

Table 1
Proteins identified by affinity enrichment on Bis8-SAM using HELA lysate

Accession number	Protein name	MW (Da)	MASCOT score	Sequence to spectrum matches	Number of peptides identified
IPI00292228.1	GSK3A	50,981	175	6	6
IPI00216190.1	GSK3B	48,034	224	8	7
IPI00848058.1	ACTG1	45,086	914	71	24
IPI00008603.1	ACTA2	42,009	593	48	16
IPI00014424.1	EEF1A2	50,470	358	36	9
IPI00003269.1	DKFZp686D0972	42,003	269	28	8
IPI00011654.2	TUBB	49,671	526	27	17
IPI00180675.4	7UBA1A	50,136	510	25	13
IPI00009342.1	IQGAP1	189,252	717	23	22
IPI00007752.1	TUBB2C	49,831	447	20	14
IPI00644079.2	HNRPU	90,584	275	9	8
IPI00219344.4	HPCAL1	22,313	338	9	9
IPI00329338.2	PCYT1A	41,732	175	7	7
IPI00022744.5	CSE1L	110,417	134	6	6
IPI00011200.5	PHGDH	56,651	242	6	6
IPI00025512.2	HSPB1	22,783	138	5	4
IPI00007402.2	IPO7	119,702	99	4	4
IPI00797001.1	MYL6	18,500	83	4	4
IPI00003865.1	HSPA8	70,898	120	4	4
IPI00782992.3	SRRM2	299,615	94	4	3
IPI00157790.7	KIAA0368	223,694	90	4	4
IPI00009790.1	PFKP	85,596	54	2	2
IPI00472102.3	HSPD1	61,213	40	2	2
IPI00453473.6	HIST1H4A	11,367	62	2	2
IPI00455976.1	LOC392557	27,869	64	2	2

Two known protein kinases are shown in *bold face*. The MASCOT score is a measure for identification quality. Only proteins with at least two identified peptides are shown

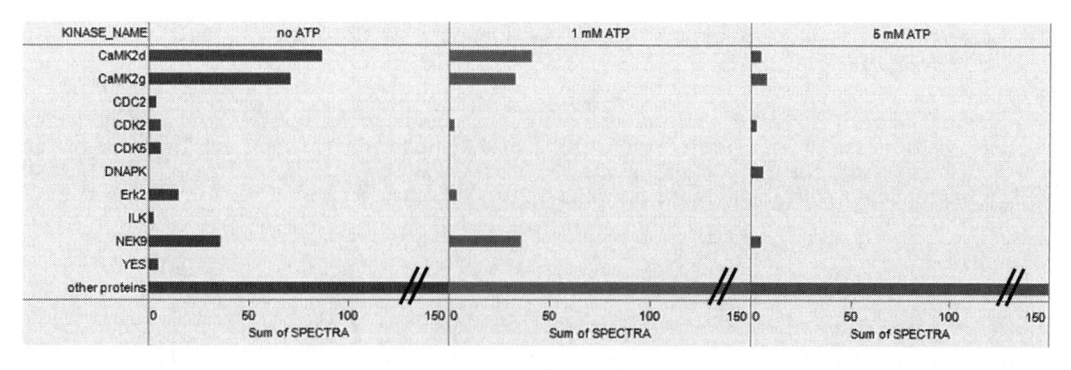

Fig. 3. Reduced binding of protein kinases to immobilized Purvalanol B in the presence of ATP. The ATP competitive binding mode of proteins binding to Purvalanol B SAMS can be confirmed by spiking ATP into the protein lysate prior to incubation with the SAM. While equal amounts of proteins binding nonspecifically to the SAM will observed in presence and absence of ATP, the amount of specific and ATP competitive binding proteins decreases with increasing ATP concentrations.

Acknowledgments

The authors thank Frank Weisbrodt for help with the figures and Gerard Drewes and Ulrich Kruse for helpful discussions.

References

1. Zhang, J., Yang, P. L., and Gray, N. S. (2009) Targeting cancer with small molecule kinase inhibitors. *Nat. Rev. Cancer* 9, 28–39.
2. Bain, J., Plater, L., Elliott, M., Shpiro, N., Hastie, C. J., McLauchlan, H., Klevernic, I., Arthur, J. S., Alessi, D. R., and Cohen, P. (2007) The selectivity of protein kinase inhibitors: a further update. *Biochem J.* 408, 297–315.
3. Bantscheff, M., Eberhard, D., Abraham, Y., Bastuck, S., Boesche, M., Hobson, S., Mathieson, T., Perrin, J., Raida, M., Rau, C., Reader, V., Sweetman, G., Bauer, A., Bouwmeester, T., Hopf, C., Kruse, U., Neubauer, G., Ramsden, N., Rick, J., Kuster, B., and Drewes, G. (2007) Quantitative chemical proteomics reveals mechanisms of action of clinical ABL kinase inhibitors. *Nat. Biotechnol.* 25, 1035–1044.
4. Fabian, M. A., Biggs, W. H., 3rd, Treiber, D. K., Atteridge, C. E., Azimioara, M. D., Benedetti, M. G., Carter, T. A., Ciceri, P., Edeen, P. T., Floyd, M., Ford, J. M., Galvin, M., Gerlach, J. L., Grotzfeld, R. M., Herrgard, S., Insko, D. E., Insko, M. A., Lai, A. G., Lelias, J. M., Mehta, S. A., Milanov, Z. V., Velasco, A. M., Wodicka, L. M., Patel, H. K., Zarrinkar, P. P., and Lockhart, D. J. (2005) A small molecule-kinase interaction map for clinical kinase inhibitors. *Nat. Biotechnol.* 23, 329–336.
5. Godl, K., Wissing, J., Kurtenbach, A., Habenberger, P., Blencke, S., Gutbrod, H., Salassidis, K., Stein-Gerlach, M., Missio, A., Cotten, M., and Daub, H. (2003) An efficient proteomics method to identify the cellular targets of protein kinase inhibitors. *Proc. Natl. Acad. Sci. USA* 100, 15434–15439.
6. Hahn, C. K., Berchuck, J. E., Ross, K. N., Kakoza, R. M., Clauser, K., Schinzel, A. C., Ross, L., Galinsky, I., Davis, T. N., Silver, S. J., Root, D. E., Stone, R. M., DeAngelo, D. J., Carroll, M., Hahn, W. C., Carr, S. A., Golub, T. R., Kung, A. L., and Stegmaier, K. (2009) Proteomic and genetic approaches identify Syk as an AML target. *Cancer Cell* 16, 281–294.
7. Rix, U., Remsing Rix, L. L., Terker, A. S., Fernbach, N. V., Hantschel, O., Planyavsky, M., Breitwieser, F. P., Herrmann, H., Colinge, J., Bennett, K. L., Augustin, M., Till, J. H., Heinrich, M. C., Valent, P., and Superti-Furga, G. (2010) A comprehensive target selectivity survey of the BCR-ABL kinase inhibitor INNO-406 by kinase profiling and chemical

proteomics in chronic myeloid leukemia cells. *Leukemia* **24**, 44–50.

8. Ha, T. K., Lee, T. G., Song, N. W., Moon, D. W., and Han, S. Y. (2008) Cation-assisted laser desorption/ionization for matrix-free surface mass spectrometry of alkanethiolate self-assembled monolayers on gold substrates and nanoparticles. *Anal. Chem.* **80**, 8526–8531.

9. Thomas, R. C., Houston, J. E., Michalske, T. A., and Crooks, R. M. (1993) The Mechanical Response of Gold Substrates Passivated by Self-Assembling Monolayer Films. *Science* **259**, 1883–1885.

Chapter 11

Kinase Inhibitor Profiling Using Chemoproteomics

Markus Schirle, Eugene C. Petrella, Scott M. Brittain, David Schwalb, Edmund Harrington, Ivan Cornella-Taracido, and John A. Tallarico

Abstract

Quantitative chemoproteomics has recently emerged as an experimental approach to determine protein interaction profiles of small molecules in a given cell line or tissue. In contrast to standard biochemical and biophysical kinase assays, application of this method to kinase inhibitors determines compound binding to endogenously expressed kinases under conditions approximating the physiological situation with regard to the molecular state of the kinase and presence of required cofactors and regulatory proteins. Using a dose-dependent, competition-based experimental design in combination with quantitative mass spectrometry approaches, such as the use of tandem mass tags (TMT) for isobaric labeling described here, allows to rank-order interactions of inhibitors to kinase by binding affinity.

Key words: Chemoproteomics, Quantitative proteomics, Target identification, Isobaric mass tags

1. Introduction

Profiling of compounds for activity or binding against protein and lipid kinases is routinely done using purified recombinant protein, which allows for tightly controlled experimental conditions (1, 2). While it is expected that such panels will cover the complete (human) kinome in the near future, correlating results to in vivo efficacy is not always straightforward (3). This is at least partially due to the fact that these results are based on inhibition of isolated, often recombinantly expressed proteins, which do not necessarily represent the cellular forms with respect to primary sequence, posttranslational modifications and lack cellular interactors required for full enzymatic activity and modulation by cellular control mechanisms. In contrast quantitative affinity proteomics-based strategies are becoming increasingly important as a means to generate testable hypotheses of compound–protein interactions for mechanism of action studies under more physiological conditions, while interrogating the full proteome in a disease-relevant cell line or tissue (4).

The conserved ATP-binding site in kinases and purine-binding proteins allows for a focused chemoproteomic strategy where a pan-kinase affinity matrix (pKAM) consisting of one or several immobilized, broad-specificity kinase inhibitors is used as the affinity tool for enrichment of kinases (5, 6). Using in-lysate competition with varying doses of free competitor (i.e., compound under investigation) prior to affinity purification, relative binding affinities can be determined by monitoring the dose-dependent reduction of kinases captured with the pKAM as measured by quantitative mass spectrometry (5, 7–9). In contrast to unbiased, i.e., not target family-focused, chemoproteomics strategies, the described approach does not require immobilization of compounds under investigation or generation of active linkable variants thereof, thus eliminating what is often the rate-limiting step in such studies. Despite the ATP-competitive nature of the pKAM components (type I inhibitors), any non-type I inhibitor that influences affinity and/or accessibility of the ATP-binding site will also give a signal in this assay. In addition, it should be noted that the described data-dependent mass spectrometry readout is by nature not limited to protein kinases but will yield quantitative information for all directly or indirectly enriched proteins, including other purine-binding proteins in the right affinity window (typically up to low µM K_D (8)) or, e.g., kinase interacting proteins.

We describe here the use of an exemplary ATP-competitive pan-kinase affinity matrix consisting of three broad specificity kinase inhibitors: Compound I, a linkable derivative of Staurosporine; Compound II, based on a published c-Src kinase inhibitor and Compound III, representing a pyrimidine diamine tyrosine kinase inhibitor scaffold (10–14) (Fig. 1a). In this example, we assessed kinase specificity and relative affinities of three further compounds (IV–VI, Fig. 1b) that originated from the same series as compound II. Each compound was used for in-lysate competition at six different concentrations (25, 2.5, 0.25, 0.025, 0.0025, and 0 µM) prior to performing 6 separate pKAM affinity enrichment experiments, protein separation by 1D SDS-PAGE, and analysis by quantitative mass spectrometry using isobaric labeling tags (Fig. 2). A 1:1 mixture of two tumor cell lines, the cervical cancer line HeLa and the chronic myelogenous leukemia line K562 was used as cellular input material, exemplifying sources rich in (activated) kinases. Ultimately, the accessibility of potential kinase targets in a given combination of input and ATP-competitive pKAM depends on a number of variables: these include binding affinities and kinetic parameters, binding site of inhibitor relative to hinge region of kinase, protein abundance, and subcellular localization. Equally important is the compatibility of cell lysate preparation methods with preservation of the binding competent state of the kinase with respect to required protein interactions, posttranslational modifications, and

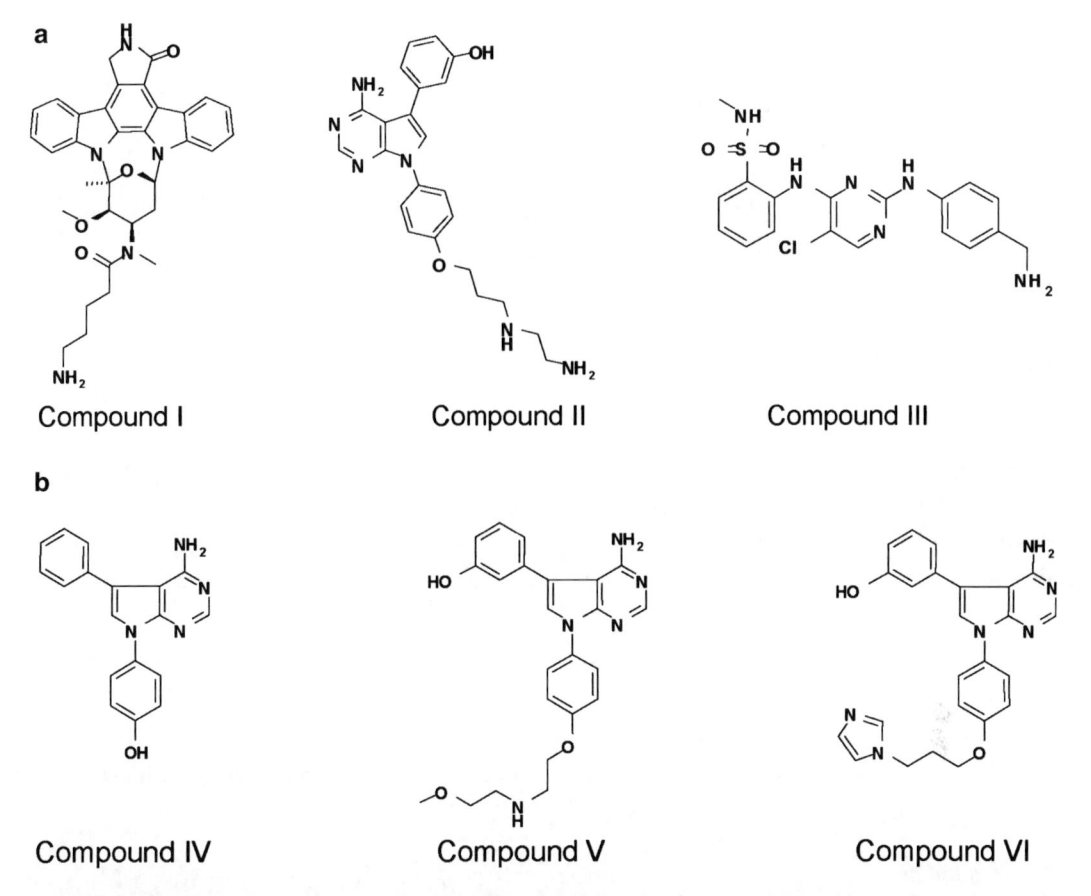

Fig. 1. (a) Components of the three-component pan-kinase affinity matrix used in this study for affinity enrichment. (b) Kinase inhibitors profiled in this study by in-lysate competition.

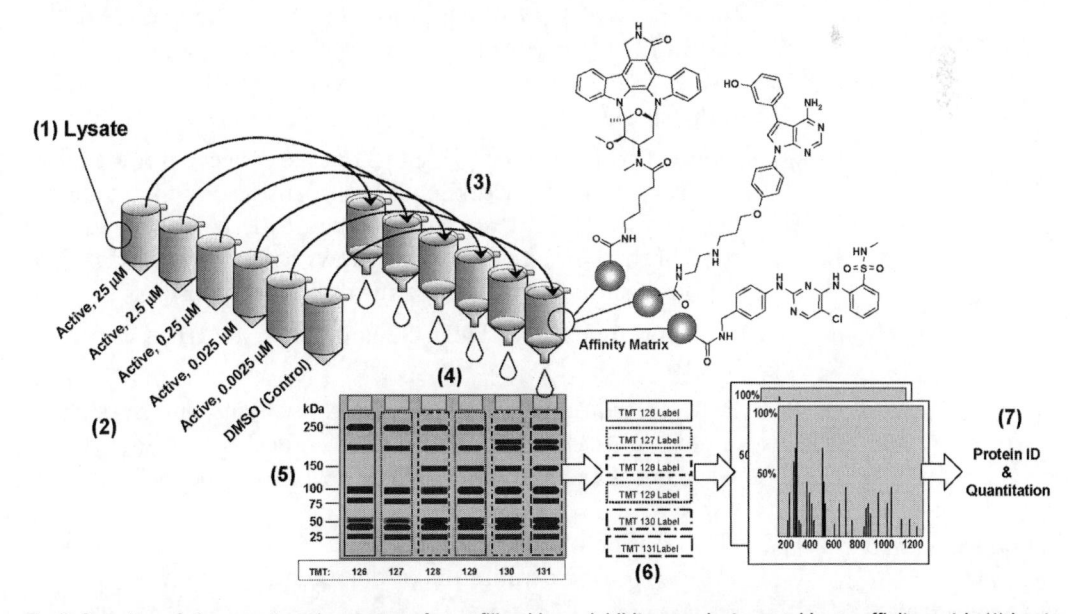

Fig. 2. Overview of chemoproteomics strategy for profiling kinase inhibitors against a pan-kinase affinity matrix (1) lysate; (2) compound *in-lysate* incubation; (3) affinity column separation; (4) protein separation by SDS-PAGE; (5) gel cutting in 16 slices per lane (not shown), in-gel digestion and TMT peptide labeling; (6) combination of digests from corresponding MW areas for nanoLC–MS/MS analysis; (7) peptide and protein identification and quantitation.

activation state. Rank ordering proteins based on the resulting affinity measurements as defined by the concentration at which 50% residual binding is observed ("RB50") has been shown to correlate by and large with reported data based on standard biochemical assays (although systematic shifts of absolute values may be observed) (5, 9).

2. Materials

2.1. Covalent Coupling of Affinity Compounds to Chromatographic Matrices

1. N-hydroxysuccinimide (NHS)-activated Sepharose™ 4 Fast Flow (GE Healthcare, Piscataway, NJ).
2. Anhydrous solvents: dimethylsulfoxide (DMSO), dimethylformamide (DMF), methanol, ethanol. Triethylamine, purity ≥ 99%; 2-aminoethanol, purity ≥ 99%.
3. Low-speed centrifuge with swinging bucket rotor, to accommodate 15-ml conical centrifuge tubes.
4. LC/MS sample vials.
5. Rotator, end-over-end, to accommodate 15 ml conical centrifuge tubes.

2.2. Preparation of Cell Lysates

1. Cell lysis buffer: 50 mM HEPES, pH 7.5, 150 mM NaCl, 1.5 mM $MgCl_2$, 1 mM Na_3VO_4. Immediately before use, add 1 mM Na_3VO_4, 25 mM NaF, 1 mM dithiothreitol (DTT), 0.8% (v/v) 2-[4-(2,4,4-trimethylpentan-2-yl)phenoxy]ethanol (CAS no. 9081-99-6, e.g., Nonidet P40 or Igepal CA-630), and an EDTA-free protease inhibitor cocktail, e.g., Complete™ EDTA-free protease inhibitor tablet (Roche Diagnostics, Indianapolis, IN).
2. Dounce homogenizer, glass, tight pestle. Select a homogenizer size such that the working cell suspension volume occupies between 30 and 50% of the volume of the narrow cylindrical tube of the homogenizer. This allows for more uniform application of shear force throughout the cell suspension.
3. Frozen cell pellets of HeLa-S3 and K562, 1×10^9 cells per cell line (see Note 1).
4. Refrigerated centrifuges: Low-speed, swinging bucket or fixed-angle, to accommodate 15 ml conical centrifuge tubes. Ultracentrifuge, fixed-angle rotor, capable of >100,000×g force.

2.3. Affinity Enrichment and Competition Experiments

1. Wash buffer I: Cell lysis buffer (see Subheading 2.2, item 1) without protease inhibitors or detergent.
2. Wash buffer II: Cell lysis buffer (see Subheading 2.2, item 1) without protease inhibitors.
3. Cell lysis buffer (see Subheading 2.2, item 1) without detergent.

4. Platform rocker.
5. Chromatography columns: Mobicol, centrifugable, 1 ml with 90-μm pore size frit and Luer-lock connector (Mobicol, MoBiTec, Göttingen, Germany).
6. Syringes: plastic disposable with Luer-lock fitting, 10 cc.
7. Heating block shaker for microcentrifuge tubes.
8. Microcentrifuge tubes, siliconized, 1.5 ml.
9. Iodoacetamide solution: 200 mg/ml in distilled deionized water (prepare freshly and protected from light).

2.4. One-Dimensional Separation of Affinity-Purified Proteins

The NuPAGE® Novex® protein gel electrophoresis system (Invitrogen Life Technologies, Carlsbad, CA) was used for the experiments described herein. Any other 1D-SDS-PAGE equipment may be used alternatively.

1. Sample buffer: 106 mM Tris–HCl, 141 mM Tris base, 2% (w/v) lithium dodecylsulfate (LDS), 10% (v/v) glycerol, 0.51 mM EDTA, 0.22 mM SERVA® Blue G250, 0.175 mM phenol red, pH 8.5 (prepared as a 4× solution).
2. Dithiothreitol (DTT): 1 M in distilled deionized water.
3. Running buffer: 50 mM MOPS, 50 mM Tris base, 0.1% (w/v) sodium dodecylsulfate (SDS), 1 mM EDTA, pH 7.7 (prepared as a 20× solution).
4. NuPAGE® antioxidant: 400× solution.
5. NuPAGE® Novex® 4–12% gradient bis–tris gels: 1.5-mm thickness, 10 wells.
6. XCell SureLock™ Mini-Cell (Invitrogen Life Technologies).
7. Unstained molecular weight standards.
8. Programmable electrophoresis power supply.
9. Microcentrifuge.
10. Gel fixing solution: 29% (v/v) Methanol, 1% (v/v) acetic acid in distilled deionized water.
11. Colloidal Blue staining kit.

2.5. Gel Cutting and In-gel Trypsinization

1. 2D iD Gel imager and cutting robot: square cutting nozzle (2 mm × 2 mm), gel-cutting tray, hydrophilic pad (Leap Technologies, Carrboro, NC).
2. Filter plate: U-bottom plate.
3. Sealing tape with 96-well pattern.
4. Pipetting robot: This method is described in combination with the Freedom EVO 200 robot equipped with vacuum block and spacers, 4-position incubator, liquid handling arm (8-tip) and trough carriers, robotic manipulator arm and fingers, purification plate, silicon preslit sealing mat, DiTi 1000-μl disposable conductive tips (Tecan, Durham, NC).

5. Destain solution: 50 mM Ammonium bicarbonate, 30% acetonitrile (v/v).
   6. Dehydration solution: 100% acetonitrile.
   7. Collection solution: 1% Formic acid–50% acetonitrile (v/v).
   8. Concentrated trypsin solution: 167 ng/μl Sequencing grade modified trypsin in 1 mM HCl.
   9. Trypsin dilution buffer: 50 mM Ammonium bicarbonate.
   10. Vacuum concentrator.

2.6. Peptide Labeling Using Isobaric Labeling Tags

   1. TMT 6plex reagent kit (Fisher Scientific).
   2. Triethylammonium bicarbonate (TEAB) solution: 100 mM in water.
   3. V-bottom 96-well plate.
   4. Heat sealer.
   5. Trifluouro acetic acid: 0.1% (v/v).

2.7. Peptide Identification and Quantitation by NanoLC–MS/MS

   1. Peptide separation column: 75 μm ID spraying capillary (In-house fabricated using a P-2000 capillary puller, Sutter Instruments, Novato, CA) packed with ReproSil-Pur 120 C18-AQ, 3 μm material (200-mm bed length, Dr. Maisch GmbH, Ammerbuch-Entringen, Germany); see Note 2 for commercially available equivalents.
   2. Kasil-fritted trapping column: 75 μm ID, packed with ReproSil-Pur 120 C18-AQ, 5 μm material (15-mm bed length) or equivalent trapping column; see Note 2 for commercially available equivalents.
   3. Liquid chromatography system: NanoLC 1D plus (Eksigent, Dublin, CA), equipped with a 10-μl loop, setup for 96-well plates (or alternative system).
   4. Mass spectrometer: LTQ-Orbitrap XL (Thermo Electron, San Jose, CA; Xcalibur 2.0.7, Tune plus 2.4 SP1 software) equipped with Picoview 550 Nanospray source (New Objective). Alternative systems may also be used.
   5. Mobile phase A: 0.1% Formic acid, 2% acetonitrile (v/v).
   6. Mobile phase B: 0.1% Formic acid, 98% acetonitrile (v/v).

2.8. Data Processing and Analysis

Other tools than the ones described may also be used.

   1. Mascot v2.2 (Matrix Science, London, UK).
   2. Transproteomic pipeline (TPP) v3.3sqall, available on the Internet from the Seattle Proteome Center at the Institute of System Biology (Seattle, WA).
   3. IPI_human v3.44 protein database (EBI, Cambridge, UK) supplemented with sequences of common nonhuman contaminants as well as reversed entries for all forward entries.

4. In-house developed software for parsing and uploading of information from TPP-derived xml files and Mascot result files to a relational database (Oracle 10g; Oracle, Redwood Shores, CA).
5. Software for curve fitting: e.g., Prism 5.

3. Methods

3.1. Covalent Coupling of Affinity Compounds to Chromatographic Matrices

1. NHS-activated Sepharose™ 4 Fast Flow is supplied as a slurry in isopropanol. Pipette the desired amount of matrix into a 15 ml graduated polypropylene centrifuge tube. Typical coupling volume is 1–2 ml packed matrix. Wash 3× with 10 ml DMSO, centrifuging at $80 \times g$ for 3 min to pellet the matrix in between washes. Resuspend in one packed matrix volume of DMSO, i.e., make a 50% slurry.

2. From a concentrated stock solution (e.g., 100 mM in DMSO or DMF), add 2 μmoles primary (or secondary) amine-containing affinity compound per ml of packed matrix. Add 40 μl triethylamine per ml of packed matrix, mix by inversion, centrifuge at $80 \times g$ for 3 min, and immediately transfer 20 μl supernatant solution to an LC/MS sampling vial containing 20 μl methanol. This sample represents a $t=0$ reaction monitoring. Set aside for final assessment of reaction completion.

3. Incubate the reaction slurry for 16 h (or overnight) at room temperature on an end-over-end rotator, protected from light.

4. Centrifuge at $80 \times g$ for 3 min. Retain 20 μl supernatant solution as in step 2 and add 50 μl 2-aminoethanol per ml packed matrix. Incubate for 16 h (or overnight) at room temperature on an end-over-end rotator, protected from light.

5. Wash matrix with 10 ml DMSO followed by 3 washes with 10 ml ethanol. Resuspend matrix in ethanol, transfer to glass vial, and store at 4°C, protected from light.

6. To assess coupling efficiency, subject $t=0$ and $t=$overnight samples obtained in steps 2 and 4 to LC/MS analysis. As a control, include an additional sample consisting of compound from the original stock solution. Typical instrumentation, column, and run parameters are Waters Micromass ZQ, Inertsil C8-3 column (3 cm × 3 mm × 3.0 μm), mobile phase: 5–95% MeCN (5 mM ammonium formate) gradient over 2 min at 2 ml/min, 3 μl injection volume. The experimenter may need to select alternative conditions to suit their particular chemistry. Coupling is deemed successful if no compound is detected in the $t=$overnight sample.

For the experiments described herein, the three matrices that were generated were combined in a 1:1:1 ratio. Each affinity enrichment utilized a total of 100 μl of this combined matrix (see Subheading 3.4, step 4).

3.2. Preparation of Lysates for Affinity Enrichment of Kinases

1. Estimate the packed cell volume (PCV) of the cells to be processed, e.g. a HeLa-S3 cell pellet containing 5×10^8 cells typically has a PCV of approximately 1.4–1.5 ml. Add two PCVs of freshly prepared cell lysis buffer and triturate to form a homogeneous cell suspension. Let stand on ice for 30 min with occasional mixing to keep cells suspended (see Note 3).

2. Transfer cell suspension to glass, tight-pestle Dounce homogenizer. Perform ten successive, even-pressured strokes, taking care to avoid foaming.

3. Transfer cells to a graduated conical polypropylene centrifuge tube. Centrifuge at $800 \times g$ for 5 min at 4°C. A swinging bucket rotor is acceptable for this step. The pellet (P0.8) includes nuclei, undisrupted cells, and some cytoskeletal components. The supernatant (S0.8), an opaque solution, is a cytoplasmic fraction containing organelles (e.g., mitochondria, endosomes, Golgi apparatus, endoplasmic reticulum, etc.).

4. Carefully remove the supernatant and centrifuge at $100,000 \times g$, 45 min at 4°C, utilizing a fixed-angle rotor. Suitable centrifuge/rotor combinations for this step are Beckman-Coulter Optima XL-100K/50.2Ti, Sorvall Discovery M150 SE/S100-AT6, or equivalent. This supernatant solution, S100 cytosol, is transparent. Often, a white-colored lipid layer will appear at the top of the liquid column. The pellet is most often small and translucent.

5. Remove the supernatant solution taking care not to aspirate the lipid layer nor disturb the pellet. Determine the total protein concentration utilizing a detergent- and reducing agent-compatible assay system, e.g., Pierce 660 nm Protein Assay. Use the S100 fraction immediately for affinity enrichments or store at −80°C.

3.3. Affinity Enrichment and Competition Experiments

Each compound concentration to be examined via in-lysate competition requires 100 μl of packed affinity matrix contacted with 25 mg protein from cell lysate. Keep lysate solutions on ice (see Notes 4 and 5).

1. Dilute the cell lysate (from Subheading 3.3, step 5) to 5 mg/ml using cell lysis buffer without detergent and adjust the detergent concentration to 0.4% (v/v). Set up the appropriate number of 25 mg aliquots in 15 ml conical polypropylene centrifuge tubes; for example, for a 6plex TMT experiment, set up six aliquots.

2. Add competition compound from a 1,000× DMSO stock to each aliquot while keeping the DMSO volume added constant, e.g., add 5 μl of 10, 1, and 0.1 mM stocks to achieve final

compound concentrations of 10, 1, and 0.1 µM, respectively. Include a vehicle (DMSO) control. Incubate for 1 h on ice.

3. Pipette appropriate amount of affinity matrix slurry into a 15 ml conical polypropylene centrifuge tube and wash twice with wash buffer I followed by one wash with wash buffer II. Resuspend matrix in one volume of wash buffer II.

4. Divide washed matrix into appropriate number of 100 µl (packed matrix volume) aliquots into individual 15 ml centrifuge tubes.

5. At the end of 1 h incubation period (step 2), add compound/lysate mixtures to individual matrix aliquots.

6. Incubate for 4 h to overnight with gentle rocking at 4°C.

7. Pellet matrix by centrifugation, remove majority of protein solution leaving behind enough solution to efficiently transfer matrix slurries to chromatography columns. Transfer slurries to individual Mobicol columns (with bottom plugs in place) mounted vertically. Mount 10 cc syringe (with plunger removed) to each column. Perform all chromatography in a cold room, 4–8°C.

8. To prevent air lock, add 1 ml wash buffer II to occupy dead volume space between matrix and bottom of syringe barrel. It may be necessary to use a syringe plunger to purge trapped air. Add an additional 9 ml wash buffer II, remove bottom column plug, and allow buffer to flow through the matrix. Add 5 ml wash buffer I, allow to flow through, and use syringe plunger to expel remaining buffer. Plug bottom of column and disconnect from syringe.

9. Place column in 1.5 ml siliconized microcentrifuge tube. Add 60 µl 2× sample buffer containing 10 mM DTT, mix, and incubate for 30 min at 55°C.

10. Carefully remove bottom plug and pulse centrifuge to expel sample into microcentrifuge tube. The volume of sample retrieved is typically about 50 µl.

11. To alkylate cysteine sulfhydryls, add 5.5 µl of 200 mg/ml iodoacetamide solution per 50 µl sample. Vortex and incubate for 30 min at room temperature, protected from light.

3.4. One-Dimensional Separation of Affinity-Purified Proteins

1. Centrifuge sample 14,000×g for 5 min. Assemble 4–12% gradient bis–tris gel(s) into electrophoresis cell. Fill outer chamber with running buffer and inner chamber with running buffer containing antioxidant (0.5 ml stock per 200 ml running buffer). Load 45 µl sample per gel lane in alternating wells. Load 4 µl of marker protein standards in remaining wells. Electrophorese at 200 V (constant) until dye front reaches 2–3 cm from bottom (approximately 45 min).

2. Place gel(s) in gel fixing solution for 1 h at room temperature with gentle shaking. Stain gel(s) with colloidal coomassie blue for 3–16 h. Destain with at least 200 ml deionized water. Gel will completely destain within 7 h.

Figure 3 shows the resulting three gels for the three separate dose–response experiments for compound IV, V and VI using 100 μl of the pKAM consisting of compounds I–III for each of the 3× 6 pulldown experiments.

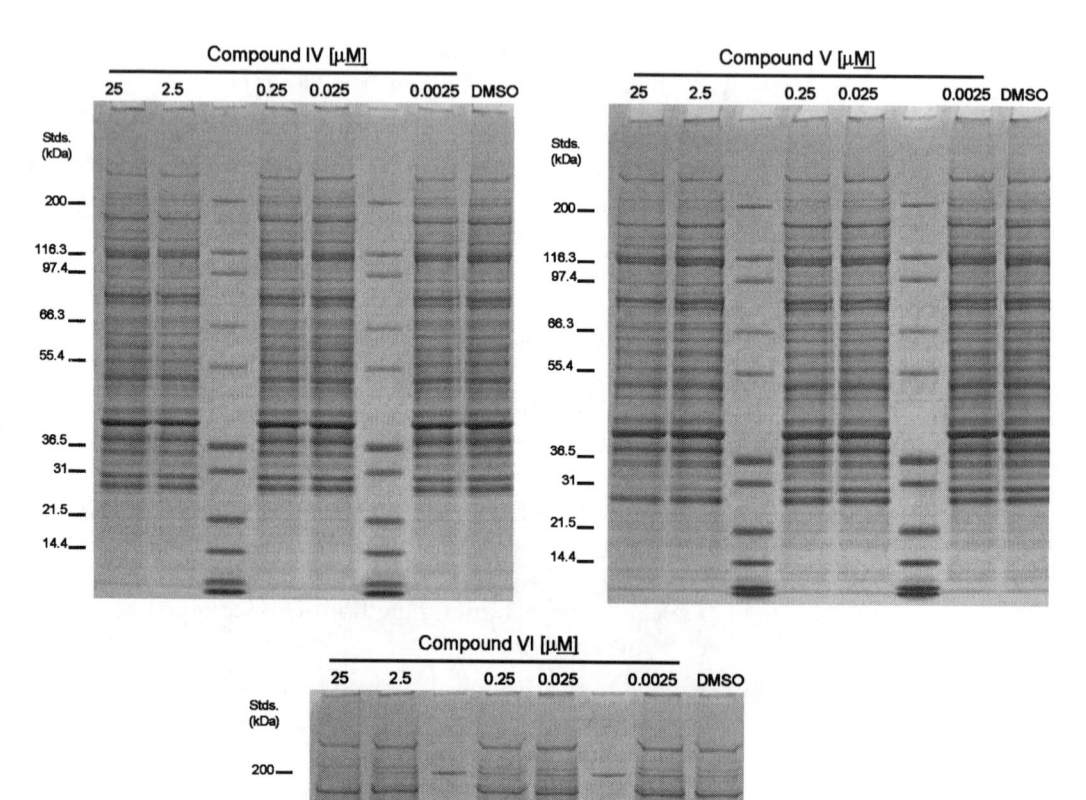

Fig. 3. Separation of affinity-enriched proteins after in-lysate competition with free compound by 1D SDS-PAGE. Each competition compound was used in separate pulldown experiments at 25, 2.5, 0.25, 0.025, 0.0025, and 0 μM, resulting in 6 pulldowns and subsequent gel separation per compound. Molecular weight markers are run in remaining lanes for orientation during gel cutting process.

3.5. Gel Cutting and In-gel Digestion

1. Moisten the hydrophilic pad in the gel cutting tray with ultrapure water, place the gel carefully in the center of the pad and secure pad with pins (see Notes 6 and 7).

2. Place a filter plate inside a U-bottom plate, secure a silicon preslit sealing mat onto the filter plate using four standard binder clips and secure the assembly in one of the positions of the robot with adhesive tape.

3. Using the 2DiD camera and software, acquire a gel picture and generate a 1D spots cutting list covering the complete lane, resulting typically per lane in 32 rows of 3 spots. Combine two consecutive rows to position 6 gel plugs in each of the 16 destination wells per lane, resulting in 96 wells in a 6plex experiment.

4. Check that gel plugs are located at the well bottom, replace silicon preslit sealing mat with a sealing tape for storage or proceed to digestion.

5. Fix filter plate covered with sealing mat in the metal purification plate for robotic handling and perform the following steps for each well on the Freedom EVO 200 robot: Destaining (3 cycles: 100 µl destain solution, 30 min, 26°C), dehydration (2 cycles: 100 µl acetonitrile, 30 min, 26°C), trypsinization (20 µl concentrated trypsin solution diluted to 10 ng/ml with trypsin dilution solution just prior to addition, incubate for 8–10 h at 37°C) and finally peptide extraction and collection of peptide digests in a total volume of 150 µl in a U-bottom plate using the vacuum block (2 cycles: 50 µl collection solution, 2 min, 20°C; 1 cycle: 50 µl dehydration solution, 20 min, 26°C) (see Note 8).

6. Evaporate to dryness in the vacuum concentrator.

3.6. Peptide Labeling Using Isobaric Labeling Tags

1. Using a different TMT reagent for each lane with 126 for highest concentration of competitor and 131 for vehicle control, allow 2 vials of each TMT reagent to come to room temperature, add 85 µl of acetonitrile to each vial, vortex several times for 30–60 s over a 5- to 10-min period (see Note 9).

2. Dissolve samples in 15 µl of 100 mM TEAB solution and shake for 10 min at 20°C and 400 rpm.

3. Add 10 µl TMT reagent to each sample, shake for 1 h at 20°C at 400 rpm, and evaporate to dryness.

4. Add 25 µl of collection solution to samples and pool corresponding samples from each lane, aspirating up and down several times before each transfer.

5. Reconstitute samples in 20 µl 0.1% trifluoroacetic acid and transfer to a V-bottom plate, then repeat and evaporate to dryness.

6. Seal the plate using the heat sealer and heat seal foil (see Note 10).

3.7. Peptide Identification and Quantitation by NanoLC–MS/MS

1. Reconstitute sample and load 8 μl of sample on the trapping column using Mobile Phase A with a flow rate of 2.5 μl/min. Eluting peptides from the trapping column in the same direction, analyze sample using a 120-min gradient elution (3% acetonitrile for 5 min, 3–28% acetonitrile in 97 min, 28–75% acetonitrile in 4 min, 3% acetonitrile for 16 min) at a flowrate of 250 nl/min and direct spraying of the eluent into the mass spectrometer (see Note 11).

2. The LTQ-Orbitrap XL mass spectrometer is operated in data-dependent mode with concurrent acquisition of full scan MS in the Orbitrap and sequential MS/MS in the linear ion trap of the five most intense ions within a mass-to-charge ratio (m/z) range of 300–1,500. Further criteria for ions to be selected for MS/MS are charge state z of 2–4, a minimum intensity of 1,500 counts, and a typical exclusion time of 30 s (repeat count 1) for ions to be selected again for MS/MS. Fragmentation in the linear ion trap is done using Pulsed-Q-dissociation (PQD) to allow for detection of TMT reporter ions (typical settings: $q=0.7$, activation time = 0.1 ms, nCE = 32; see Note 12), using the following scan parameters: 2 microscans; "target value" 50,000 ions; maximum accumulation time 1,000 ms; isolation width 2 m/z. For high accuracy m/z determination of intact peptides in survey scans, the Orbitrap is operated at 30,000 resolution (R) at $m/z=400$ using a "target value" for accumulation in the linear ion trap of 1,000,000 ions. Spray voltage is set to 3 kV, heated capillary temperature is 170°C and no sheath or auxiliary gas flow is applied.

3.8. Data Processing and Analysis

1. Conversion of Xcalibur Rawfiles to Mascot-compatible mgf-files as well as subsequent generation of mzXML, pepXML, protXML, and Interact files is done using the corresponding TPP-modules.

2. Mgf-files are searched using Mascot with 10 ppm tolerance for precursor ions and 0.8 Da tolerance for fragment ions. Carbamidomethylation of cysteine is set as fixed modification, S, T, Y phosphorylation, methionine oxidation, and TMT-modification of N-termini and lysine residues are set as variable modifications.

3. Data validation of peptide and protein identifications is done at the level of the complete dataset consisting of combined Mascot search results for all 16 samples per experiment via the PeptideProphet and ProteinProphet modules in TPP using the decoy database function and a peptide probability threshold of 0.

4. TPP output (Interact) files containing peptide and protein information and corresponding TMT reporter ion peak intensity information for each peptide–to-spectrum match (as parsed

from the Mascot result files) are uploaded to Oracle using in-house software (see Note 13).

5. For each peptide sequence and modification state, reporter ion signal intensities from all spectral matches are summed for each reporter ion type to account for lower precision of reporter ion ratios at low absolute signal intensities and potential variations in protein migration across the gel and gel processing. Summed intensities are corrected according to the isotope correction factors given by the manufacturer for each batch of TMT reagent to account for isotope impurities. Only peptide-to-spectrum matches that are unique assignments to a given identified protein within the total dataset are considered for protein quantitation.

6. Proteins are reported based on protein probability cut-off values based on a false-positive prediction of <1% by ProteinProphet.

7. For each concentration of competitor compound, raw peptide fold changes over vehicle (DMSO) are calculated and subsequently renormalized using the median fold change of all quantified peptides to compensate for differences in total protein yield for each affinity purification. Protein fold changes over control are derived as median peptide fold change per protein and curve fitting in Prism 5 is used for determination of compound concentrations where 50% residual binding is observed (unconstrained four-parameter dose–response curve: $Y = \text{Bottom} + (\text{Top} - \text{Bottom})/(1 + 10((\text{LogIC50} - X) \times \text{HillSlope}))$ where Y is set to 50% and X is the Log of the RB50 concentration). Values in Fig. 4a are reported for proteins with at least four unique peptide-to-spectrum matches (see Note 14). Figure 4b shows dose–response curves for selected kinases.

4. Notes

1. For the experiments described herein, frozen cell pellets (HeLa-S3 and K-562) were obtained from a contract research organization. Both of these cell lines grow in suspension culture and as such can be scaled up readily by the investigator if required (see Subheading 2.2).

2. Commercially available alternatives we have used successfully are PicoFrit spraying capillaries (75 μm ID, 10 μm tip ID, packed, for example, with ProteoPep 5 μm material, 100 mm bed) and IntegraFrit sample trap inserts (75–150 μm ID packed, for example, with ProteoPep 5 μm material) for use with a trap cartridge assembly (all New Objective, Woburn, MA) (see Subheading 2.7).

a

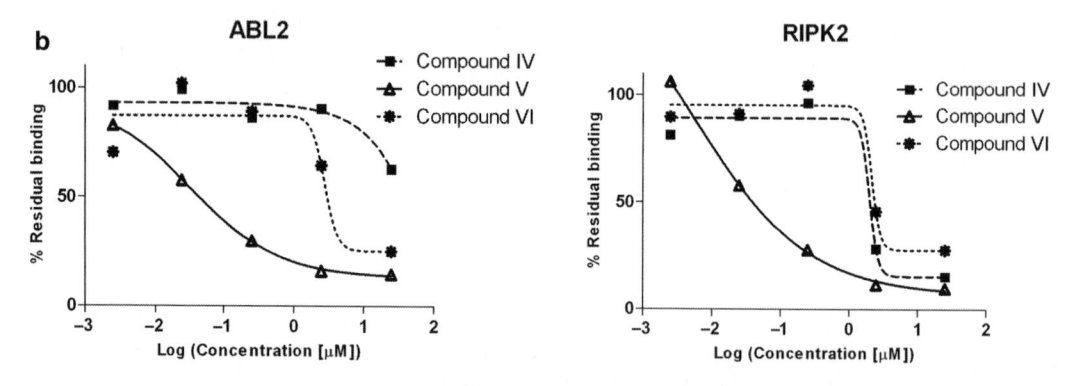

Kinase	RB50 Compound IV [µM]	RB50 Compound V [µM]	RB50 Compound VI [µM]	Kinase	RB50 Compound IV [µM]	RB50 Compound V [µM]	RB50 Compound VI [µM]
AAK1	>25	>25	>25	LOK	2.60	>25	>25
ABL1	>25	0.05	2.54	LYN	>25	0.23	>25
ABL2	>25	0.05	2.56	MAP2K1	>25	2.65	>25
ALK2	>25	0.05	>25	MAP2K3	>25	>25	>25
AMPKa1	>25	>25	>25	MAP2K6	>25	>25	>25
AMPKa2	>25	>25	>25	MAP3K1	>25	>25	>25
AurA	>25	>25	>25	MAP3K2	>25	>25	>25
AurB	>25	>25	>25	MAP3K5	>25	>25	>25
AurC	>25	>25	>25	MAP3K5	>25	>25	>25
BCR	>25	0.06	2.51	MAP3K6	>25	>25	>25
BIKE	>25	>25	>25	MARK3	>25	>25	>25
BMPR1A	2.76	0.26	9.42	MELK	>25	2.62	>25
BRK	2.72	2.49	6.86	MET	>25	>25	>25
BTK	>25	>25	>25	MPSK1	>25	>25	>25
CaMKK1	>25	>25	>25	MSK2	>25	>25	>25
CaMKK2	>25	>25	>25	MST1	>25	>25	>25
CDC2	>25	>25	>25	MST2	>25	>25	>25
CDK2	>25	>25	>25	NEK2	>25	>25	>25
CDK5	>25	>25	>25	NEK6	>25	>25	>25
CDK7	>25	4.77	>25	NEK9	>25	>25	>25
CDK9	>25	2.66	>25	PAK4	>25	>25	>25
CHK1	>25	>25	>25	PCTAIRE1	>25	>25	>25
CK1a	2.54	0.02	2.73	PDK1	>25	>25	>25
CK2a1	>25	>25	>25	PIM1	>25	>25	>25
CK2a2	>25	>25	>25	PKCb	>25	>25	>25
CRIK	>25	0.22	2.77	PKD2	>25	>25	>25
CRK7	>25	>25	>25	PKD3	>25	>25	>25
DDR1	>25	2.01	>25	PKN1	>25	>25	>25
DNAPK	>25	>25	>25	PKN2	>25	>25	>25
EGFR	>25	0.11	>25	PLK4	>25	>25	>25
EphA2	>25	1.60	4.38	PRPK	>25	0.40	2.50
EphB4	>25	0.03	2.45	PYK2	>25	>25	>25
Erk1	>25	>25	>25	RIPK2	2.34	0.03	2.47
Erk2	>25	>25	>25	RSK2	>25	>25	>25
FAK	>25	>25	>25	RSK3	>25	19.70	>25
FER	>25	>25	>25	SLK	>25	>25	>25
FRAP	>25	>25	>25	SRC	>25	0.06	>25
FYN	>25	0.07	>25	STK33	>25	>25	>25
GAK	5.85	0.03	2.12	TAO3	>25	>25	>25
GSK3A	>25	>25	>25	TBK1	>25	>25	>25
GSK3B	>25	>25	>25	TEC	>25	>25	>25
IGF1R	>25	>25	>25	TGFbR1	>25	0.29	16.90
INSR	>25	>25	>25	TNK1	>25	>25	>25
IRAK4	>25	>25	>25	TRKA	>25	>25	>25
JAK1	>25	>25	>25	TYK2	>25	>25	>25
JAK2	>25	>25	>25	ULK3	>25	>25	>25
JNK1	>25	>25	>25	Wee1	>25	2.51	>25
JNK2	>25	>25	>25	YES	>25	0.05	2.80
KHS1	>25	>25	>25				

Fig. 4. (**a**) Table of kinases quantified with ≥4 spectra for unique peptide assignments in all three experiments and determined concentrations of free compound at which 50% residual binding was observed (RB50). *Black*: RB50 < 0.25 µM; *dark gray*: RB50 < 2.5 µM; *light gray*: RB50 < 25 µM. (**b**) Dose–response curves for selected kinases.

3. Although we routinely affinity enrich a number of membrane-associated kinases (e.g., receptor tyrosine kinases), the reader should note that this lysate preparation is ideally suited for cytosolic proteins. To obtain sufficient protein to conduct the

number of experiments described herein, start with 1×10^9 of each cell line (see Subheading 3.2).

4. It is essential to keep all solutions, cell suspensions, and lysates ice-cold for the duration of this procedure. Use precooled buffers and equipment. Perform all centrifugations at 4°C using precooled rotors (see Subheading 3.3).

5. Keratins from hair and skin are frequent contaminants in mass spec samples. Use gloves, tie back hair, and wear full-length lab coat during all following procedures and sample handling. Use fresh buffers whenever possible (see Subheading 3.3).

6. Gel cutting can be done manually in a clean environment such as a clean bench with a standard scalpel using a gel illumination box and a shield (as used in work with radioactivity) to minimize keratin contamination during the cutting process. Slicing all excised gel bands into smaller pieces (~3-mm side length) will ensure constant digestion/extraction efficiencies (see Subheading 3.5).

7. When handling gradient gels, grasp bottom portion of gel which is less prone to ripping; keep gel well moisturized during cutting process (see Subheading 3.5).

8. All robotic liquid steps, especially when involving vacuum steps in combination with solutions of varying viscosity, have to be optimized carefully to minimize cross-contamination due to spraying. Coloring solutions with food coloring can be used for visualization during test runs. Plotting molecular weight of identified proteins over sample will identify cross-contamination in adjacent wells (see Subheading 3.5).

9. If low labeling efficiencies are observed (<95%), check that lyophilized TMT reagents are fully solubilized and the pH is ~8 throughout the reaction. We have found that a quenching step by adding glycine in 100 mM TEAB or 8 μl 5% hydroxylamine in 20 mM TEAB as suggested by the manufacturer is optional but can help if, for example, high levels of side reactions (e.g., tyrosine modification) are observed (see Subheading 3.6).

10. Give sealed plates a final spin (~500 rpm) to remove air bubbles and ensure proper location of sample in well (see Subheading 3.6).

11. In order to prevent sample losses, we routinely omit the cation exchange chromatography step recommended by the manufacturer for sample cleanup. In order to minimize ions suppression from label-derived background, it is crucial to wash samples extensively after loading on the trapping column (e.g., 5–10 trapping column volumes) (see Subheading 3.7).

12. PQD settings have been found to vary considerably between instruments and need to be optimized by scanning activation

time and normalized collision energy one at a time for one or more labeled peptide standards to achieve optimal absolute and relative response for fragment ions spanning the total m/z range (reporter ions as well as low/high mass backbone fragments) (15) (see Subheading 3.7).

13. In Xcalibur, raw signal intensities are normalized by accumulation time; denormalization of intensities can be achieved by accessing accumulation time values per spectrum via the Xcalibur Developers kit (see Subheading 3.8).

14. Data-dependent analyses for a given pKAM and input material can be supplemented using, for example, high mass accuracy, inclusion-list based targeted analyses (16) to increase identification confidence and accuracy of quantitation for low-level kinases (see Subheading 3.8).

Acknowledgments

We thank Heather Contant and Lindsay Nolitt for expert technical assistance and John Damask and Ioannis Moutsatsos for their crucial role in building the data processing and analysis environment.

References

1. Fabian, M. A., Biggs, W. H., III, Treiber, D. K., Atteridge, C. E., Azimioara, M. D., Benedetti, M. G., Carter, T. A., Ciceri, P., Edeen, P. T., Floyd, M., Ford, J. M., Galvin, M., Gerlach, J. L., Grotzfeld, R. M., Herrgard, S., Insko, D. E., Insko, M. A., Lai, A. G., Lelias, J. M., Mehta, S. A., Milanov, Z. V., Velasco, A. M., Wodicka, L. M., Patel, H. K., Zarrinkar, P. P., and Lockhart, D. J. (2005) A small molecule-kinase interaction map for clinical kinase inhibitors. *Nat.Biotechnol.* **23**, 329–336.

2. Vesely, J., Havlicek, L., Strnad, M., Blow, J. J., Donella-Deana, A., Pinna, L., Letham, D. S., Kato, J., Detivaud, L., and Leclerc, S. (1994) Inhibition of cyclin-dependent kinases by purine analogues. *Eur.J. Biochem.* **224**, 771–786.

3. Hall, S. E. (2006) Chemoproteomics-driven drug discovery: addressing high attrition rates. *Drug Discovery Today* **11**, 495–502.

4. Rix, U. and Superti-Furga, G. (2009) Target profiling of small molecules by chemical proteomics. *Nat. Chem. Biol.* **5**, 616–624.

5. Bantscheff, M., Eberhard, D., Abraham, Y., Bastuck, S., Boesche, M., Hobson, S., Mathieson, T., Perrin, J., Raida, M., Rau, C., Reader, V., Sweetman, G., Bauer, A., Bouwmeester, T., Hopf, C., Kruse, U., Neubauer, G., Ramsden, N., Rick, J., Kuster, B., and Drewes, G. (2007) Quantitative chemical proteomics reveals mechanisms of action of clinical ABL kinase inhibitors. *Nat. Biotechnol.* **25**, 1035–1044.

6. Oppermann, F. S., Gnad, F., Olsen, J. V., Hornberger, R., Greff, Z., Keri, G., Mann, M., and Daub, H. (2009) Large-scale proteomics analysis of the human kinome. *Mol.Cell Proteomics.* **8**, 1751–1764.

7. Graves, P. R., Kwiek, J. J., Fadden, P., Ray, R., Hardeman, K., Coley, A. M., Foley, M., and Haystead, T. A. (2002) Discovery of novel targets of quinoline drugs in the human purine binding proteome. *Mol.Pharmacol.* **62**, 1364–1372.

8. Ong, S. E., Schenone, M., Margolin, A. A., Li, X. Y., Do, K., Doud, M. K., Mani, D. R., Kuai, L., Wang, X., Wood, J. L., Tolliday, N. J., Koehler, A. N., Marcaurelle, L. A., Golub, T. R., Gould, R. J., Schreiber, S. L., and Carr, S. A. (2009) Identifying the proteins to which small-molecule probes and drugs bind in cells. *Proc. Natl. Acad. Sci. USA* **106**, 4617–4622.

9. Sharma, K., Weber, C., Bairlein, M., Greff, Z., Keri, G., Cox, J., Olsen, J. V., and Daub, H. (2009) Proteomics strategy for quantitative protein interaction profiling in cell extracts. *Nat. Methods* **6**, 741–744.

10. Garcia-Echeverria, C., Kanazawa, T., Kawahara, E., Masuya, K., Matsuura, N., Miyake, T., Ohmori, O., and Umemura, I. (2004) Preparation of novel 2,4-di(phenylamino) pyrimidines useful in the treatment of neoplastic diseases, inflammatory and immune system disorders. *PCT Int. Appl.* WO2004080980 A1 20040923.

11. Baenteli, R., Zenke, G., Cooke, N. G., Duthaler, R., Thoma, G., Von Matt, A., Honda, T., Matsuura, N., Nonomura, K., Ohmori, O., Umemura, I., Hinterding, K., and Papageorgiou, C. (2003) Pyrimidine derivatives. *PCT Int. Appl.* WO 2003078404 A1 20030925.

12. Duthaler, R., Gerspacher, M., Holzer, P., Streiff, M., Thoma, G., Waelchli, R., and Zerwes, HG. (2007) Preparation of 2,4-di(arylamino)-pyrimidine-5-carboxamides as JAK kinases inhibitors. *PCT Int. Appl.* WO 2008009458 A1 20080124.

13. Garcia-Echeverria, C., Kanazawa, T., Kawahara, E., Masuya, K., Matsuura, N., Miyake, T., Ohmori, O., Umemura, I., Steensma, R., Chopiuk, G., Jiang, J., Wan, Y., Zhang, Q., Gray, N. S., and Karanewsky, D. (2004) Preparation of 2,4-pyrimidinediamines useful in the treatment of neoplastic diseases, inflammatory and immune system disorders. *PCT Int. Appl.* WO2005016894 A1 20050224.

14. Argade, A., Singh, R., Li, H., Carroll, D., and Catalano, S. (2004) 2,4-pyrimidinediamine compounds and uses as antiproliferative agents. *PCT Int. Appl.* WO 2005013996 A2 20050217.

15. Bantscheff, M., Boesche, M., Eberhard, D., Matthieson, T., Sweetman, G., and Kuster, B. (2008) Robust and sensitive iTRAQ quantification on an LTQ Orbitrap mass spectrometer. *Mol. Cell Proteomics.* **7**, 1702–1713.

16. Jaffe, J. D., Keshishian, H., Chang, B., Addona, T. A., Gillette, M. A., and Carr, S. A. (2008) Accurate inclusion mass screening: a bridge from unbiased discovery to targeted assay development for biomarker verification. *Mol. Cell Proteomics.* **7**, 1952–1962.

Chapter 12

Covalent Cross-Linking of Kinases with Their Corresponding Peptide Substrates

Alexander V. Statsuk and Kevan M. Shokat

Abstract

Protein phosphorylation represents the most dominant and evolutionary conserved posttranslational modification for information transfer in cells and organisms. The human genome encodes >500 protein kinases, and thousands of phosphorylation sites are present in mammalian proteome. To develop a global view of phosphorylation network, there is a need to map the connectivity between kinases and phosphoproteome. We developed a chemical kinase–substrate cross-linker 1 that converts transient kinase–substrate interactions into a covalently linked kinase–substrate complex in vitro and in the presence of cell lysates. The method can be applied to identify unknown upstream kinases responsible for phosphorylation events in cell lysates.

Key words: Kinase, Substrate, Kinase inhibitor, Thiophene-2,3-dialdehyde, Covalent cross-link

1. Introduction

The human genome encodes more than 500 kinases, and thousands of protein phosphorylation sites have been identified. Given the spacial and temporal regulation of protein phosphorylation, mapping the connectivity between kinases and the phosphoproteome represents a daunting task. To this end, we and others have developed methods that enable the identification of protein kinase substrates (1–8). The inverse problem, however, that is identification of unknown kinases responsible for known phosphorylation events, has proven to be much more challenging. Examples of phosphorylation sites with unknown upstream kinases include the following: Ser-170 of the protein BAD which enhances its antiapoptotic activity (9), Ser-497 of the natriuretic peptide receptor, which is responsible for desensitization of the receptor's antihypertensive activity (10), and Ser-325 of the tumor suppressor LKB1, which is phosphorylated in response to the biguanide antidiabetic agent metformin (11, 12). These examples, as well as the thousands of other phosphorylation sites in the mammalian proteome (13), highlight the need to develop new tools for mapping phosphorylation networks. We have previously reported that Akt1 kinase and cysteine-containing fluorescent substrate peptide can be covalently cross-linked by an adenosine-based o-phthaldialdehyde reagent in vitro shown in Fig. 1 (14). However, the initially developed adenosine based o-phthaldialdehyde reagent failed to cross-link the kinase with the cysteine-containing fluorescent substrate peptide in the presence of cell lysate. To improve the selectivity of the cross-linker, we replaced the weak, kinase-binding adenosine moiety with a promiscuous kinase inhibitor scaffold, and replaced the highly reactive o-phthaldialdehyde moiety with the less-reactive

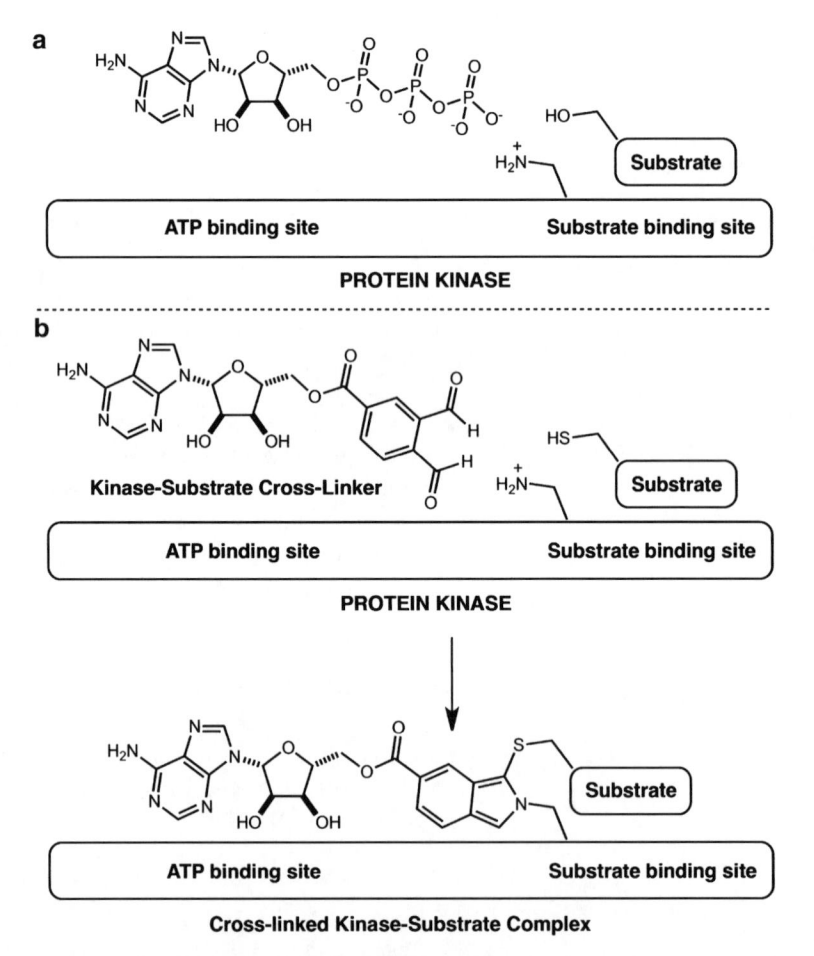

Fig. 1. Kinase–substrate cross-linking strategy. (a) Phosphorylation of the protein substrate by an upstream kinase. (b) The serine of the kinase is replaced with a reactive cysteine moiety that facilitates kinase–substrate cross-link by cross-linker.

thiophene-2,3-dialdehyde fragment. The combination of those two structural modifications that we describe in this chapter led to the development of a new reagent **1** capable of cross-linking Akt1 kinase with its substrate peptide **2** (Fluorescein-ZZRPRTSCF-OH, Z = 6-aminohexanoic acid) both in vitro and in the presence of competing cellular lysate proteins (15).

2. Materials

2.1. Synthesis of Cross-Linker 1

1. 2,4-Dichloropyrimidine: ≥98% purity.
2. 3-Cyclopropyl-1H-pyrazol-5-amine.
3. *p*-Phenylenediamine: ≥97% purity.
4. 2,3-Thiophenedicarboxaldehyde.
5. Ethylene glycol: ≥99% purity.
6. *n*-Butyllithium: 2.5 M solution in hexane.
7. *N,N*-Dimethyl formamide (DMF): anhydrous.
8. Sodium cyanoborohydride: 95% purity.
9. Trifluoroacetic acid (TFA): 98% purity.
10. Benzene: ≥99% purity.
11. Tetrahydrofuran (THF): anhydrous, ≥99.9% purity, inhibitor free.
12. Methanol: ≥99% purity.
13. Acetonitrile: ≥99.9% purity.

2.2. Synthesis of Akt1 Substrate Peptide Fluorescein-ZZRPRTSCF-OH, 2

1. Fmoc-Phe-Wang resin: 100–200 mesh.
2. Fmoc-Cys(Trt)-OH.
3. Fmoc-Ser(tBu)-OH.
4. Fmoc-Thr(tBu)-OH.
5. Fmoc-Arg(Pbf)-OH.
6. Fmoc-e-Ahx-OH.
7. 5-Carboxyfluorescein.
8. 2-(1H-benzotriazol-1-yl)-1,1,3,3-tetramethyluronium-hexafluorophosphat (HBTU).
9. *N,N*-Diisopropylethylamine.

2.3. Reagents and Equipment for Cross-Linking Experiments

1. Recombinant active Akt1/PKBα.
2. Fluorescein-ZZRPRTSCF-OH (Z = 6-aminohexanoic acid, peptide is prepared via solid phase synthesis).
3. Cross-linker **1** (prepared via synthesis).

4. Flourescent imager: e.g., Typhoon 9400, variable mode imager, 490 nm excitation band, 520 nm emission band.

5. Buffer for kinase–substrate cross-linking experiments: 25 mM (4-(2-hydroxyethyl)-1-piperazineethanesulfonic acid (HEPES)), pH 6.5, 150 mM NaCl, 2 mM $MgCl_2$, 1 mM β-mercaptoethanol.

2.4. SDS-Polyacrylamide Gel Electrophoresis

1. Running buffer (1×): 0.025 M Tris base, 0.19 M Glycine, 0.004 M SDS, pH 8.5.

2. Polyacrylamide gel: 12% acrylamide, Tris–HCl, 50-μL well, 10 wells.

3. Prestained molecular-weight markers.

4. Laemmli loading buffer (5×): 1.5 g SDS, 3.75 mL of 1 M tris(hydroxymethyl)aminomethane (Tris–HCl) pH 6.8, 0.015 g of bromophenol blue, 1.16 g of DTT, 7.5 mL of water, and 7.5 mL of glycerol.

2.5. Equipment for Chromatographic Purifications

An automated chromatography purification system (Intellyflash 280) was used throughout our experiments to purify chemical intermediates. Alternatively, any other such device or regular glass chromatography columns may be used for chromatographic purifications.

3. Methods

The covalent cross-linking reaction of Akt1 kinase with the fluorescently labeled cysteine-containing substrate peptide is very rapid and is generally completed within 20 min at room temperature. The extent of the cross-linking reaction can be monitored by visualizing the covalently cross-linked fluorescent kinase–substrate complex by direct in-gel fluorescence scanning. Our studies indicate that pH < 7 is optimal for the cross-linking reaction (see Fig. 2a). The cross-linking reaction of Akt1 kinase with the cysteine-containing substrate peptide is resistant toward competing external sulfur nucleophiles, tolerating up to 1,000-fold excess of β-mercaptoethanol relative to Akt1 substrate peptide 2 (see Fig. 2b). Boiling the cross-linked Akt1-peptide substrate complex induces its decomposition, thus it is not recommended to boil samples containing covalently cross-linked kinase–substrate complex prior to loading on polyacrylamide gel (see Fig. 1c). The kinase–substrate cross-linker 1 should always be added at the very last step to the reaction mixture. Cross-linker 1 cross-linked Akt1 kinase with the fluorescent, cysteine-containing substrate peptide in the presence of HeLa cell lysates (see Fig. 3).

12 Covalent Cross-Linking of Kinases with Their Corresponding Peptide Substrates 183

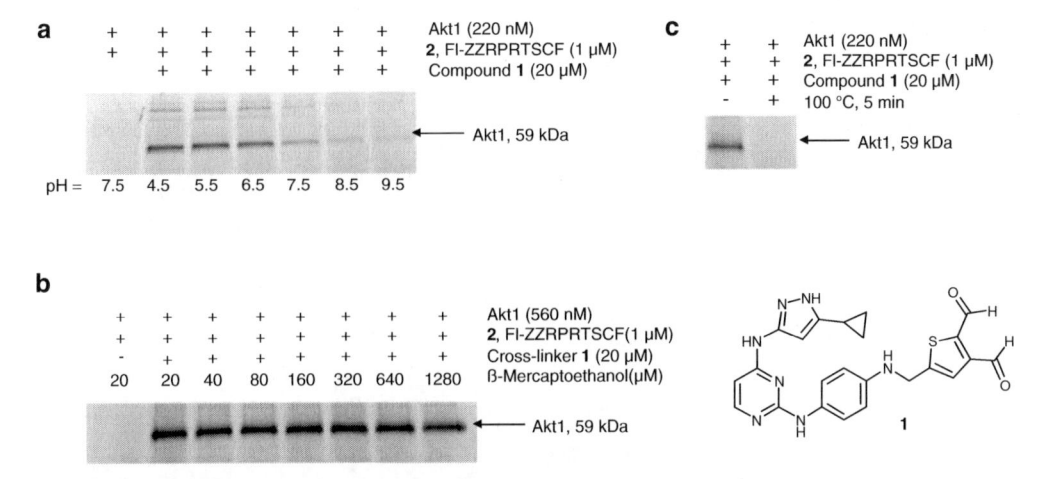

Fig. 2. Cross-linking of kinase Akt and a model peptide substrate 2. (**a**) Cross-linking of Akt1 and fluorescent substrate peptide Fl-ZZRPRTSCF-OH (2) with cross-linker 1 at different pH values. Akt1 (220 nM) and fluorescent peptide 2 (1 μM) are treated with cross-linker 1 (20 μM) for 20 min at r.t. at different pH values, followed by SDS-PAGE and in-gel scanning fluorescence. (**b**) Akt1 (560 nM) and fluorescent peptide 2 (1 μM) were treated with cross-linker 1 (20 μM) for 20 min at r.t. in the presence of increasing concentrations of β-mercaptoethanol, followed by SDS-PAGE and in-gel fluorescence scanning. (**c**) Decomposition of the cross-linked product upon heating. Akt1 (220 nM) and fluorescent peptide 2 (1 μM) were treated with cross-linker 1 (20 μM) for 20 min at r.t., then boiled for 5 min, followed by SDS-PAGE and in-gel scanning fluorescence.

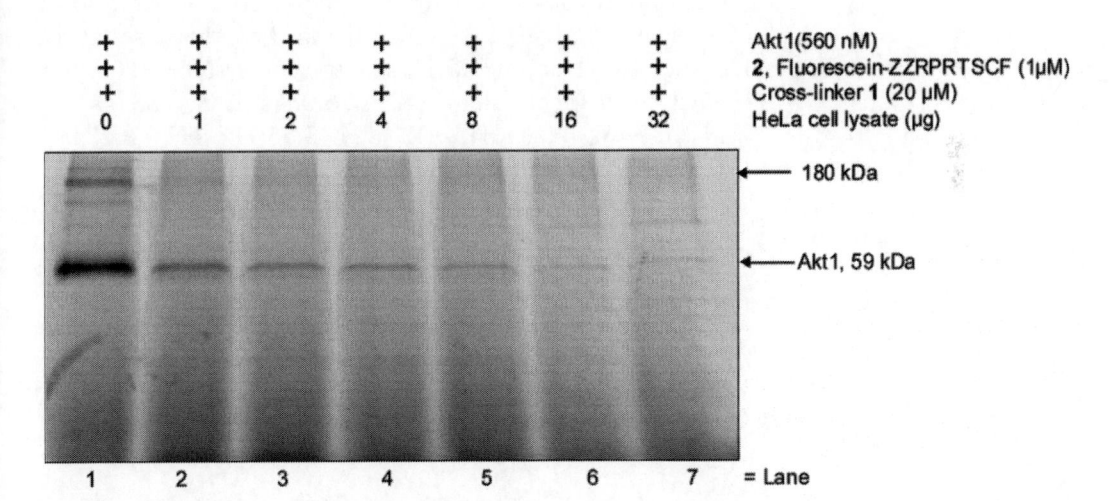

Fig. 3. Cross-linking of Akt1 and fluorescent peptide substrate 2 with cross-linker 1 in the presence of increasing amounts of HeLa cell lysate proteins. Akt1 and substrate peptide 2 were treated with cross-linker 1 for 20 min at r.t., followed by SDS-PAGE and in-gel scanning fluorescence.

3.1. Synthesis of Chemical Cross-Linker 1

Unless specified otherwise, all reactions were performed in dry solvents and under nitrogen atmosphere.

3.1.1. Synthesis of Compound 4

1. Charge a 500-mL round-bottom flask equipped with a reflux condenser and a Dean-Stark trap with 2,3-thiophene dicarboxaldehyde **3** (5.35 g, 38 mmol), p-toluenesulfonic acid monohydrate (0.1 g), ethylene glycol (11.73 g, 190 mmol), and benzene (80 mL).
2. Reflux the resulting mixture for 2 h with simultaneous removal of water into the Dean-Stark trap.
3. Quench the reaction mixture with a 5% aqueous solution of Na_2CO_3 (100 mL).
4. Separate organic layers and extract the aqueous layer with ethyl acetate (100 mL).
5. Wash combined organic fractions with saturated sodium chloride solution (100 mL), dry over $MgSO_4$, filter, and evaporate.
6. Purify the resulting oily residue on the Intelliflash 280 using disposable SF65-400g columns (Gradient, Hexane–ethyl acetate = 100:0 → 0:100, over 30 min, flow rate = 100 mL/min) to afford 2,3-Bis(1,3-dioxolan-2-yl)thiophene **4** as the major elution peak (7 g, 85% yield). Alternatively, purification can be done using regular glass chromatography columns and 300 g of regular silica gel. It is recommended in this case to use Hexane: Ethyl acetate = 2:1 as a solvent system. ^{1}H NMR ($CDCl_3$) 4.03 (t, 2H), 4.11 (t, 2H), 6.05 (s, 1H), 6.33 (s, 1H), 7.11 (d, J = 5.2 Hz, 1H), 7.27 (d, J = 5.55 Hz, 1H) (Fig. 4).

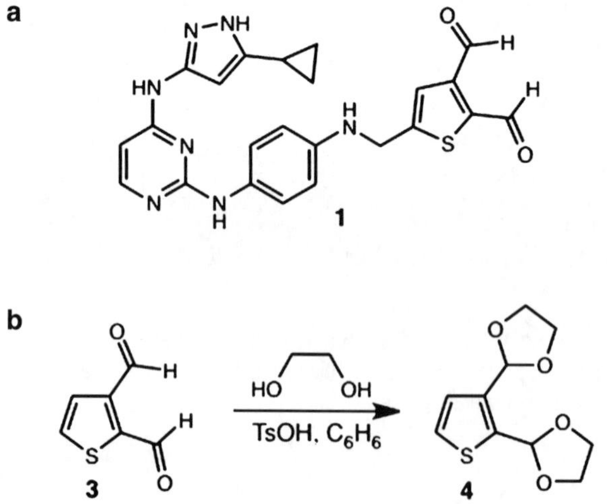

Fig. 4. Synthesis of compound 4. (**a**) Structure of the kinase–substrate cross-linker 1. (**b**) Synthesis of compound 4.

3.1.2. Synthesis of Compound 5

1. Charge a 250 mL Round-bottom flask with 2,3-Bis(1,3-dioxolan-2-yl)thiophene **4** (2.6 g, 11.40 mmol) and tetrahydrofurane (50 mL), and cool down to −78°C.

2. Add *n*-BuLi (5 mmol) dropwise at −78°C.

3. Raise the temperature to 0°C and stir the reaction mixture for an additional 30 min.

4. Add dimethyl formamide (DMF) (5 mmol, 0.971 mL) to the reaction mixture at 0°C.

5. Stir the reaction mixture at ambient temperature for 30 min followed by quenching with water (50 mL) (see Note 1).

6. Separate organic layers and extract the aqueous layer with ethyl acetate (100 mL). Wash the combined organic extracts with saturated sodium chloride solution (100 mL), dry over MgSO$_4$, filter, and evaporate. Purification of the resulting residue on Intelliflash 280 using disposable SF25-40g columns (Gradient, Hexane–ethyl acetate = 100:0 → 0:100, over 30 min, flow rate = 40 mL/min) affords aldehyde **5** (2.2 g, 75% yield) as the major elution peak. Alternatively, purification can be done using regular glass chromatography columns charged with 60 g of regular silica gel. It is recommended in this case to use Hexane–Ethyl acetate (1:1) as a solvent mixture. ^{1}H NMR (400 MHz, CDCl$_3$) δ 9.80 (s, 1H), 7.74 (s, 1H), 6.32 (s, 1H), 5.98 (s, 1H), 4.10-4.05 (m, 4H), 4.05-3.95 (m, 4H). ^{13}C NMR (100 MHz, CDCl$_3$) δ 183.4, 150.5, 142.2, 138.8, 136.1, 98.8, 98.6, 65.8, 65.5. MS calculated for C$_{11}$H$_{12}$O$_5$S 256.04, found 257.03 (Fig. 5).

3.1.3. Synthesis of Compound 8

1. Charge a round-bottom flask equipped with a reflux condenser with 2,4-dichloropyrimidine **6** (3.2 g, 21.6 mmol), 5-cyclopropyl-2H-pyrazol-3-ylamine **7** (2.65 g, 21.5 mmol), KOAc (30 eq., 64 g) and dissolve in THF–water 1:1 (140 mL).

2. Keep the resulting reaction mixture at 55°C for 48 h.

3. After 48 h, remove heating and separate organic layers. Evaporate the organic layer and dissolve residue in CH$_2$Cl$_2$ (30 mL) and keep at −20°C for 3 h. Collect the precipitated pyrimidine chloride **8** by filtration. To collect additional amounts of pyrimidine chloride, evaporate filtrates, redissolve

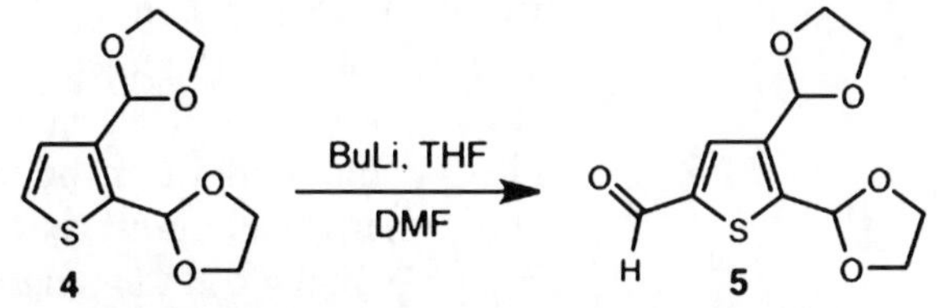

Fig. 5. Synthesis of compound 5.

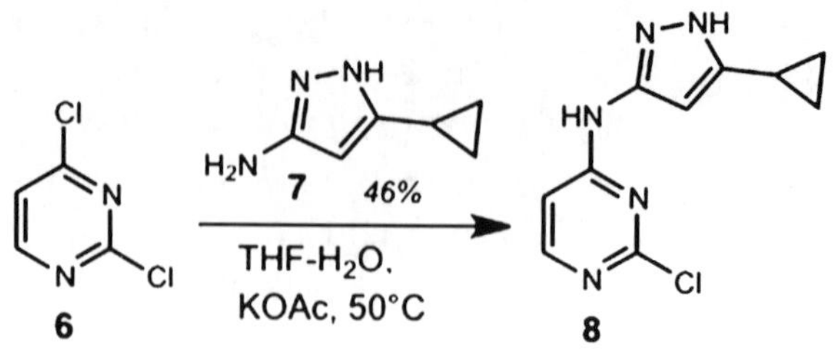

Fig. 6. Synthesis of compound 8.

in CH$_2$Cl$_2$ (25 mL) and keep at –20°C for another 3 h followed by filtration. Purification of the combined solids on Intelliflash 280 using disposable SF25-80g columns (Gradient, CHCl$_3$–CH$_3$OH (100:0→92:8), over 30 min, flow rate = 85 mL/min) affords compound **8** as the major elution peak (46% yield, 2.32 g). Alternatively, purification can be done using regular glass chromatography columns charged with 60 g of regular silica gel. It is recommended in this case to use CHCl$_3$–CH$_3$OH (9:1) as a solvent mixture. ^{1}H NMR (400 MHz, DMSO) δ 12.14 (s, 1H), 10.23 (s, 1H), 8.10 (s, 1H), 1.84 (m, 1H), 0.88 (m, 2H), 0.64 (m, 2H). ^{13}C NMR (100 MHz, DMSO) δ 161.4, 160.7, 160.0, 153.9, 148.6, 147.8, 146.8, 8.4, 8.2. MS calculated for C$_{10}$H$_{10}$ClN$_5$ 235.06 (M$^+$), found 236.15 (M$^+$) (Fig. 6).

3.1.4. Synthesis of Compound 10

1. Charge a round-bottom flask equipped with a reflux condenser with pyrimidine monochloride **8** (1.6 g, 6.8 mmol), *p*-phenylenediamine **9** (0.74 g, 6.8 mmol) and *n*-BuOH (60 mL). Treat the resulting mixture with concentrated HCl (0.1 mL) and keep at 100°C overnight.

2. Collect purple precipitates by filtration, wash with 20 mL of *n*-BuOH and dry at 50°C under vacuum overnight, to afford amine **10** (1.5 g, 73% yield), which is used in the next step without further purification (see Note 2). MS calculated for C$_{16}$H$_{17}$N$_7$ 307.15, found 308.17 (Fig. 7).

3.1.5. Synthesis of Compound 11

1. Charge a round-bottom flask with amine **10** (0.06 g, 195 μmol), aldehyde **5** (0.048 g, 187 μmol), and CH$_3$OH (5 mL).

2. Treat the resulting mixture with solid NaBH$_3$CN (0.01 g, 168 μmol), stir at ambient temperature overnight and evaporate. Purification on Intelliflash 280 using disposable SF10-4g columns (Gradient, CH$_2$Cl$_2$ (1% NEt$_3$)– CH$_3$OH (1% NEt$_3$) (100:0→92:8), over 30 min, flow rate = 18 mL/min) affords compound **11** as the major elution peak (0.064 g, 63% yield). Alternatively, purification can be done using regular glass chromatography columns charged with 10 g of regular silica gel. It is recommended in this case to use CHCl$_3$–CH$_3$OH (9:1) containing 1% NEt$_3$ as a solvent mixture. ^{1}H NMR (400 MHz,

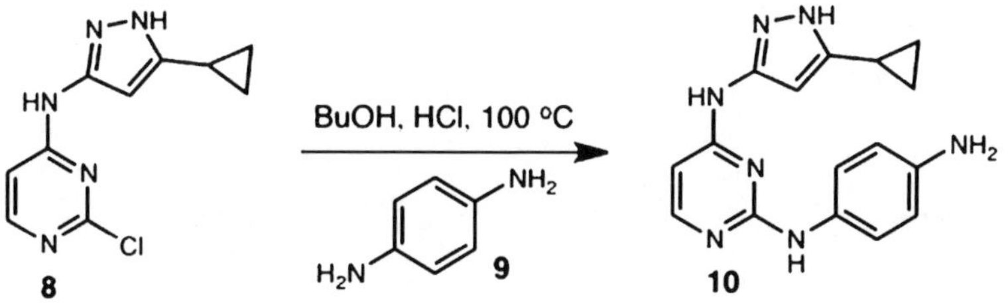

Fig. 7. Synthesis of compound 10.

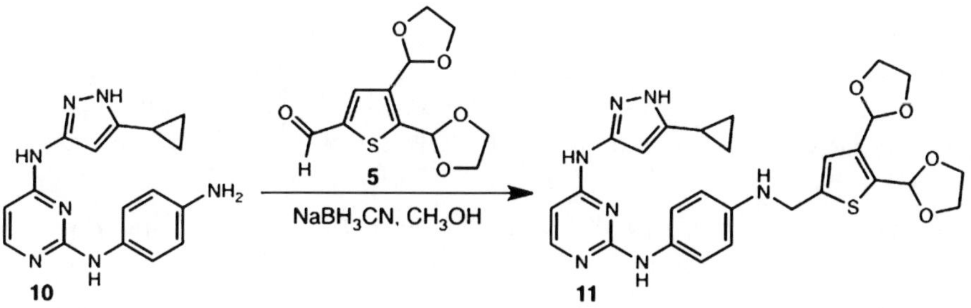

Fig. 8. Synthesis of compound 11.

CDCl$_3$) δ 9.13 (bs, 1H), 7.78 (m, 2H), 7.17 (m, 2H), 6.90 (s, 1H), 6.51 (m, 2H), 6.15 (m, 1H), 5.73 (m, 1H), 4.27 (s, 2H), 3.99 (m, 4H), 3.87 (m, 4H), 1.74 (m, 1H), 0.80 (m, 2H), 0.56 (m, 2H). ^{13}C NMR (100 MHz, CDCl$_3$) δ 160.2, 155.6, 144.3, 143.9, 143.6, 139.1, 138.9, 137.5, 136.1, 130.2, 125.0, 124.3, 123.7, 113.6, 99.1, 98.6, 97.5, 65.5, 65.4, 46.5, 9.0, 8.3. MS calculated for C$_{27}$H$_{29}$N$_7$O$_4$S 547.2, found 548.07 (Fig. 8).

3.1.6. Synthesis of Cross-Linker 1

1. Charge a round bottom flask with compound **11** (0.035 g, 64 μmol) and dissolve in a 1:1 mixture of CH$_3$CN–H$_2$O (3 mL) followed by treatment with trifluoroacetic acid (50 μL, 10 eq.).

2. Stir the reaction mixture overnight (see Note 3) and purify directly *via* reverse phase HPLC CH$_3$CN/H$_2$O containing 0.1% TFA (Gradient, CH$_3$CN (0.1% TFA)–H$_2$O (0.1% TFA) = 2:98→98:2, over 40 min, flow rate = 20 mL/min) followed by lyophilization to afford cross-linker **1** (13 mg, 45% yield). ^{1}H NMR (400 MHz, DMSO-d_6) δ 11.94 (bs, 1H), 10.38 (s, 1H), 10.34 (s, 1H), 9.54 (bs, 1H), 8.73 (bs, 1H), 7.81 (m, 1H), 7.53 (s, 1H), 7.31 (s, 1H), 7.21 (s, 1H), 6.54 (s, 1H), 6.52 (s, 1H), 4.49 (s, 2H), 1.76 (bs, 1H), 0.83 (m, 2H), 0.59 (m, 2H). MS calculated for C$_{23}$H$_{21}$N$_7$O$_2$S 459.15, found 459.99.

3. Dissolve the resulting cross-linker **1** in DMSO to make a 20 mM DMSO stock solution, and store at −80°C until further use. It is recommended to avoid freeze–thaw cycles, since the cross-linker **1** may decompose (Fig. 9).

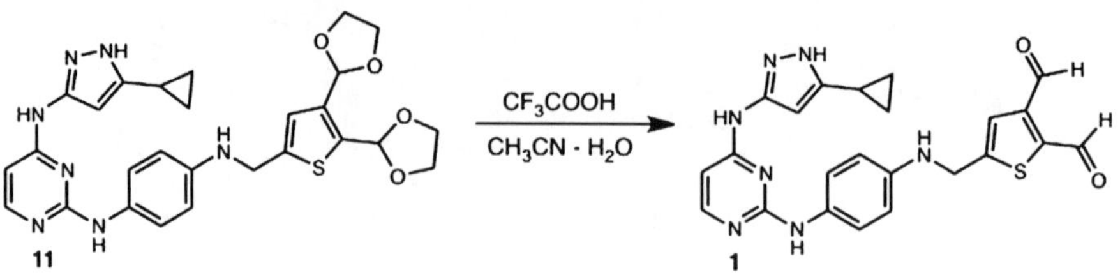

Fig. 9. Synthesis of kinase–substrate cross-linker 1.

3.2. Solid Phase Synthesis of Fluorescent Cysteine Containing Akt1 Peptide Substrate Fluorescein-ZZRPRTSCF-OH, 2

3.2.1. Fluorescein-Ahx-Ahx-Arg-Pro-Arg-Thr-Ser-Cys-Phe-OH (2)

1. Prepare the substrate peptide 2 i according to the general solid phase peptide synthesis procedure using Fmoc-Phe-Wang resin. Perform each coupling step for 2 h with 2 mmol of corresponding amino acid dissolved in 5 mL of DMF, in the presence of HBTU (2 mmol, 0.758 g) and iPr$_2$NEt (4 mmol, 0.695 mL).

2. Carry out Fmoc deprotection in 20% piperidine/DMF for 20 min at room temperature.

3. Cap the N-terminus of the peptide by agitating the resin overnight in the presence of 6-carboxyfluorescein (0.5 mmol), HBTU (0.5 mmol, 0.189 g), and i-Pr$_2$NEt (1 mmol, 0.173 mL) overnight.

4. Prior to cleavage, wash the resin with DMF (3×5 mL), CH$_2$Cl$_2$ (3×5 mL), CH$_3$OH (3×5 mL), and CH$_2$Cl$_2$ (3×5 mL).

5. Cleave the peptide from the resin by treatment with 94:2:2:2 TFA–1,2-ethanedithiol–H$_2$O–triisopropylsilane for 3 h. Remove the solvent in vacuo and purify the resulting crude product by C18 reverse-phase HPLC (CH$_3$CN/H$_2$O/0.1% TFA). Following lyophilization, the peptide is obtained as a yellow solid. MS (ESI), m/z calcd for C$_{69}$H$_{91}$N$_{15}$O$_{18}$S: 1,449.6. Found: m/z 1,450.8 (M+H)$^+$. Dissolve the resulting solid peptide in water to prepare a 1 mM stock solution and store at −80°C until further use.

3.3. General Protocol for Cross-Linking of AKT1 Substrate Peptide 2 with AKT1

Final concentrations of reaction components are the following: cross-linker 1 20 μM, substrate peptide 2 1 μM, Akt1 kinase 400 ng/30 μL.

1. Prepare a 600 μM stock solution of cross-linker 1 in water.

2. Prepare a 30 μM stock solution of Akt1 substrate peptide 2 in water.

3. Dissolve 400 ng of Akt kinase (0.4 mg/mL) in 30 μL of reaction buffer (25 mM HEPES, pH=6.5, 150 mM NaCl, 2 mM MgCl$_2$, 1 mM β-mercaptoethanol).

4. Add 1 μL of Akt1 substrate peptide 2 (30 μM stock solution in water) and mix well by pipetting it up and down.

5. Add 1 μL of cross-linker 1 (600 μM stock solution in water), mix well with the reaction mixture by pipetting up and down (see Note 4).

6. Incubate reaction mixture for 20 min at room temperature.
7. After 20 min, quench the reaction with 6 μL of 5× Laemmli buffer. Remember not to boil the sample.
8. Load the samples (30 μL) onto polyacrylamide gels, followed by SDS-Polyacrylamide Gel Electrophoresis (SDS-PAGE) and direct in-gel scanning fluorescence measurements (490 nm excitation band, 520 nm emission band).
9. The same procedure should be used to cross-link Akt1 kinase with the substrate Akt1 peptide **2** in the presence of HeLa cell lysate. In this case, one should premix Akt1 kinase with the substrate peptide **2** and 5 μg of HeLa cell lysate in the reaction buffer, adding chemical cross-linker **1** last. Representative cross-linking experiments with or without HeLa cell lysates are presented in Fig. 3.

4. Notes

1. Chemical transformations that involve organolithium intermediates are usually quenched with acidic aqueous media such as 1 M HCl. In the case of compound **5**, however, this must be avoided because the 1,3-dioxolane protective group is easily removed under acidic conditions. This will liberate a dialdehyde moiety that will interfere with the subsequent reductive amination step (Subheading 3.1.2).
2. The LCMS trace of compound **11** should show one elution peak. Thus no additional purification should be needed. Compound **11** is very polar and insoluble in a variety of solvents, such as $CH_3OH/CH_3CN/DMSO$, which makes chromatographic purifications hard to perform (see Subheading 3.1.4).
3. The final deprotection step in the synthesis of cross-linker **1** is usually completed within 10–14 h, but it is important to check the progress of the deprotection reaction by LCMS before purifying it. In the case of incomplete conversion, the reaction mixture should be evaporated on a rotary evaporator, redissolved in $CH_3CN–H_2O$ (1:1), and treated with trifluoroacetic acid (10 eq., 50 μL) and stirred until full conversion of the starting material **12** (see Subheading 3.1.5).
4. When performing the cross-linking reaction between Akt1 kinase and the peptide substrate **2**, cross-linker **1** should be added at the very last step. We have noticed that Akt1 kinase can be nonspecifically cross-linked with the cross-linker **2** in the absence of the peptide **2**, forming nonspecifically cross-linked higher molecular weight intermediates (see Subheading 3.3).

Acknowledgments

KMS thanks NIH RO1-EB001987 for funding as well as a grant from Eli Lilly. The authors thank Beatrice Wang for helpful comments on the manuscript. Dustin Maly and Megan Riel-Mehan are acknowledged for their contributions to the project.

References

1. Manning, B.D.; Cantley, L.C. (2002) Hitting the Target: Emerging Technologies in the Search for Kinase Substrates. *Sci. STKE*, *2002*:pe49.
2. Ptacek, J.; Snyder, M. (2006) Charging it up: global analysis of protein phosphorylation. *Trends Genet.* **22**, 545–554.
3. Ptacek, J., Devgan, G., Michaud, G., Zhu, H., Zhu, X., Fasolo, J., Guo, H., Jona, G., Breitkreutz, A., Sopko, R., McCartney, R.R., Schmidt, M.C., Rachidi, N., Lee, S.J., Mah, A.S., Meng, L., Stark, M.J., Stern, D.F., De Virgilio, C., Tyers, M., Andrews, B., Gerstein, M., Schweitzer, B., Predki, P.F., Snyder, M. (2005) Global analysis of protein phosphorylation in yeast. *Nature* **438**, 679–684.
4. Songyang, Z.; Blechner, S.; Hoagland, N.; Hoekstra. M.F.; Piwnica-Worms, H.; Cantley, L.C. (1994) Use of an oriented peptide library to determine the optimal substrates of protein kinases. *Curr. Biol.* **4**, 973–982.
5. Obenauer, J.C.; Cantley, L.C.; Yaffe, M.B. (2003) Scansite 2.0: proteome-wide prediction of cell signaling interactions using short sequence motifs. *Nucleic Acids Res.* **31**, 3635–3641.
6. Berwick, D.C.; Tavare, J.M. (2004) Identifying protein kinase substrates: hunting for the organ-grinder's monkeys. *Trends Biochem. Sci.* **29**, 227–232.
7. Allen, J.J.; Li, M.; Brinkworth, C.S.; Paulson, J.L.; Wang, D.; Hübner, A.; Chou, W.H..; Davis, R.J.; Burlingame, A.L.; Messing, R.O.; Katayama, C.D.; Hedrick, S.M.; Shokat, K.M. (2007) A semisynthetic epitope for kinase substrates. *Nat. Methods* **4**, 511–516.
8. Blethrow, J.D.; Glavy, J.S.; Morgan, D.O.; Shokat K.M. (2008) Covalent capture of kinase-specific phosphopeptides reveals Cdk1-cyclin B substrates. *Proc. Natl. Acad. Sci. USA* **105**, 1442–1447.
9. Dramsi, S.; Scheid, M.P.; Maiti, A.; Hojabrpour, P.; Chen, X.; Schubert, K.; Goodlett, D.R.; Aebersold, R.; Duronio, V. (2002) Identification of a Novel Phosphorylation Site, Ser-170, as a Regulator of Bad Pro-apoptotic Activity. *J. Biol. Chem.* **277**, 6399–6405.
10. Potter, L.R.; Hunter, T. (1998) Phosphorylation of the Kinase Homology Domain Is Essential for Activation of the A-Type Natriuretic Peptide Receptor. *Mol. Cell. Biol.* **18**, 2164–2172.
11. Forcet, C.; Billaud, M. (2007) Dialogue Between LKB1 and AMPK: A Hot Topic at the Cellular Pole. *Sci. STKE* 404, pe51.
12. Sapkota, G.P.; Boudeau, J.; Deak, M.; Kieloch, A.; Morrice, N.; Alessi, D.R. (2002) Identification and characterization of four novel phosphorylation sites (Ser^{31}, Ser^{325}, Thr^{336} and Thr^{366}) on LKB1/STK11, the protein kinase mutated in Peutz–Jeghers cancer syndrome. *Biochem. J.* **362**, 481–490.
13. Beausoleil, S.A.; Jedrychowski, M.; Schwartz, D.; Elias, J.E.; Villén, J.; Li, J.; Cohn, M.A.; Cantley, L.C.; Gygi, S.P. (2004) Large-scale characterization of HeLa cell nuclear phosphoproteins *Proc. Natl. Acad. Sci. USA* **101**, 12130–12135.
14. Maly, D.J.; Allen, J.A.; Shokat, K.M. (2004) A Mechanism-Based Cross-Linker for the Identification of Kinase-Substrate Pairs. *J. Am. Chem. Soc.* **126**, 9160–9161.
15. Statsuk, A.V.; Maly, D.J.; Seeliger, M.A.; Fabian, M.A.; Biggs III, W.H.; Lockhart, D.J.; Zarrinkar, P.P.; Kuriyan, J.; Shokat, K.M. (2008), Tuning a three-component reaction for trapping kinase substrate complexes. *J. Am. Chem. Soc.* **130**, 17568–17574.

Chapter 13

Receptor Tyrosine Kinase Inhibitor Profiling Using Bead-Based Multiplex Sandwich Immunoassays

Oliver Pötz, Nicole Schneiderhan-Marra, Tanja Henzler, Thomas Herget, and Thomas O. Joos

Abstract

Receptor tyrosine kinases (RTK) are important targets in drug discovery processes. Studying the phosphorylation pattern of RTKs enables the determination of their activation and inactivation states. Multiplex bead-based sandwich immunoassays are powerful tools for measuring the phosphorylation state of key regulators within cellular signalling networks. Here, we describe the analysis of the phosphorylation state of receptor tyrosine kinases using the epidermal growth factor receptor (EGFR) as an example. We provide a protocol for a bead-based sandwich immunoassay that enables a relative quantification of the EGFR and its generic tyrosine phosphorylation. We also present data from a kinase inhibitor experiment using 96-well cell-culture plates and a commercially available kit for the analysis of seven receptor tyrosine kinases.

Key words: Receptor tyrosine kinases, Multiplex bead-based sandwich immunoassay, Antibody array

1. Introduction

Receptor tyrosine kinases (RTK) are important entry points through which a cell transmits information across the cellular membrane (1, 2). The extracellular binding of a growth factor results in a conformational change, kinase activation, and subsequent intracellular autophosphorylation of the receptor. This event then triggers cellular responses via activating signalling cascades.

The aberrant activation of a signalling pathway is a common event for many tumours (3). Mutations or duplications of the RTK genes or the genes for their ligands can lead to overexpression and result in the hyperactivation of the respective pathway. Two well-known examples of the RTK gene family are the epidermal growth factor receptor (EGFR, ErbB1) and Her2 (ErbB2), which are overexpressed in over 30% of breast and colon cancers, respectively, and which can drive uncontrolled cell proliferation (3). Hence, the analysis of expression and activation of receptor tyrosine kinases plays a central role in tumour diagnosis and treatment. Consequently, the determination of RTKs' concentration and their degree of phosphorylation are of great interest for medical research to develop novel compounds for targeted therapy (1).

A snapshot of the activation state of one kinase might only provide limited information within the context of such highly branched pathways, especially with regard to any potential side effects of kinase inhibitor drugs. Multiplexed sandwich immunoassay systems enable the detection of dozens of analytes in one reaction (4, 5).

In this protocol, RTK-specific kinase antibodies as capture reagents are immobilised on fluorophor-coded polystyrene beads (6, 7). Whole extracts from tissue or inhibitor-treated cell lines are incubated with these beads and the RTKs in the sample are captured by the respective antibody on the beads. Generic tyrosine phosphorylation of the RTKs can be detected using biotinylated phosphotyrosine-specific antibodies and phycoerythrin-conjugated streptavidin as the reporter molecule. Moreover, the total number of RTKs can be determined in parallel using a second biotinylated RTK-specific detection antibody recognising the RTK independent of its phosphorylation status. In special flow cytometers (Luminex 100, Luminex 200 or FlexMap3D), the results are deconvoluted through the use of two laser detector combinations: one for bead classification and one for the reporter signal detection, reflecting the amount of protein bound to the antibody-coated bead.

Here, we give an example of how to set up a sandwich assay to measure the total amount of EGFR and how to detect the generic tyrosine phosphorylation of EGFR (shown in Fig. 1). We also show the determination of the specificity of a known inhibitory compound (8) tested in 96-well cell-culture experiments using a commercially available panel of multiplex sandwich immunoassays (shown in Fig. 2).

2. Materials

Commercially available kits provide straightforward protocols for the analysis of RTKs and intracellular signalling events. A list of kit distributors can be found on the Luminex Corporation Web page (http://www.luminexcorp.com/partners/index.html). Protocols for the WideScreen™ Receptor Tyrosine Kinase Assay Kits used here can be found on the EMD chemicals Web page (http://www.emdchemicals.com/life-science-research).

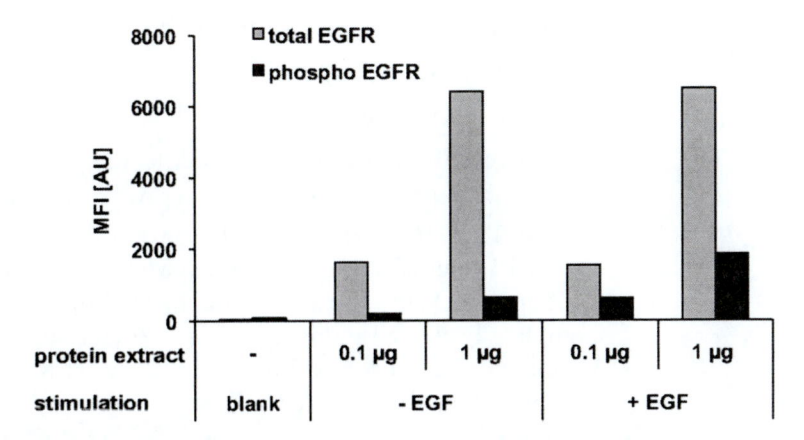

Fig. 1. A431 cells were either stimulated with EGF (100 ng/ml) or mock treated. Proteins were extracted and analysed for total EGFR and tyrosine-phosphorylated EGFR using bead-based sandwich immunoassays. Total EGFR concentration remained constant after EGF stimulation, whereas the signal for phospho-EGFR increased. In the A431 cell lysates, a high basic phosphorylation level was observed (see panel labelled "EGF").

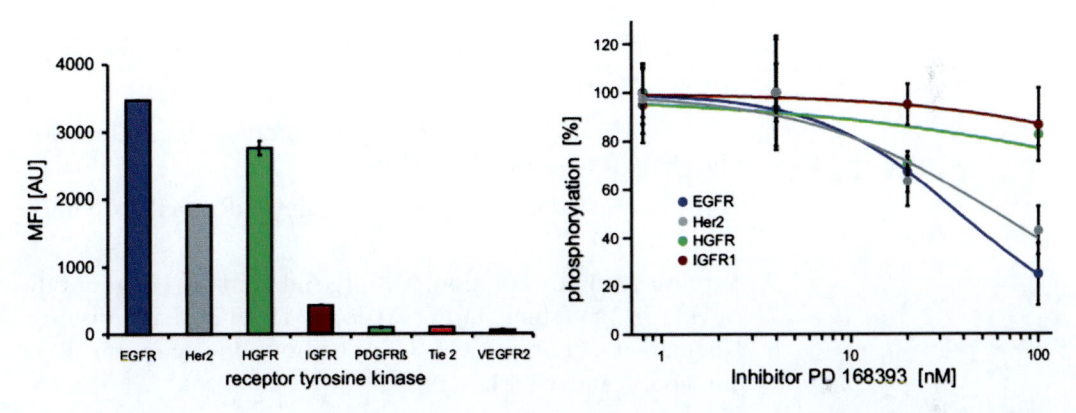

Fig. 2. Specificity analysis of a kinase inhibitor for RTKs. HT-29 cells were cultivated in 96-well plates. After 24 h starvation, the cells were treated with different concentrations of the kinase inhibitor PD 168393 (1 nM, 5 nM, 20 nM, and 100 nM) for 1 h. The cells were subsequently stimulated for 10 min with a growth factor cocktail containing 100 ng/ml EGF, 100 ng/ml heregulin, 100 ng/ml IGF, 50 ng/ml HGF, 100 ng/ml VEGF, and 100 ng/ml PDGF α/β. Protein extracts were analysed for the relative amount of EGFR, HER2, HGFR, IGFR1, Tie2, VEGFR2, and PDGFRβ (*left panel*) and for their relative phosphorylation (*right panel*) using WideScreen™ Receptor Tyrosine Kinase Assay Kits. EGFR, Her2, HGFR, and IGFR were detectable in HT-29 (results shown are averaged median fluorescence intensities from duplicate cell culture wells). PD 168393 reduced the degree of EGFR and HER2 phosphorylation in a concentration-dependent manner (data are normalised by setting the signal obtained from maximal stimulated cells without inhibitor to 100%). Only a slight inhibition of PD 168393 on IGFR and HGFR phosphorylation was observed in IGF- and HGF-treated cells.

2.1. Cell Culture and Sample Preparation

1. 96-well filter plates.
2. Ultrafree-MC filter units, 0.65 μm Durapore.
3. Ordinary cell culture plates.
4. Cell line of interest: e.g. HT-29.
5. Medium: Mc Coy's 5A modified liquid medium supplemented with 5 mM glutamine and 10% foetal bovine serum (FBS).
6. Starvation medium: Mc Coy's 5A modified liquid medium.

7. Protein kinase inhibitor: e.g. PD 168393.
8. Dimethylsulfoxid (DMSO).
9. Growth factor: e.g. epidermal growth factor (EGF).
10. Phosphate-buffered saline (PBS): sterile, pH 7.4.
11. Lysis buffer: 150 mM NaCl, 1 mM $MgCl_2$, 1 mM $CaCl_2$, 50 mM Tris–HCl, pH 7.4, 1% Triton, Phosphatase Inhibitor Cocktail I (Sigma Aldrich, St. Louis, MO, USA), Phosphatase Inhibitor Cocktail II (Sigma Aldrich, St. Louis, MO, USA), Complete Protease Inhibitor Cocktail (Roche Applied Science, Mannheim, Germany), Benzonase® Nuclease (EMD Chemicals Inc., San Diego, CA, USA).
12. Protein Assay Reagent: e.g. bicinchoninic acid (BCA).

2.2. Coupling of Capture Antibody

1. Activation buffer: 100 mM sodium phosphate (Na_2HPO_4), pH 6.2.
2. Coupling buffer: 50 mM 2-(N-morpholino)ethanesulfonic acid (MES), pH 5.0.
3. Wash buffer: sterile PBS, pH 7.4, 0.05% (v/v) Tween 20.
4. Sterile PBS, pH 7.4.
5. 1-Ethyl-3-[3-dimethylaminopropyl]carbodiimide hydrochloride (EDC): 50 mg/ml in DMSO.
6. N-hydroxysulfosuccinimide sodium salt (Sulfo-NHS): 50 mg/ml in DMSO.
7. Capture antibody solution: 100 µg/ml Anti-EGFR antibody Ab-11 in coupling buffer (Clone 199.12, Lab Vision/Neomarkers, Fremont, CA, USA; without bovine serum albumin (BSA) and azide).
8. Carboxylated Luminex xMap microspheres (Luminex Corp., Austin, TX, USA): local distributors are listed on the Luminex Web page (http://www.luminexcorp.com).
9. 1.5 ml microcentrifuge tubes (STARLAB GmbH, Hamburg, Germany): for bead handling disposables please follow the suggestions given on http://www.luminexcorp.com/support/recommendedmaterials/index.html.
10. Ultrafree-MC filter units, 0.65 µm Durapore.
11. 96-well microtitre plate: half well (flat bottom, non-binding surface, non-sterile, polystyrene, Corning Inc.).

2.3. Biotinylation of Detection Antibody

1. EZ-Link™ Sulfo-NHS-LC-LC-Biotin (Pierce, Rockford, IL, USA): 10 mg/ml in PBS.
2. Detection antibody: 1 mg/ml in PBS; anti-EGFR antibody Ab-10 (Clone 111.6, Lab Vision/Neomarkers, Fremont, CA, USA, without BSA and azide).
3. Phosphate-buffered saline (PBS): pH 7.4.

4. Centri-Spin-10 columns (Princeton Separations INC., Adelphia, NJ, USA).

5. Glycerol.

2.4. Sandwich Immunoassay and Detection

The equipment and reagents listed below are of crucial importance to the success of the described protocol.

1. Luminex L100 reader (alternatively L200 or FlexMap3D): local distributors are listed on the Luminex Web page (http://www.luminexcorp.com).

2. Thermomixer comfort exchangeable MTP thermoblock, (Eppendorf GmbH, Hamburg, Germany).

3. 96-well membrane filter plates MultiScreen (Millipore Corp., Billerica, MA, USA).

4. Vacuum manifold.

5. Wash buffer: PBS, pH 7,4, 0.1% (v/v) Tween 20.

6. Assay buffer: Roche Blocking Reagent for ELISA (Roche Applied Science), 0.1% (v/v) Tween.

7. Detection antibody mix: 0.2–1 µg/ml biotinylated antibody specific for each analyte (here biotinylated anti EGFR Ab-10) or biotinylated anti-phosphotyrosine clone 4G10 (Millipore Corp., Billerica, MA, USA) in Roche Blocking Reagent for ELISA (Roche Applied Science, Mannheim, Germany), 0.1% v/v Tween (Merck KGaA, Darmstadt, Germany).

8. Phycoerythrin-conjugated streptavidin.

3. Methods

A workflow for the detection of phosphorylation of the EGFR receptor is given here. Activation or inhibition of the EGFR can be measured by evaluating the tyrosine phosphorylation of the receptor using bead-based sandwich immunoassays (see Fig. 1). Potential off-target effects on other tyrosine kinase receptors can be detected using the WideScreen™ Receptor Tyrosine Kinase Assay Kits (EMD Chemicals Inc., San Diego, CA, USA) (see Fig. 2).

3.1. Coupling of Capture Antibodies to Microspheres

1. COOH-bead activation: Vortex the bead stock provided by the vendor thoroughly for at least 10 s. Take 3.75×10^6 beads per coupling reaction. Transfer 300 µl beads from the bead stock (1.25×10^7 beads/ml) to an Ultrafree-MC filter unit. Centrifuge the filter unit briefly at $3,000 \times g$ and discard the flow-through. Wash beads by adding 300 µl activation buffer, vortex, and centrifuge again as described above. Discard the flow-through and repeat the wash step.

2. Prepare the EDC and sulfo-NHS solutions (50 mg/ml) during the last wash step and add 15 µl EDC solution and 15 µl sulfo-NHS solution to 120 µl activation buffer (activation mix). Incubate the beads with 150 µl activation mix for 20 min at RT on a shaker (800 rpm). Protect the beads from light during incubation.

3. Wash beads in an Ultrafree-MC filter with 400 µl coupling buffer, vortex, and centrifuge briefly and discard the flow-through. Repeat the wash step twice.

4. Couple antibodies to activated beads by adding 250 µl of the prepared anti-EGFR Ab-11 antibody solution to the filter unit (100 µg/ml, see Notes 1 and 2). Mix the beads thoroughly and incubate for 150 min at RT in the dark on a shaker.

5. Wash beads with 400 µl coupling buffer, vortex, and centrifuge and discard the flow-through. Repeat the wash step four times in total.

6. Add 100 µl of Roche ELISA Blocking Reagent containing 0.05% (w/v) Na-azide to the filter unit (handle with care, Na-azide is toxic) and vortex. Resuspend the beads by pipetting up and down and transfer the bead suspension to a Starlab microcentrifuge tube. Repeat this step and pool the bead suspensions in one microcentrifuge tube. The remaining volume of bead solution is 200 µl. For long-term storage, keep the beads at 4°C in the dark.

7. Determine recovery of antibody-coated beads: Dilute the antibody-coated bead stock 1:500 in a Starlab microcentrifuge tube. Vortex for at least 10 s. Take 100 µl of the dilution and transfer to a microtitre plate (two replicates). Place the microtitre plate for 30 min at 650 rpm on a shaker at RT (e.g. Eppendorf Thermomixer with a plate module). The settings for determining the bead concentration in the stock solution with the Luminex 100 system are as follows: sample size 50 µl, time-out 80 s, and total beads 10,000. Calculate the bead concentration as follows: beads per µl = number of beads divided by 30 and multiplied by a dilution factor of 500. The recovery is usually over 90% (see Note 3).

3.2. Biotinylation of Detection Antibodies

1. Prepare the Centri-Spin-10 columns at least 30 min before use. Rehydrate dry column gel with 650 µL PBS. Vortex carefully to avoid bubbles (alternative: moderate sonication). Hydrate the material in the columns for at least 30 min at RT. Keep the same orientation of the column in all subsequent centrifugation steps.

2. Biotinylation reaction: Warm the Sulfo-NHS-LC-LC-Biotin to room temperature. Dilute 100 µg Ab10 in 100 µl PBS and biotinylate with a 35-fold molar excess of Sulfo-NHS-LC-LC-Biotin.

Freshly prepare a 10 mg/ml solution of Sulfo-NHS-LC-LC-Biotin in PBS and pipette 2 µl of this solution to the antibody and mix carefully. Place the reaction tube on ice for 2 h (see Notes 1, 4 and 5).

3. Remove excess biotinylation reagent: Spin the Centri-Sin-10 column inserted in a wash tube at 750×*g* for 2 min to remove interstitial fluid. Important: Always position the column in the centrifuge in the same direction. Observe the orientation mark of the column.

4. Replace the wash tube with the sample collection tube and pipette the biotinylated antibody directly onto the centre of the gel bed at the top of the column without disturbing the gel surface.

5. Centrifuge at 750×*g* for 2 min. The purified sample collects at the bottom of the sample collection tube. Determine the protein content of the sample. Thereafter, determine the volume of the sample and dilute 1:2 with glycerol to enable long-term storage at −20°C (see Note 6).

3.3. Cell Stimulation and Sample Preparation Using a 96-Well Format Cell Culture

1. Seed cells at the appropriate density in a 96-well tissue culture plate (e.g. 2×10^4 HT-29 cells in 200 µl) and cultivate the cells for 24 h. The growth rate depends considerably on cell line and incubation parameters.

2. Replace the cultivation medium by medium lacking FBS and starve cells for 12–16 h.

3. Reconstitute inhibitor (e.g. PD 168393) in DMSO.

4. Prepare inhibition medium by diluting the inhibitor stock to the desired concentrations in 1 ml tissue culture medium lacking FBS. For mock control, prepare serum-free tissue culture medium lacking inhibitors, but including an equivalent volume of DMSO.

5. Following serum starvation, remove medium. Replace with 100 µL inhibition medium (or mock control medium). Immediately return cells to incubator.

6. Incubate cells at 37°C and 5% CO_2 for 1 h.

7. Prepare induction medium by diluting all growth factor stocks to a final concentration of for example 200 ng/ml EGF in tissue culture medium lacking FBS. This results in a 2× solution.

8. Add 2× induction medium (or mock medium lacking EGF) directly to inhibitor-treated cells. Immediately return cells to incubator.

9. Incubate cells at 37°C and 5% CO_2 for 10 min.

10. Prepare 120 µl lysis buffer per cell culture well. Add protease and phosphatase inhibitors and Benzonase to the lysis buffer immediately before use (see Note 7). Keep lysis buffer on ice.

11. Cool plate with cells on ice directly after treatment and remove the medium with a multichannel pipette. Wash treated cells twice using ice-cold PBS.
12. Remove all liquid and add 120 µl cold lysis buffer per well.
13. Incubate for 20 min at 4°C with gentle agitation on a rocking platform.
14. Dislodge and solubilise all adherent cells by repeated pipetting. Extracts should be clear and non-viscous.
15. Pre-wet one 96-well filter plate with 100 µl wash buffer for a minimum of 30 min. Remove liquid on the vacuum manifold.
16. Clear lysates: Transfer 100 µl lysate into a pre-blocked 96-well filter plate and centrifuge at $1,500 \times g$ for 1 min at 4°C into a pre-blocked 96-well receiver plate.
17. Either proceed immediately with the bead-based sandwich immunoassay protocol or store samples at −70°C until further use. Avoid multiple freeze–thaw cycles.
18. Determine protein concentration using the BCA method.

3.4. Cell Stimulation and Sample Preparation Using a Six-Well Format Cell Culture

1. Seed cells at the appropriate density in a six-well tissue culture plate (e.g. 3×10^5 HT-29 in 2 ml) and cultivate cells for 24 h. Optimal growth varies considerably between cell lines and labs. See above.
2. Replace the growth medium by medium lacking FBS and starve cells for 12–16 h.
3. Reconstitute inhibitor (e.g. PD 168393) in DMSO.
4. Prepare inhibition medium by diluting the inhibitor stock to the desired concentrations in 1 ml tissue culture medium lacking FBS. For mock inhibitions, prepare serum-free tissue culture medium lacking inhibitors, but including an equivalent volume of DMSO.
5. Following serum starvation, remove medium. Replace with inhibition medium (or mock control medium). Immediately return cells to incubator.
6. Incubate at 37°C and 5% CO_2 for 1 h.
7. Prepare induction medium by diluting all growth factor stocks to a final concentration of e.g. 200 ng/ml EGF in tissue culture medium lacking FBS. This results in a 2× solution.
8. Add 1 ml 2× induction medium (or mock induction medium) directly to inhibitor-treated cells. Immediately return cells to incubator.
9. Incubate at 37°C and 5% CO_2 for 10 min.
10. Prepare 200 µl lysis buffer per cell culture well. Add protease and phosphatase inhibitors and Benzonase to the lysis buffer immediately before use (see Note 7). Keep lysis buffer on ice.

11. Cool cells on ice directly after treatment and remove the medium with a multichannel pipette. Wash treated cells twice using ice-cold PBS.

12. Remove all liquid and add 200 µl cold lysis buffer per well.

13. Incubate for 20 min at 4°C with gentle agitation on a rocking platform.

14. Dislodge and solubilise all adherent cells by repeated pipetting. Extracts should be clear and non-viscous.

15. Clear lysates: Transfer 200 µl lysate into a pre-wetted 96-well filter plate and centrifuge at 1,500×*g*, 1 min, and 4°C into a 96-well-receiver plate.

16. Determine protein concentration using the BCA Method.

17. Either proceed immediately with the bead-based sandwich immunoassay protocol or store samples at −70°C. Avoid multiple freeze–thaw cycles.

3.5. Bead-Based Sandwich Immunoassay

1. Pre-wet 96-well filter plate wells with 50 µl assay buffer for a minimum of 5 min. Remove liquid by applying a gentle vacuum (3 in.Hg/76 mmHg) to filter plate. Tap drains of the filter plate onto a paper towel to remove any buffer (see Note 8).

2. Transfer 50 µl of the filtered lysate from the 96-well sample plate (from step 17 in Subheading 3.3) to each well (see Note 9).

3. Thoroughly vortex bead solution from step 6 in Subheading 3.1 and prepare a working solution containing 50,000 beads per ml. Add 50 µl bead solution to each well (corresponding to 2,500 beads).

4. Incubate overnight at 4°C or 3 h at 37°C at 750 rpm on a platform plate shaker (e.g. Eppendorf Thermomixer with a plate module). Use aluminium foil or a lid to protect the beads from light and to avoid evaporation.

5. Remove liquid by applying a gentle vacuum (3 in.Hg/76 mmHg) to filter plate. Wash beads by adding 100 µl washing buffer per well. Perform a total of two wash steps (see Note 8).

6. Add 50 µl of either biotinylated anti-EGFR (3 µg/ml in assay buffer) from step 5 in Subheading 3.2 or biotinylated anti-phosphotyrosine antibody (2 µg/ml in assay buffer) (see Note 10).

7. Incubate for 1 h at RT at 750 rpm on a platform plate shaker with a plate module. Use aluminium foil or a lid to protect the beads from light.

8. Remove liquid by applying a gentle vacuum (3 in.Hg/76 mmHg) to filter plate. Wash beads by adding 100 µl washing buffer per well. Perform a total of two wash steps.

9. Add 50 μl of phycoerythrin-conjugated streptavidin (5 μg/ml) to each well.
10. Remove liquid by applying a gentle vacuum (3 in.Hg/76 mmHg) to filter plate. Wash beads by adding 100 μl washing buffer per well. Perform a total of two wash steps.
11. Place plate in the Luminex reader (LX 100, LX 200, or FlexMap3D) and read assay. Standard settings are as follows: doublet discriminator 7,500–15,000, sample volume 100 μl, and minimal bead count per region 100.
12. All results generated by this method represent a relative quantification. Absolute concentration can be calculated by using recombinant EGFR protein as a reference (see Note 11).

4. Notes

1. It is important that the antibody solutions used for the immobilisation and biotinylation procedures are free of primary amine-containing compounds, e.g. glycine buffer (see Subheadings 3.1 and 3.2).
2. If novel sandwich immunoassays are to be developed, different antibody concentrations for the coupling procedure need to be tested to define the best assay conditions (see Subheading 3.1).
3. Coupling efficiency can be controlled by the detection of the immobilised IgG using Phycoerythrin-conjugated anti-species specific antibodies, e.g. R-Phycoerythrin-conjugated goat-anti-mouse IgG (Jackson ImmunoResearch Laboratories, West Grove, PA, USA), (see Subheading 3.1).
4. In order to define the best biotinylation conditions, test different ratios of the biotinylation reagent to the given antibody amount. A typical antibody–biotin ratio is 1:50 (see Subheading 3.2).
5. Biotinylation reagents containing spacers with different lengths and hydrophobicity are available on the market. They may also influence the signal intensity in the sandwich immunoassay (see Subheading 3.2).
6. The efficacy of the biotinylation reaction can be controlled by capturing different concentrations of the biotinylated antibody with anti-species-IgG-coated beads, followed by detection with R-Phycoerythrin-conjugated streptavidin (see Subheading 3.2).
7. The type of detergent used for cell lysis has a major impact on extraction efficiency, especially on that of membrane-bound

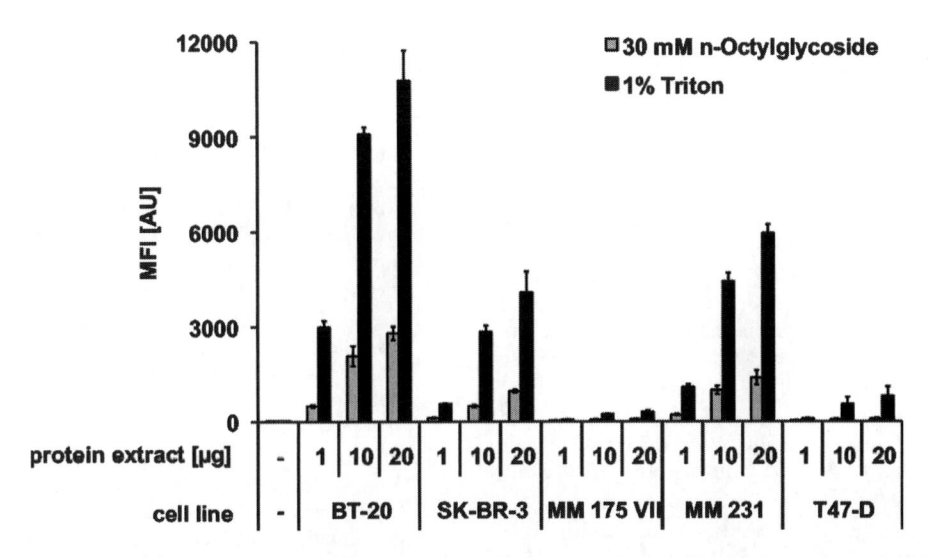

Fig. 3. Different detergents utilised for cell lysis have a major impact on the extraction efficiency of membrane-bound proteins such as RTKs. Here, proteins from various breast cancer cell lines were extracted using either 1% Triton X-100 or 30 mM *n*-octylglycopyranoside (*n*-OG). Total EGFR was analysed using a bead-based sandwich immunoassay. 1% Triton (*black bars*) is a more efficient detergent to solubilise EGFR than 30 mM *n*-OG (*grey bars*).

proteins such as RTKs (see Fig. 3). Various detergents need to be tested to give the optimum results for protein extraction if a novel assay has to be developed (see Subheadings 3.3 and 3.4).

8. Ensure that buffer does not remain in the drains of the filter plate. If buffer remains, it may cause well draining due to capillary forces (see Subheading 3.5).

9. Amount of expressed EGFR or other RTKs varies considerably between cell lines. Therefore, the amount of protein extract or protein concentration of the sample has to be adjusted (see Subheading 3.5).

10. Generic tyrosine phosphorylation and protein quantity must be determined in separate experiments (wells) and cannot be multiplexed together (see Subheading 3.5).

11. The given protocol does not include the generation of a standard. Therefore, all results generated using this method represent a relative quantification of phosphorylation. If available, a standard may be used for absolute quantification (see Subheading 3.5).

Acknowledgements

We would like to thank Thomas Schreiber and Jutta Bachmann for proofreading this manuscript.

References

1. Gschwind, A., Fischer, O. M., and Ullrich, A. (2004) The discovery of receptor tyrosine kinases: targets for cancer therapy, *Nat Rev Cancer* **4**, 361–370.
2. Schlessinger, J. (2000) Cell signaling by receptor tyrosine kinases. *Cell* **103**, 211–225.
3. Venter, D. J., Tuzi, N. L., Kumar, S., and Gullick, W. J. (1987) Overexpression of the c-erbB-2 oncoprotein in human breast carcinomas: immunohistological assessment correlates with gene amplification. *Lancet* **2**, 69–72.
4. Carson, R. T., and Vignali, D. A. (1999) Simultaneous quantitation of 15 cytokines using a multiplexed flow cytometric assay. *J. Immunol. Methods* **227**, 41–52.
5. Fulton, R. J., McDade, R. L., Smith, P. L., Kienker, L. J., and Kettman, J. R., Jr. (1997) Advanced multiplexed analysis with the FlowMetrix system. *Clin. Chem.* **43**, 1749–1756.
6. Du, J., Bernasconi, P., Clauser, K. R., Mani, D. R., Finn, S. P., Beroukhim, R., Burns, M., Julian, B., Peng, X. P., Hieronymus, H., Maglathlin, R. L., Lewis, T. A., Liau, L. M., Nghiemphu, P., Mellinghoff, I. K., Louis, D. N., Loda, M., Carr, S. A., Kung, A. L., and Golub, T. R. (2009) Bead-based profiling of tyrosine kinase phosphorylation identifies SRC as a potential target for glioblastoma therapy. *Nat. Biotechnol.* **27**, 77–83.
7. Poetz, O., Henzler, T., Hartmann, M., Kazmaier, C., Templin, M. F., Herget, T., and Joos, T. O. (2010) Sequential multiplex analyte capturing for phosphoprotein profiling. *Mol. Cell Proteomics* **9**, 2474–2481.
8. Fry, D. W., Bridges, A. J., Denny, W. A., Doherty, A., Greis, K. D., Hicks, J. L., Hook, K. E., Keller, P. R., Leopold, W. R., Loo, J. A., McNamara, D. J., Nelson, J. M., Sherwood, V., Smaill, J. B., Trumpp-Kallmeyer, S., and Dobrusin, E. M. (1998) Specific, irreversible inactivation of the epidermal growth factor receptor and erbB2, by a new class of tyrosine kinase inhibitor. *Proc. Natl. Acad. Sci. USA* **95**, 12022–12027.

Chapter 14

Monitoring Phosphoproteomic Response to Targeted Kinase Inhibitors Using Reverse-Phase Protein Microarrays

Gabriela Lavezzari and Mark R. Lackner

Abstract

Phosphoproteomic networks mediated by protein kinases are the key drivers of proliferative and survival signals underlying human cancers, and as such a number of kinases have been the subject of intensive drug discovery efforts. A key question that must be answered during clinical development is whether a kinase inhibitor is effectively inhibiting its appropriate target kinase and pathway in the tumor. Reverse-phase protein arrays (RPMAs) offer the ability to analyze behavior of entire signaling networks in response to drug treatment and thus have promise as a technology for monitoring cellular response to kinase inhibitors. We have shown that it is possible to use RPMAs to detect phosphorylation changes in key multiple signaling pathway proteins in response to targeted inhibitors of EGFR, MEK, and PI3 kinase.

Key words: MEK inhibitor, PI3 Kinase inhibitor, Reverse-phase protein array, Pharmacodynamic biomarker

1. Introduction

Almost all signal transduction pathways involved in proliferation and survival of cancer cells contain networks of cascading and interconnected phosphorylation events; hence, disrupting key nodes of these networks with inhibitors targeting specific kinases has great conceptual appeal in the treatment of cancer. Indeed, the diverse family of protein kinases encoded by the human genome have become the subject of intensive drug discovery efforts in recent years and therapeutics targeting kinases such as EGFR (erlotinib, gefinitinib), HER2 (trastuzumab, lapatinib), and BCR-Abl (imatinib) have all received FDA approval for the treatment of various solid tumor and hematological malignancies (reviewed in ref. 1). In addition to already approved agents, one recent estimate suggests that novel agents targeting at least 30 of the 515 or so human kinases have currently progressed to at least the phase I stage of clinical development (2). Two pathways that are currently the subject of particularly intense efforts are the EGFR/RAS/MEK/ERK pathway (3) and the PI3 kinase/Akt pathway (4), since these two pathways are thought to play fundamental roles integrating and transducing signals from multiple extracellular receptors (see Fig. 1) and are also frequently dysregulated through mutation or other genetic alterations in neoplasms (3, 5).

A key factor that will enhance success of drug discovery efforts targeting these pathways is the development of tools that will allow assessment of target pathway modulation in response to kinase inhibition in small amounts of patient tumor material. Such readouts would be invaluable during early drug development in that they would allow confirmation that the intended kinase target and corresponding pathway was being modulated at the dose and schedule being tested. With this in mind, we have developed a protocol that uses reverse-phase protein microarrays (RPMAs) to profile and monitor multiple components of signaling pathways and have demonstrated its utility in cell lines treated with selective kinase inhibitors that target EGFR (6), MEK (7), and PI3 kinase (8).

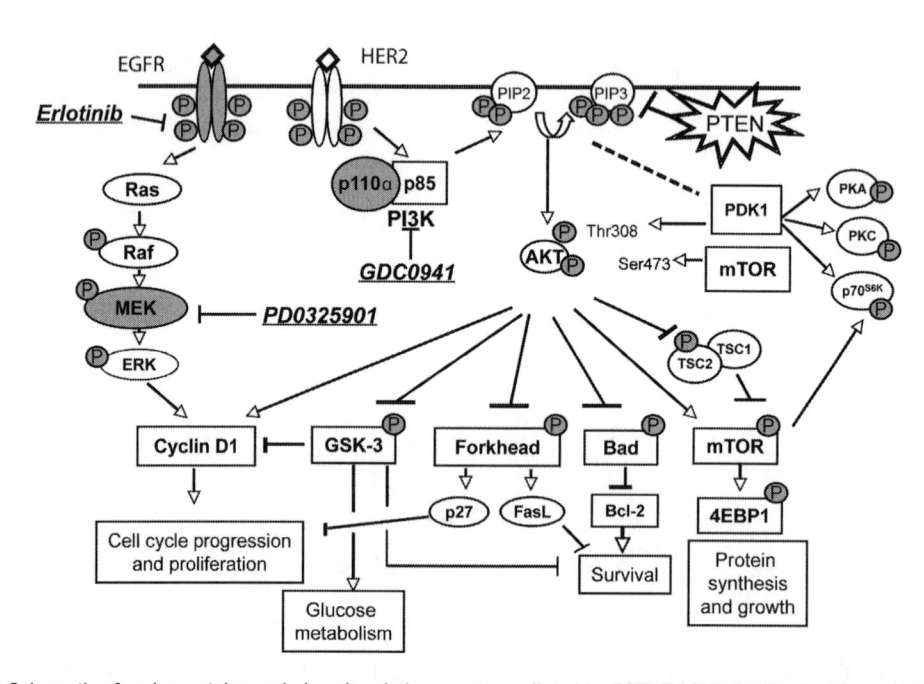

Fig. 1. Schematic of major proteins and phosphorylation events mediated by EGFR/RAS/RAF/MEK signaling and PI3K/Akt signaling in tumor cells. Drugs used to inhibit EGFR, MEK, and PI3 kinase are *underlined* and *italicized* (adapted with permission from ref. 12).

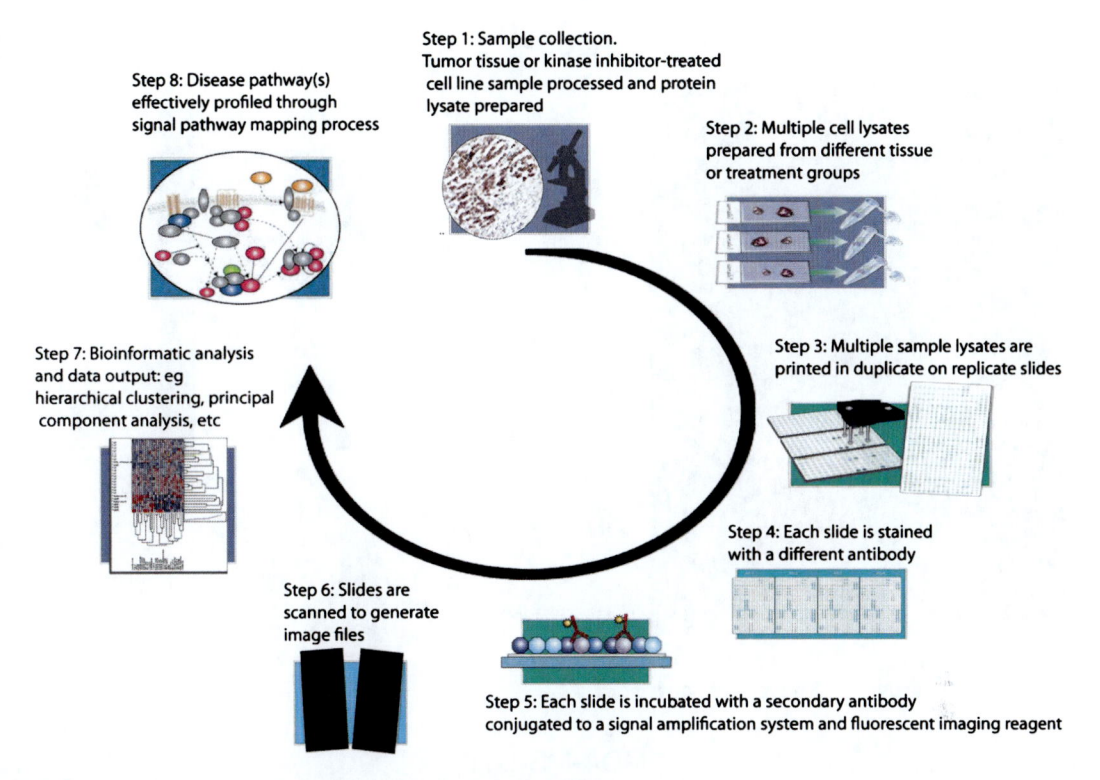

Fig. 2. Schematic of the reverse-phase protein microarray workflow.

The basis of the technology is to immobilize small amounts of lysate from a cell line or tumor sample in serial dilution on a microarray slide. Multiple samples are thus arrayed on a slide and can be probed with antibodies that detect a particular phosphoepitope (9, 10) (see Fig. 2 for overview). A key advantage of RPMAs is that they offer the potential to profile and measure potentially hundreds of phosphorylation events in very small quantities of tumor material such as one that might be obtained from laser capture microdissection from a biopsy (11), so RPMA pathway mapping should also have utility in the clinical setting.

Through these studies, we have shown that an inhibitor of all isoforms of the class I catalytic subunit of PI3 kinase, GDC-0941, results in potent and selective inhibition of multiple nodes in the PI3K/Akt pathway, and that a selective MEK inhibitor results in potent downregulation of pErk1/2 and actually increases signaling through the PI3K/Akt axis (12) (Fig. 3). Thus, RPMAs not only can be used to confirm expected pathway effects and specificity for a given kinase target but may also enable discovery of novel feedback loops that may have clinical implications. Here we describe a detailed protocol that can be used to monitor in vitro phosphoproteomic response to kinase inhibitors through profiling lysates on reverse-phase protein arrays.

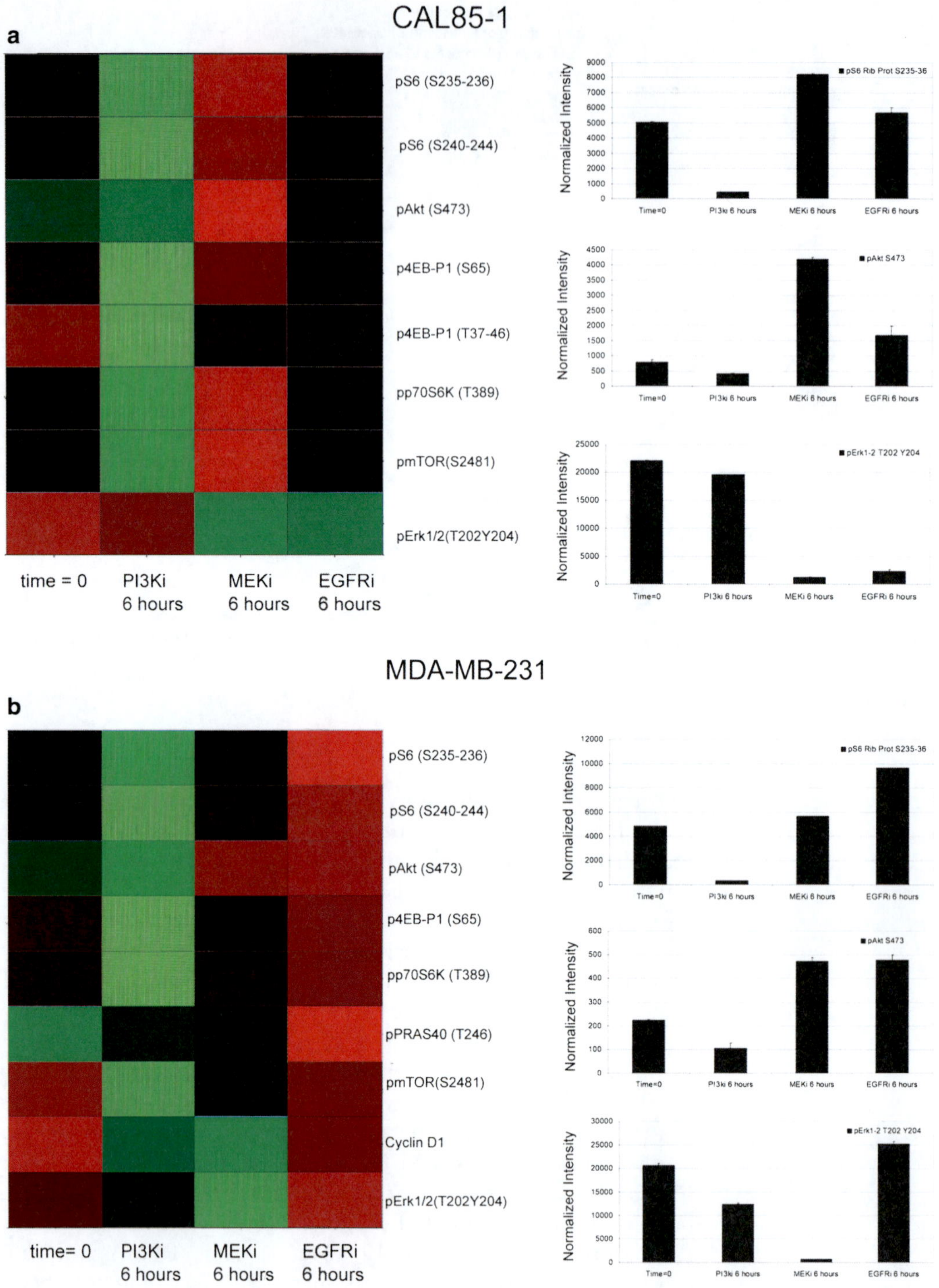
CAL85-1
a
pS6 (S235-236)
pS6 (S240-244)
pAkt (S473)
p4EB-P1 (S65)
p4EB-P1 (T37-46)
pp70S6K (T389)
pmTOR(S2481)
pErk1/2(T202Y204)
time = 0
PI3Ki 6 hours
MEKi 6 hours
EGFRi 6 hours
Normalized Intensity
pS6 Rib Prot S235-36
pAkt S473
pErk1-2 T202 Y204
Time=0
PI3ki 6 hours
MEKi 6 hours
EGFRi 6 hours
MDA-MB-231
b
pS6 (S235-236)
pS6 (S240-244)
pAkt (S473)
p4EB-P1 (S65)
pp70S6K (T389)
pPRAS40 (T246)
pmTOR(S2481)
Cyclin D1
pErk1/2(T202Y204)
time= 0
PI3Ki 6 hours
MEKi 6 hours
EGFRi 6 hours
Normalized Intensity
pS6 Rib Prot S235-36
pAkt S473
pErk1-2 T202 Y204

2. Materials

2.1. Cell Lines and Kinase Inhibitors

1. The breast cancer cell lines MDA-MB-231 and CAL-85-1 were obtained from American Type Culture Collection (ATCC, Manassas, VA) and the Deutsche Sammlung von Mikroorganismen und Zellkulturen GmbH (DSMZ, Braunschweig, Germany), respectively.

2. Culture conditions medium: Dulbecco's Modified Eagle's Medium (DMEM) supplemented with 10% fetal bovine serum, nonessential amino acids, and 2 mM L-glutamine.

3. Kinase inhibitors: 10 mM in 0.1% dimethyl sulfoxide (DMSO); MEK1/2 inhibitor PD0325901, PI3 kinase inhibitor GDC-0941, and EGFR inhibitor Erlotinib. Store in aliquots at −80°C.

4. Lysis buffer (components per 1 ml): 913 μl T-PER Reagent (includes 25 mM bicine, 150 mM sodium chloride, pH 7.6 and an unknown quantity of a detergent proprietary to Pierce), 60 μl of a 5 M NaCl solution, 10 μL of a 100 mM orthovanadate solution, 10 μL of a 200 mM PEFABLOC (4-(2-Aminoethyl)-benzensulfonylfluorid) solution, 1 μL of a 5 mg/mL Aprotinin solution, 5 μL of a 1 mg/mL Pepstatin A solution, and 1 μL of a 5 mg/mL Leupeptin solution. Note that the final concentration of NaCl is 450 mM. Just prior to use, add 2-mercaptoethanol to a final concentration of 2.5% (v/v).

2.2. Sample Arraying

1. Nitrocellulose coated glass slides.

2. 384 well plates.

3. Drierite drying material and zip-lock bags for storing printed nitrocellulose slides.

4. Kitchen plastic wrapping foil.

5. Phosphate-buffered saline (PBS): 137 mM NaCl, 2.7 mM KCl, 100 mM Na_2HPO_4, 2 mM KH_2PO_4, adjusted to pH 7.4 using HCl or NaOH.

Fig. 3. Pharmacodynamic modulation of signaling pathways by targeted kinase inhibitors. The heat map shows end points with at least a twofold change in intensity between pretreatment and 6 h treatment with at least one inhibitor in CAL85-1 cells (**a**) and MDAMB231 cells (**b**). *Green* indicates low and *red* high levels of phosphorylation. *Graphs to the right* show normalized intensity values for select end points that were modulated by compound treatment. Treatment with the PI3 kinase inhibitor GDC-0941 resulted in downregulation of multiple components of the PI3K/mTOR axis in both cell lines, including pAkt(S473), pp70S6K(T389), 4EBP1, and pS6 ribosomal protein. By contrast, treatment with the MEK inhibitor resulted in decreased levels of pErk1/2 and upregulation of key nodes in the PI3K pathway such as pAkt and pS6. This finding suggests the existence of a feedback loop whereby inhibition of the MEK/ERK axis causes upregulation of signaling in the PI3K/AKT pathway. Finally, treatment with the EGFR inhibitor had little or no effect on downstream pathway components such as pErk1/2 in the erlotinib unresponsive, KRAS mutant cell line MDAMB231, but did dramatically reduce pErk1/2 levels in the sensitive cell line CAL85-1 (reprinted with permission from ref. 12).

6. Dulbecco's phosphate-buffered saline (DPBS): 130 mM NaCl, 7.5 mM Na_2HPO_4, 1.5 mM KH_2PO_4, 0.5 mM $MgSO_4$, 1 mM $CaCl_2$, 0.03 mM KCl, and 5 mM glucose, adjusted to pH 7.4 using HCl or NaOH.

2.3. Slide Staining

1. Primary antibody for protein of choice.
2. Hydrogen peroxide: 3% (v/v) in water.
3. ReBlot mild antibody stripping solution: 10× stock.
4. I-block reagent.
5. Dako Catalyzed Signal Amplification Kit (CSA).
6. Biotin Blocking System.
7. DAKO Catalyzed Signal Amplification (CSA) System: Streptavidin Biotin Complex consisting of Reagent A and Reagent B.
8. Dako antibody diluent with background reducing components.
9. Fluorophor: IRDYE 680 Streptavidin.
10. Wash buffer: TBST, 20 mM Tris, 137 mM Sodium Chloride, 0.1% Tween-20, pH 7.6.
11. SYPRO Ruby protein blot stain.

3. Methods

Disruption of key signaling pathway nodes with kinase inhibitors is expected to perturb phosphorylation of multiple components of signaling pathways and yield a proteomic signature unique to each inhibitor. Identification and evaluation of such signatures could have use both in preclinical target pathway validation and ultimately in the clinical setting to determine assess target modulation at clinically achievable doses. We determined the quantitative in vitro pharmacodynamic effects of small-molecule kinase inhibitors of MEK1/2, PI3 kinase, and EGFR on a subset of 24 signaling pathway components using RPMAs (12). We evaluated relative phosphorylation levels of all 24 end points pre and post (6 h) treatment with each compound in the breast cancer cell lines CAL85-1 and MDA-MB-231 (see Note 1) and were able to identify distinct patterns of pathway modulation in response to the different inhibitors in both cell line. Here, we describe a general approach to in vitro pharmacodynamic analyses of phosphoproteomic networks using RPMA technology.

3.1. Sample Preparation for RPMA

1. Cells are maintained in DMEM until use.
2. The cells are plated in six-well plates and allowed to adhere overnight, and should be checked the next day to ensure 60–80% confluence (see Note 2). For the cell lines used in this study,

a split ratio of 1:2 will typically yield the appropriate confluence the following day, but this should be empirically determined for other cell lines.

3. Upon confirmation of appropriate confluence, the cells are then lysed either immediately or after 6 h incubation in the presence of 1 µM of each inhibitor or a DMSO control (see Note 3).

4. Cell lysis is accomplished directly in six well plates by addition of lysis buffer.

5. Determine protein concentration of each lysate using your preferred method.

6. Dilute all lysates in lysis buffer to a final protein concentration of 0.5 mg/ml and then print 30 µL of each sample, arrayed in a series of sixfold dilutions, in duplicate on slides as described in Subheading 3.2. Control lysates derived from, for example, Hela cells or Hela cells treated with pervanadate may also be printed on each slide as low and high phosphorylation controls, respectively (see Notes 4 and 5).

3.2. Arraying Samples on Nitrocellulose Slides

1. Make sure to prepare a sufficient number of slides including one as negative control (see Subheadings 3.4 and 3.5).

2. These instructions assume the use of the Aushon 2470 arrayer. Any other arrayer may be used but optimizations may apply.

3. Turn on power. If the arrayer is not switched on prior to starting the Aushon software, the communication with the arrayer will not be established and the computer will be unable to download the control instructions to the instrument when the run is started.

4. Perform the necessary housekeeping processes by emptying the waste carboy and by filling wash carboy and the humidifier with deionized water (see Note 6).

5. Load the samples plates in the Well Plate Elevator and the nitrocellulose slides into the Substrate Hotel. The loading order is from top to bottom on the left side of the Well Plate Hotel and then from top to bottom on the right side of the Well Plate Hotel.

6. If slides have labels, the slide must be positioned so that the label is located at the "finger-hole end" of the slide position on the platen.

7. Up to ten slides can be loaded on a platen. Please note that there should not be any breaks or gaps between slides on the platens. However, empty platens can be left in the hotel during a print run because the user specifies during programming which platens have slides present.

8. Program the arrayer. Define the type of well plates to be used, which wells in each plate should be used for sample extraction and the location of the well plates in the Well Plate Hotel.
9. Define the Array and Substrate by entering the characteristics of the array to be printed on the slide. There are five areas for entering information: Substrate Parameters, Feature Parameters, Sub Array Parameters, Super Array Parameters, and Replicate Parameters. User must customize each of these parameters.
10. Review the graphical representation of the slide in the lower right section of the screen. The arrays will be shown in the locations that they will be printed on a slide. Once the layout is acceptable, proceed to the next programming step, which will allow you to enter the length of time for the pins to be washed between samples to avoid any carryover. The user should customize this parameter based on the matrix of his/her samples. Some samples might be more viscous and require stricter protocol to avoid contamination.
11. Run the instrument preparation checklist, and once everything is set, start the deposition of lysates onto nitrocellulose slides.
12. When deposition is complete, the arrayer displays the message "Quit or Continue". Select "Continue" to continue printing more slides or select "Quit" if you have printed the desired number of slides.
13. Remove slides from platens. Remove the slides in the opposite order that they were loaded on the platens so that there is less chance of touching the nitrocellulose surface.
14. Store the slides in small slide boxes. Place the slide boxes in zip-lock plastic bags with several scoops of Drierite. Close the zip-lock bags and store the slide boxes in the −20°C.
15. Remove the well plates from the well plate holders. Place the well plates on the bench top, remove the lid and place the sticky side of a small piece (approximately 5 in. by 7 in.) of kitchen plastic wrapping foil on the surface of the well plate covering the surface completely and overlapping the sides. Smooth out any wrinkles to seal all wells. Wrap the excess foil over toward the underside of the well plate. Place the lid back in place on the well plate. Repeat the same process for all well plates and store at −20°C.
16. Empty the waste from the Waste Carboy, exit the operating software by choosing "Quit" in the file menu. Turn the power off.

3.3. Stripping and Blocking Nitrocellulose Slides

Protein immobilized on nitrocellulose coated slides may be used for protein characterization. Nonspecific binding sites on the nitrocellulose cause high background staining and must be blocked prior to addition of primary antibody to prevent nonspecific binding of the antibody to nitrocellulose membrane. Blocking is achieved via a two-step process using an antigen recovery step in the addition to a blocking step. Antigen recovery utilizes a mild stripping reagent to expose the antigenic sites. Blocking is performed with conventional protein-based reagents.

1. Remove the microarray slides from freezer. Place them in a petri dish or a slide box in case there are many slides to process.
2. Add sufficient mild antibody stripping reagent (ReBlot) to cover each slide in the container and rock gently for exactly 14 min. Please note that this step is critical. Therefore, do not exceed or cut short the 14-min time. This is a very strict requirement for the protocol.
3. Decant the ReBlot reagent and rinse the slides with (1×) DPBS.
4. Pour 1× PBS without calcium and magnesium into the container, enough to just cover the microarray slides. Allow to gently rock for 5 min.
5. Decant the 1× DPBS.
6. Repeat steps 4 and 5.
7. Add sufficient I-Block reagent to cover the slides in the container; allow rocking for at least 1 h prior to immunostaining (see Note 7).

3.4. Immunostaining of Slides

The DAKO CSA System is an extremely sensitive immunohistochemical (IHC) staining procedure that incorporates a signal amplification method based on a peroxidase-catalyzed deposition of a biotinylated phenolic compound, followed by a secondary reaction with a fluorescent dye conjugated with streptavidin. This protocol is optimized for use with an automated DAKO Autostainer. However, this procedure can be carried out manually or with any other kind of autostainer but may have to be adapted or optimized on a case by case basis.

1. Prepare reagents, optimized antibody dilution, required amount of wash buffer and load them in the autostainer. After the blocking step, load the slides in the autostainer and keep them wet with wash buffer until you are ready to start the autostainer.
2. The first step is to block endogenous peroxidase. Incubate the slides for 10 min in 3% hydrogen peroxide.
3. Wash with wash buffer for 3–5 min.
4. Block endogenous avidin and biotin by adding the avidin and biotin blocking solutions respectively and incubate for 5 min.
5. Wash with wash buffer 3–5 min.

6. Add protein blocking solution to suppress the nonspecific binding and incubate for 10–20 min.

7. Wash with wash buffer 3–5 min.

8. Add the first antibody (except for negative control slide) which has been diluted to an optimal dilution in antibody diluents and incubate for 30 min. Each slide is immunostained with only one antibody. Each antibody must have been previously validated (see Note 8). The phosphoproteins we have analyzed are described in reference (12).

9. After three washes of 3–5 min each to remove the first antibody solution, add the biotin-conjugated secondary antibody to all slides (including the negative control slide) and incubate for 15 min. Make sure to use the appropriate species.

10. Wash thoroughly (3× 3–5 min) with wash buffer to remove the secondary antibody solution.

11. Add the Streptavidin Biotin Complex consisting of Reagent A and Reagent B diluted in Streptavidin Biotin Complex Diluent and incubate for 15 min.

12. Wash thoroughly with wash buffer for 3× 3–5 min.

13. Add the amplification reagent and incubate for 15 min.

14. Wash thoroughly with wash buffer for 3× 3–5 min to remove the amplification reagent solution.

15. Add the streptavidin-conjugated fluorophore and incubate for 15 min.

16. Wash with deionized water and dry the slides at ambient temperature; store the slides at room temperature in the dark (the slides are now light sensitive) until further use.

17. Scan the slides using any fluorescent slide scanner, preferably at 2,540 dots per inch (dpi). Each detected spot will be associated with a raw intensity value.

3.5. Image Acquisition and Data Normalization

1. Each detected spot is associated with a raw intensity value. To allow normalization of total protein on printed arrays, one to two slides in each print run are stained with SYPRO Ruby protein blot stain (see Note 9) and the value obtained from these stained arrays are used for normalization of all analyte end-point values.

2. Subject the phosphoprotein analyte intensity values for each slide to local background subtraction and check the intensity values for saturation effects and the limit of detection.

3. Subject intensity values to nonspecific binding subtraction using the data from the negative control slide, in which the primary antibody was omitted and only the secondary antibody applied.

4. Normalize each value relative to the total protein intensity value obtained from the SYPRO Ruby stained slide. Samples

may additionally be normalized to lysates from ligand/chemical-stimulated cell lines that contain high levels of phosphoproteins (e.g., Hela cells ± pervandate for 30 min) that are printed on every slide and provide for high or low phosphorylation controls. These lysates ensure for process QA/QC as well as provide for bridging cases so that relative comparisons of data generated from different experimental runs can be performed.

3.6. Statistical Analysis of RPMA Data

1. Data analysis in our laboratory is performed with Partek Genomics Suite software version 6.3 but may also be performed with any other appropriate software.

2. RPMA data are preprocessed by Log2 transformation and further linear scaling (z-score conversion) to ensure data normality and linearity. The log transformed data are useful for Principle Component Analysis (PCA) and other statistical analyses and the z-scores may be used in hierarchical cluster analysis (HC). Examples of data visualization for multiple pathway components using a heat-map representation as well as bar charts showing normalized signal intensity in treated and untreated cells are shown in Fig. 3.

4. Notes

1. Cell lines have been characterized previously for both molecular subtype (12) and sensitivity to targeted kinase inhibitors (11). CAL85-1 is a basal-like breast cancer cell line with submicromolar in vitro EC_{50} sensitivity to all three compounds (0.33 μM for GDC0941, 0.11 μM for PD0325901, and 0.23 μM for erlotinib) in a standard ATP-based viability assay (see Subheading 3).

2. It is essential that cells are still in log phase growth and actively cycling through the cell cycle to assess biological effects of kinase inhibitors, thus such analyses should not be conducted on overconfluent cultures which may have a majority of quiescent and nonresponsive cells (see Subheading 3.1).

3. A DMSO control is essential for these experiments to ensure effects are due the specific inhibitor being tested (see Subheading 3.1).

4. Pervanadate is an irreversible protein tyrosine phosphatase inhibitor (13) that results in global cellular increase in protein phosphorylation and hence pervanadate treatment provides a useful high phosphorylation control (see Subheading 3.1).

5. The use of low and high phosphorylation controls printed on each array is important to allow comparison of data from arrays

run at different times and is discussed in detail in reference (8) (see Subheading 3.1).

6. The water used in all procedures has a resistance of 18.2 MΩ cm and it is filtered with a 0.22-μm filter (see Subheading 3.2).

7. The slides should remain rocking for the entire blocking period. Blocking times can range from 1 h to overnight. If overnight blocking is performed, the microarray slides should be blocked at 2–4°C (see Subheading 3.3).

8. Prior to use, antibodies should undergo validation for both phosphorylation detection and protein specificity using criteria such as single band detection at the appropriate molecular weight by immunoblotting. Each antibody should also be titrated to find the most appropriate concentration for RPMA applications (see Subheading 3.4).

9. SYPRO ruby is a ruthenium-based florescent stain for the detection of proteins separated by polyacrylamide gel electrophoresis (PAGE) or on blotted membranes. It is useful for quantitation of total protein, since it has a linear quantitation range of over three orders of magnitude and detects the majority of the cellular proteome (14) (see Subheading 3.5).

References

1. Grant, S. K. (2009) Therapeutic Protein Kinase Inhibitors, *Cell. Mol. Life Sci*, **66**(7), 1163–1177.
2. Zhang, J., Yang, P. L., and Gray, N. S. (2009) Targeting cancer with small molecule kinase inhibitors. *Nat. Rev. Cancer* **9**, 28–39.
3. Kohno, M., and Pouyssegur, J. (2006) Targeting the ERK signaling pathway in cancer therapy. *Ann. Med.* **38**, 200–211.
4. Ihle, N. T., and Powis, G. (2009) Take your PIK: phosphatidylinositol 3-kinase inhibitors race through the clinic and toward cancer therapy. *Mol. Cancer Ther.* **8**, 1–9.
5. Carnero, A., Blanco-Aparicio, C., Renner, O., Link, W., and Leal, J. F. (2008) The PTEN/PI3K/AKT signalling pathway in cancer, therapeutic implications. *Curr. Cancer Drug Tar.* **8**, 187–198.
6. Bareschino, M. A., Schettino, C., Troiani, T., Martinelli, E., Morgillo, F., and Ciardiello, F. (2007) Erlotinib in cancer treatment., *Ann. Oncol.* **18 Suppl 6**, vi35–41.
7. Brown, A. P., Carlson, T. C., Loi, C. M., and Graziano, M. J. (2007) Pharmacodynamic and toxicokinetic evaluation of the novel MEK inhibitor, PD0325901, in the rat following oral and intravenous administration. *Cancer Chemoth. Pharm.* **59**, 671–679.
8. Folkes, A. J., Baker, S. J., Chuckowree, I. S., Eccles, S. A., Hayes, A., Hancox, T. C., Latif, M. A., Olivero, A. G., Patel, S., and Shuttleworth, S. J. (2008) The discovery of GDC-0941: A potent, selective, orally bioavailable inhibitor of class I PI3 kinase for the treatment of cancer. in *AACR Annual Meeting*, San Diego.
9. Espina, V., Wulfkuhle, J., Calvert, V. S., Liotta, L. A., and Petricoin, E. F., 3rd. (2008) Reverse phase protein microarrays for theranostics and patient-tailored therapy. In *Methods in molecular biology (Clifton, N.J)* **441**, 113–128.
10. Wulfkuhle, J. D., Edmiston, K. H., Liotta, L. A., and Petricoin, E. F., 3 rd. (2006) Technology insight: pharmacoproteomics for cancer – promises of patient-tailored medicine using protein microarrays. *Nat. Clin. Pract. Oncol.* **3**, 256–268.
11. Espina, V., Wulfkuhle, J. D., Calvert, V. S., Petricoin, E. F., 3rd, and Liotta, L. A. (2007) Reverse phase protein microarrays for monitoring biological responses. In *Methods in molecular biology (Clifton, N.J)* **383**, 321–336.

12. Boyd, Z. S., Wu, Q. J., O'Brien, C., Spoerke, J., Savage, H., Fielder, P. J., Amler, L., Yan, Y., and Lackner, M. R. (2008) Proteomic analysis of breast cancer molecular subtypes and biomarkers of response to targeted kinase inhibitors using reverse-phase protein microarrays. *Mol. Cancer Ther.* **7**, 3695–3706.

13. Secrist, J. P., Burns, L. A., Karnitz, L., Koretzky, G. A., and Abraham, R. T. (1993) Stimulatory effects of the protein tyrosine phosphatase inhibitor, pervanadate, on T-cell activation events. *J. Biol. Chem.* 1993 Mar 15;**268**(8), 5886–5893.

14. Steinberg, T. H., Jones, L. J., Haugland, R. P., and Singer, V. L. (1996) SYPRO orange and SYPRO red protein gel stains: one-step fluorescent staining of denaturing gels for detection of nanogram levels of protein, *Anal Biochem.* **239**(2), 223–237.

Chapter 15

Measuring Phosphorylation-Specific Changes in Response to Kinase Inhibitors in Mammalian Cells Using Quantitative Proteomics

Nurhan Özlü, Marc Kirchner, and Judith Jebanathirajah Steen

Abstract

Many cancers have been associated with the deregulation of kinases, and thus, kinases have become a prime target for the development of cancer treatments. This focus on kinases has resulted in the approval of several small-molecule kinase inhibitors for cancer treatments. Further, the use of these inhibitors as tools to study cancer has provided valuable information about biological mechanisms. However, to date, not much is known about the global effects of kinases on the proteome or phosphoproteome. In this protocol, we describe methodology to study the impact of kinase inhibitors on the proteome and phosphoproteome using mass spectrometry-based quantitative proteomics. More specifically, we focus on the effects of Aurora B kinase inhibitors on the proteome, cytoskeleton proteome, the phosphoproteome, and the cytoskeleton phosphoproteome during cell cycle. This methodology is easily extended to other biological studies whose aim is to study the global proteomic effects of a kinase inhibitor.

Key words: Quantitative mass spectrometry, Kinase inhibitors, Aurora kinase, Phosphoproteome, Microtubulome

1. Introduction

Posttranslational modifications are important hallmarks of protein function including cellular signaling activities, energy metabolism, cell division, and cell death. Phosphorylation is the most ubiquitous protein modification that has been conserved throughout evolution. The reversible and transient nature of protein phosphorylation allows tight regulation of diverse cellular functions. Various complex cellular events are orchestrated by several kinase families, which catalyze protein phosphorylation. It is often technically very challenging to dissect the role of a kinase using traditional genetic approaches

Bernhard Kuster (ed.), *Kinase Inhibitors: Methods and Protocols*, Methods in Molecular Biology, vol. 795,
DOI 10.1007/978-1-61779-337-0_15, © Springer Science+Business Media, LLC 2012

or RNAi techniques. This is because kinase activities often trigger a cascade of phosphorylation events that require a temporal control of kinase inhibition to access the downstream events. A particularly explicit case is the study of kinases that are active during cell division. Several kinases, such as Aurora B and Polo-like kinase, are active during several stages of mitosis; thus, it is difficult to study these kinases in all stages of mitosis using RNAi, as the cells arrest in the first stages of mitosis that the kinase is active (1). Thus, one does not learn much about the role of that kinase in subsequent stages of cell division. Partial knockdown of a kinase may also not be very effective as the residual kinase would be sufficient to trigger enzymatic activities. Therefore, small molecules have proved to be powerful tools for elucidating the role of different kinases and the mechanism of their action by providing potent, selective, prompt and often reversible inhibition of a kinase activity. Kinase inhibitors not only are great research tools to understand biology but can also serve as drugs to treat diseases where the misregulation of a kinase is responsible (2). For example, a synthetic inhibitor of a tyrosine kinase, BCR-ABL is used as an anticancer drug for treatment of chronic myeloid leukemia. Similarly, various synthetic inhibitors of CDK kinases – master regulators of cell cycle – have been proved to be promising for various cancer treatments (3).

Mass spectrometry (MS)-based techniques are becoming important tools to expand the picture of regulatory mechanism of phosphorylation. The ultimate goal of identifying phosphorylation sites is (a) to identify substrate and to (b) elucidate the function of the modification. The identification of the kinase and the substrate is theoretically addressable using MS and bioinformatics methods, whereas the latter involves specific biological experiments. Phosphorylation analysis using mass spectrometry provided large-scale data sets of phosphorylation sites in many different model organisms, tissues, and cultured cells (4). These data sets are useful resources that document specific phosphorylation sites under a particular biological condition. One of the next challenges in phosphoproteomics is to establish new methods to understand the effect of a specific kinase on the phosphoproteome. This is also important for therapeutic purposes: a drug (i.e., kinase inhibitor) may not have one particular molecular target, thus MS-based techniques can analytically examine all targets in an in-depth and unbiased manner which would be useful for further optimization of the drug by medical chemistry (5). For example, a study using nonselective kinase inhibitors immobilized on beads identified novel targets of therapeutic kinase inhibitors when used in competitive proteomic assays (6).

Here, we describe a quantitative method to study the effect of kinase inhibitors by monitoring the changes on the phosphoproteome in response to kinase inhibitors. By this method, targets of a kinase can be identified in the whole proteome. Our interest underlies on an important mitotic kinase, Aurora kinase.

15 Measuring Phosphorylation-Specific Changes in Response to Kinase Inhibitors... 219

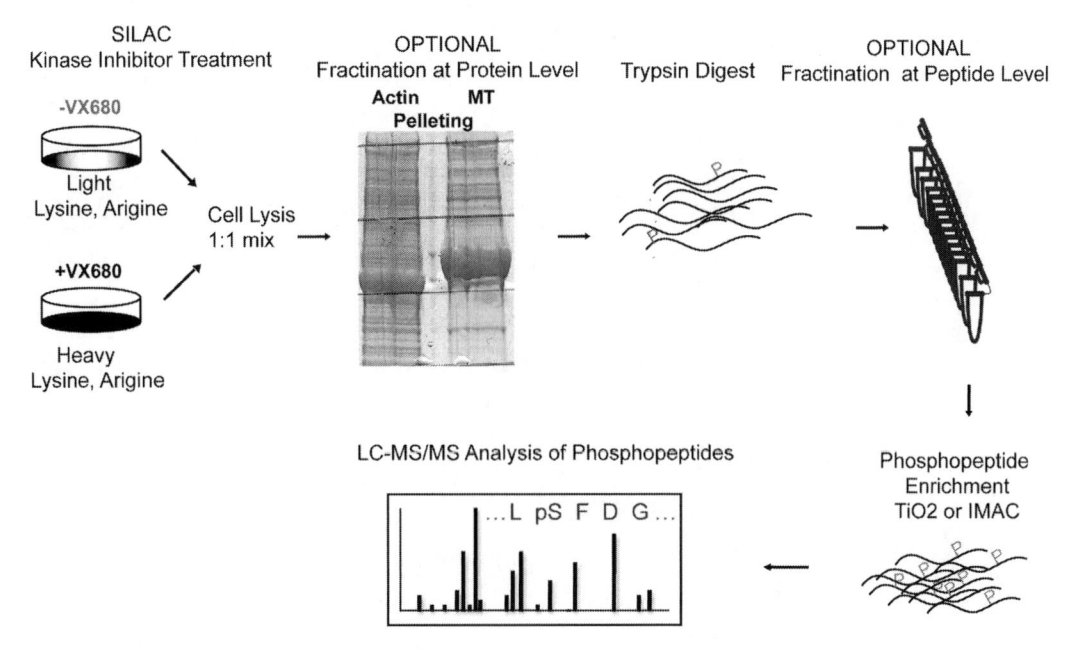

Fig. 1. Work flow of SILAC-based phosphoproteomic analysis of kinase inhibitor-treated cells.

Aurora kinases are required for spindle assembly, which is a microtubule based structure that segregates the duplicated chromosomes during cell division (7). Given the fact that many anticancer drugs target microtubules, Aurora kinases have garnered attention and various small molecules that inhibit Aurora kinases are in clinical trials for anticancer treatments (3, 8). Here we used VX-680, a potent inhibitor of Aurora kinases (IC_{50} VX-680: Aurora B = 18 nM, Aurora A = 36 nM, and Aurora C = 25 nM) (9) as an example to examine the effect of Aurora kinases on the phosphoproteome and microtubulome. Typical steps of this experiment, which we describe here, are as follows: (1) growing tissue culture cells in SILAC media for quantitative analysis of kinase inhibition, (2) cell lysis, (3) fractionation of complex protein mixture (optional), (4) proteolysis, (6) enrichment of phosphopeptides, (7) analysis by LC–MS/MS, and (8) data evaluation (see Fig. 1).

2. Materials

2.1. Cell Culture and SILAC Media

1. Cell line: this study used HeLa S3 suspension cells, which are easy to grow in bulk for cell structure isolations or other biochemical experiments which require more starting material. Many other cell lines may also be used.

2. Cell culture medium: Dulbecco's modified Eagle's medium (DMEM) without L-lysine and L-arginine.

3. Dialyzed fetal bovine serum (FBS).
4. Amino acids: "Light" (^{12}C, ^{14}N) L-Lysine and L-Arginine and "heavy" (^{13}C, ^{15}N) L-Lysine and L-Arginine for SILAC labeling. In this study, ^{13}C$_6$, ^{15}N$_2$ L-Lysine and ^{13}C$_6$, ^{15}N$_4$ L-Arginine were used resulting in mass differences of 8 and 10 Da between heavy and light isoforms for Lysine and Arginine, respectively.
5. Antibiotics: Streptomycin (10.000 µg/ml) and penicillin (10,000 µg/ml).
6. Trypsin–EDTA: 0.25% Trypsin (w/v), 2.21 mM ethylenediaminetetraacetic acid (EDTA) in Hank's balanced salt solution (HBSS) without sodium bicarbonate, calcium, and magnesium.
7. Phosphate-buffered saline (1×): sterile, without magnesium and calcium.
8. S-Trityl-L-cysteine: 1 mM in dimethylsulfoxide (DMSO).
9. Nocodazole: 1 mM in dimethylsulfoxide (DMSO).
10. Vincristine: 1 mM in dimethylsulfoxide (DMSO).
11. Thymidine: 100 mM stock solution in sterile PBS, filtered through 0.22-µm pore size filter prior to use.
12. Particle Count and Size Analyzer or Hemocytometer for counting cells.

2.2. Cell Lysis

1. Lysis buffer for in-solution digest: 6 M urea, 2 M thiourea, 50 mM Tris–HCl, 10% glycerol, 2% *n*-octylglucoside.
2. Lysis buffers for in-gel digest (see Subheading 2.4).
3. Protease inhibitor cocktail tablet, EDTA free.
4. Phosphatase inhibitors: See Table 1 and Note 1.
5. SDS-Page sample buffer: 100 mM Tris–HCl(hydroxymethyl)-aminomethane (Tris), pH 6.8, 50 mM dithiothreitol (DTT), 2% SDS, 15% glycerol (see Note 2).
6. Coomassie blue stain.
7. Sonicator.

2.3. Protein Concentration Determination

1. Protein standard: Bovine serum albumin (BSA).
2. Protein assay reagent: Bicinchoninic acid (BCA).
3. Spectrophotometer.

2.4. Cytoskeleton Pelleting

2.4.1. Actin Pelleting

1. Lysis buffer: 20 mM HEPES, pH 7.4, 100 mM KCl, 2 mM ethylene glycol tetraacetic acid (EGTA), 2 mM MgCl$_2$, 10% glycerol, 1% NP-40 (see Note 3).
2. F buffer: 20 mM HEPES, pH 7.4, 100 mM KCl, 2 mM MgCl$_2$.

Table 1
List of phosphatase inhibitors used in the lysis buffer (see Note 1)

Inhibitor	Stock concentration	Stock solvent	Final concentration
Okadaic acid	1 mM	DMSO	1 µM
Microcystin-LR	1 mM	DMSO	1 µM
Sodium fluoride	500 mM	Water	10 mM
Sodium orthovanadate	100 mM	Water	1 mM
β-Glycerol phosphate	1 M	Water	20 mM
Sodium pyrophosphate	100 mM	Water	1 mM

3. Phalloidin: 1 mg/ml Stock in DMSO. Phalloidin is used to stabilize actin polymers.
4. Glycerol cushion: 40% (v/v) Glycerol in F Buffer.

2.4.2. Microtubule Pelleting

1. Lysis buffer: 100 mM potassium 1,4-piperazinediethanesulfonate (K-Pipes), pH 6.8, 1 mM MgCl$_2$, 2 mM EGTA, 1% NP-40 (see Note 4).
2. CM buffer: 100 mM K-Pipes, pH 7.0, 1 mM EGTA, 2 mM MgCl$_2$.
3. Paclitaxel (Taxol): 2 mM stock in DMSO. Taxol is used to stabilize microtubules.
4. 40% Glycerol cushion in BRB80: 40% (v/v) glycerol in 80 mM 4-piperazinediethanesulfonate (Pipes), pH 6.8, 1 mM MgCl$_2$, 1 mM EGTA.

2.5. Reduction, Alkylation, and Digestion of Protein Samples

1. HPLC-grade water.
2. HPLC-grade acetonitrile (ACN).
3. Ammonium bicarbonate: 1 M in water (see Note 5).
4. Iodoacetamide: 500 mM in water (see Note 6).
5. Trypsin: Sequencing grade.

2.6. Enrichment of Phoshopeptides

1. HPLC-grade water.
2. Trifluoroacetic acid (TFA).
3. HPLC-grade ACN.
4. TiO$_2$ Toptip columns.
5. Binding buffer: 5% (v/v) TFA, 40% (v/v) ACN in water.
6. Wash buffer: 1% TFA (v/v), 80% (v/v) ACN in water.
7. Elution buffer: 0.4 M NH$_4$OH in water.

2.7. LC–MS Analysis

1. Loading buffer: 4% Formic acid, 4% ACN in HPLC-grade water.
2. HPLC buffer A: 95:5 (v/v) water–ACN 0.2% formic acid.
3. HPLC buffer B: 5:95 (v/v) water–ACN 0.2% formic acid.
4. Nano HPLC: In this study, an Eksigent nanoLC•2D™ HPLC system was used. Alternative systems may also be used.
5. HPLC column: Magic C18 (5 U, 100 A) reversed-phase nano-column packed in-house into FS360-100-15-N-5-C30 PicoTips.
6. Mass spectrometer: In this study, an LTQ-Orbitrap mass spectrometer was used. Alternative systems may also be used.

3. Methods

3.1. Preparation of Cell Culture Medium for SILAC

1. Prepare a 100× stock solution of labeled amino acids (both light and heavy isoforms) in sterile 1× PBS and store at –20°C. The concentration of amino acids should be calculated such that they are at the concentration of the original medium. For DMEM media, add Lysine and Arginine amino acids to a final concentration of 0.146 and 0.084 g/l concentration, respectively (see Note 7).
2. Prepare Light and Heavy DMEM media (for HeLa S3 cells) by adding light and heavy labeled amino acids, respectively. The following should be added to the media: dialyzed fetal bovine serum (FBS) to a 10% concentration and 1% of streptomycin and penicillin. Filter both heavy and light media through a 0.22-μm filter. Store the media at 4°C.

3.2. Growing Cells in SILAC Media

1. Grow equal amounts of cells (from the same clonal stock) in light and heavy media. For complete incorporation of the SILAC amino acids, 6–8 cell passages (with 1:5 split ratio) are recommended. Starting with a small amount of cells (~10^6) minimizes the amount of media needed for complete labeling (see Note 8).
2. Once full incorporation of the isotopic labeled amino acids has been achieved, grow HeLa S3 cells to a density of 10^6 cells/mL in suspension using Erlenmeyer culture flasks with a 0.22-μm vented cap.

3.3. Synchronization of HeLa S3 Cells

Before treating cells with a kinase inhibitor it may be necessary to synchronize cells at a certain cell stage. For proteomic analysis, it is very important to generate robust synchronization protocols and homogenous cell populations to minimize noise between different biological replicates. In our case, we are interested in the cell cycle dependent activity of Aurora B, thus we established protocols that produce cells that are 90–100% synchronous. To synchronize cells at G1/S, follow the protocol established by Fang et al. using a double thymidine block (10). For Mitotic Cell Synchronization, a single thymidine block followed by a mitotic block is recommended.

1. Treat HeLa S3 suspension cells grown in SILAC labeled DMEM media with Thymidine added to a final concentration of 2 mM for 18 h.
2. Centrifuge cells at $300 \times g$ for 5 min.
3. Wash cells twice with sterile PBS (at 37°C) by resuspending cells in PBS followed by pelleting cells in a centrifuge at $300 \times g$.
4. After the last wash, resuspend the cells in fresh SILAC medium for 3–4 h (see Note 9).
5. Block cells at mitosis using media containing 10 µM of the kinesin-5 inhibitor S-Trityl-L-cysteine (STC) for 12 h. Alternative drugs for mitotic arrest are as follows: 0.1 µg/ml nocodazole for 12 h, 10 nM vincristine for 18 h, 20 nM taxol for 20 h (11, 12) (see Note 10).

3.4. Treatment of Cells with Kinase Inhibitor

Prior to performing SILAC experiments, it is imperative to determine the correct concentration of the kinase inhibitor for cell culture. It should be low enough to selectively inhibit the kinase of interest and avoid nonspecific inhibition of other kinases, but it should also be potent enough for large scale experiments to affect the biochemistry of the bulk cell population homogenously. For this purpose it is important to evaluate the kinase inhibitor selectivity, i.e., IC_{50}s of the kinase of interest versus irrelevant kinases. Also, if the kinase inhibitor affects other kinases that are active in the cell cycle phase that you are studying, it is beneficial to use an alternative inhibitor to distinguish off-target effects. It is recommended to perform a series of experiments in which the concentration of the kinase inhibitor is titrated and the kinase treatment is preformed in a time course manner to determine the most effective and selective condition. A practical way of evaluating different conditions is to perform western blotting analyses against known phosphorylation sites (see Fig. 2). After the conditions for the particular kinase inhibitor have been determined, SILAC samples are prepared as above to analyze global changes.

1. Count the number of cells grown in suspension in heavy and light media using a hemocytometer or coulter counter. Ensure that there are equal numbers of cells from both conditions; if not, adjust the cell amount.
2. Split the cells grown in heavy and light media into two equal amounts.

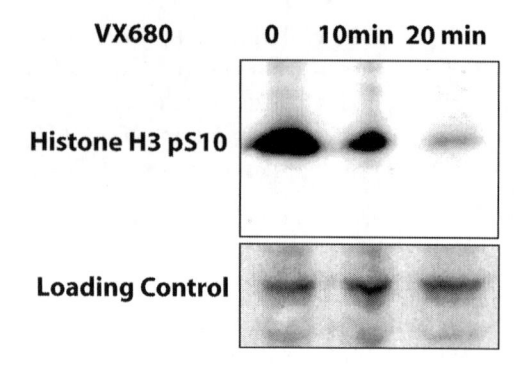

Fig. 2. Time course inhibition of an Aurora-B phosphorylation site using the Aurora kinase Inhibitor VX680. Mitotic cells were treated with 400 nM VX680 for 0, 10 and 20 min. Western blotting against a phoshoserine residue on Histone H3, a known Aurora-B phosphorylation site, showed a dramatic inhibition by VX680 treatment after 20 min (*top panel*). The loading control from the same blot is shown at the *bottom panel*.

3. Treat half of the heavy cells and half of the light cells with the kinase inhibitor and the other halves with mock (the same volume of DMSO, if the inhibitor was dissolved in DMSO) or a generic, nonselective inhibitor (see Note 11).

4. Wash both mock- and inhibitor-treated heavy and light cells with ice-cold PBS twice by resuspending the cells in PBS followed by cell pelleting in a refrigerated centrifuge at $300 \times g$.

5. Snap-freeze the cells in liquid nitrogen.

3.5. Cell Lysis and Protein Digestion

3.5.1. Cell Lysis for In-gel Digest

1. Lyse frozen cells in lysis buffer (see Subheading 2.4.1 or 2.4.2) containing protease inhibitors and phosphatase inhibitors (see Note 12). The lysis buffer should be twice the volume of the cell pellet. Incubate for 20 min on ice.

2. Centrifuge cell lysates at $2,800 \times g$ for 10 min at 4°C.

3. Measure the protein concentration of supernatants using the BCA assay. Use BSA (50–2,000 µg/ml) as a standard.

4. Mix cell lysates in 1:1 ratio (v/v): Mix inhibitor-treated heavy cells (+) with mock-treated light cells (−). To swap the metabolic label, mix mock-treated heavy cells (−) with inhibitor-treated light cells (+).

5. Add SDS-PAGE buffer to each sample. Add iodoacetamide to a final concentration of 50 mM and incubate and incubate in the dark for 30 min.

6. Separate the protein mixture via SDS-PAGE. Stain the gel with a Coomassie stain.

3.5.2. In-gel Digest

For further details on the digestion procedure, refer to (13).

1. Cut the gel into ten or more slices and wash gel slices in HPLC water (see Note 13).

2. Wash the gel slices with 0.1 M ABC followed by acetonitrile (ACN). Repeat this washing procedure three times.

3. After the last ACN wash, add trypsin to 12.5 ng/µl in 100 mM ABC to cover gel slices. Leave on ice for 30 min, remove excess trypsin solution and add enough 0.1 M ABC to cover gel pieces (see Note 14).

4. Incubate at 37°C for 8 h.

5. Extract the peptides using 0.1 M ABC and ACN in a 1:1 (v/v) ratio and perform a final extraction using 100% ACN. Lyophilize the digested samples and store at −20°C until use.

3.5.3. Cell Lysis for In-solution Digest

1. Add five volumes of cell lysis buffer per volume of frozen cell pellet. Incubate for 20 min on ice.

2. Mix cell lysates in 1:1 ratio (v/v): Mix inhibitor-treated heavy cells (+) with mock-treated light cells (−). To swap the metabolic label, mix mock-treated heavy cells (−) with inhibitor-treated light cells (+) (see Note 15).

3. Sonicate cells on ice at 40% maximal sonicator output with three time intervals, 15 s on, 45 s off.

4. Centrifuge cell lysates at 2,800×g for 10 min at room temperature (RT).

5. Add DTT to a final concentration of 20 mM to each supernatant and incubate at RT for 30 min.

3.5.4. In-solution Digest

1. Add 40 mM iodoacetamide to the sample generated the last step of Subheading 3.5.3, incubate for 30 min at RT in the dark.

2. Dialyze the lysates overnight against 1 l of 10 mM ammonium bicarbonate (ABC).

3. Raise the ABC concentration to 50 mM using the 1 M stock solution.

4. Add trypsin at a protein to enzyme ratio of 100:1 and incubate at 37°C for 6–8 h.

3.6. Fractionation of Cell Content After Inhibitor Treatment

It is useful to reduce the complexity of the proteome prior to the enrichment of phosphorylated peptides. This is especially useful if one is interested in a particular molecular pathway. Treatment of cells with a kinase inhibitor may promote global affects in different cellular compartments. However, it is not always feasible to obtain an in-depth analysis of these changes as excessive fractionation must be performed, which would require many hours of instrument time and several LC/MS runs. Depending on the purpose of the experiment, it may not be necessary to cover the whole proteome, but rather focus on a specific cellular compartment where the kinase's substrates are mostly localized. For example, Aurora kinases are mainly involved in cell division and cytoskeleton regulation. Therefore, the isolation of the cytoskeleton (14) or chromosomes will likely enrich the substrates of the Aurora B. One disadvantage of cellular enrichment is that kinase inhibitors will also affect the binding efficiency of substrates to the cytoskeleton. Therefore, the phosphorylation difference for each protein should be normalized by the amount of protein in each condition.

3.6.1. Actin Cytoskeleton Pelleting

1. Use the lysis buffer listed in Subheading 2.4.1 and follow the first four steps described in Subheading 3.5.1 (see Note 16).
2. After mixing cell lysates, clear the lysate by centrifugation for 25 min at 80,000×g. Recover the middle layer and avoid collecting the white, fluffy lipid layer on top.
3. To stabilize actin filaments, add 10 µg/ml phalloidin and incubate on ice for 20 min.
4. Pellet actin through a 40% glycerol cushion in F buffer (supplemented with 10 µg/ml phalloidin as well as protease and phosphatase inhibitors) with twice the volume of the supernatant for 25 min at 80,000×g at 4°C.
5. Discard the supernatant and the cushion. Resuspend the pellet in 1/4 of the original volume of F buffer. Load the sample onto a second 40% glycerol cushion as described above and centrifuge at 80,000×g for 25 min.
6. Discard the supernatant and cushion and resuspend the pellet in SDS-PAGE buffer, and separate protein mixture via SDS-PAGE.
7. Perform tryptic digestion as described in Subheading 3.5.2.

3.6.2. Microtubule Pelleting

1. Use the lysis buffer listed in Subheading 2.4.2 and follow the first four steps described in Subheading 3.5.1 (see Note 16).
2. After mixing cell lysates, clear the supernatant by centrifugation for 25 min at 80,000×g. Recover the middle layer and avoid the white, fluffy lipid layer on top.
3. Take supernatant, add 5 µM taxol and 0.5 mM GTP, mix well, and incubate for 2–3 min before adding additional 20 µM taxol (final taxol concentration is 25 µM). Incubate for 20 min at RT.
4. Pellet the microtubules using two volumes of a 40% glycerol cushion in 1× BRB80 (+protease inhibitors, phosphatase inhibitors, 1 mM DTT, 25 µM taxol, 1 mM GTP). Centrifuge for 25 min at 80,000×g at 20°C.
5. Discard supernatant and cushion. Resuspend pellet in 1/4 original volume of 50 µl CM buffer, wash tube with an additional 50 µl of CM buffer, and load the sample onto another cushion (same as above). Centrifuge again for 25 min at 20°C at 80,000×g. Discard supernatant and cushion as above.

6. Discard the supernatant and cushion and resuspend the pellet in SDS-PAGE buffer, and separate protein mixture via SDS-PAGE.
7. Perform tryptic digestion as described in Subheading 3.5.2.

3.7. Phosphopeptide Enrichment

1. Dissolve lyophilized tryptic digests in 50 µl binding buffer.
2. Equilibrate the TiO_2 column with binding buffer.
3. Load samples slowly onto the TiO_2 column.
4. Wash the column twice with 50 µl of binding buffer each and once with HPLC water.
5. Elute phosphopeptides first with 30 µl of 100 mM ammonium bicarbonate and then with 30 µl of 0.4 M NH_4OH/40% acetonitrile. Acidify the eluate using 3 µl of TFA (see Note 17).
6. Optional: Lyophilize the eluate and reload onto the same TiO_2 column as described above (see Note 18).

3.8. Liquid Chromatography and Mass Spectrometry

Reversed-Phase high performance liquid chromatography (RP-HPLC) is the most common peptide separation technique prior to MS acquisition because of its high compatibility with MS. For accurate quantification of isotopic peptide ratios, it is necessary to acquire the data on a high mass accuracy instrument. The protocol described here uses an Eksigent nanoLC•2D™ chromatography system coupled on-line to an LTQ Orbitrap mass spectrometer (other LC–MS instruments can also be used). Protein digests are separated at 400 nl/min via 60 min linear gradient from 5 to 35% acetonitrile in 0.2% formic acid. Up to six of the most intense ions per peptide mass spectrum are fragmented and analyzed in the linear trap. The resulting MS files are converted into peak lists. For each MS/MS spectrum, the 200 most intense fragment ions are selected and formatted into a Mascot generic file (mgf). The mgf files are submitted to the search engine MASCOT specifying 10 ppm (for precursor ion) and 0.8 Da (for product ion) mass tolerance respectively. Standard search criteria are cysteine carbamidomethylation as fixed modification, and acetyl (N-terminal), deamidation (N and Q), oxidation (M), phosphorylation (S, T, and Y) as variable modifications. In addition, $^{13}C/^{15}N$-labeled Arg and Lys are specified as variable modifications to account for the SILAC labeling. Up to two missed tryptic cleavages are allowed (see Note 19).

3.9. Data Analysis

3.9.1. Peptide Level Analysis

Example quantification data of a phosphopeptide SILAC ratio in kinase inhibitor- and mock-treated cells are shown in Fig. 3. Isotope ratios using inverse labeled cells were analyzed in parallel (for further details of quantification of SILAC data see (15, 16)). If we compare ratios a_i^L / a_i^H of the light and heavy peptide SILAC pair intensities a_i^L and a_i^H, ratios with $a_i^L < a_i^H$ will fall into the interval (0,1) and ratios with $a_i^L > a_i^H$ will fall into (1,∞). To account for this asymmetry, it is necessary to log-transform the SILAC ratios prior to statistical analysis (17), yielding $z_i = \log(a_i^L / a_i^H)$. For testing if a *peptide* has

Vimentin LRpSpSVPGVR

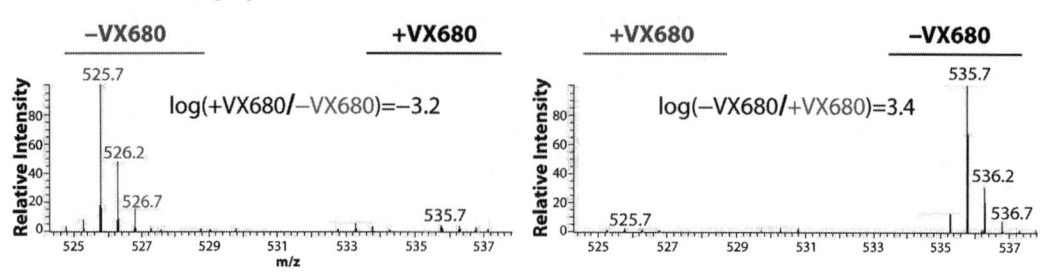

Fig. 3. Example for phosphopeptide quantitation following kinase inhibitor treatment. SILAC quantification of the doubly phosphorylated peptide (S71, S72) from Vimentin between VX680-treated (heavy) versus mock-treated (light) cells. The log isotope ratio of VX680 (heavy) versus Mock (light) reveals a log ratio of –3.2 (*left panel*). Quantification of the same phosphopeptide with inversely labeled cells (*right panel*) shows a log ratio of 3.4. The SILAC ratios for this phosphopeptide from both experiments show significant deviations from the distribution of the majority of peptide ratios ($p < 0.001$).

a SILAC ratio that is significantly different from the majority of peptides is desired, one can derive an empirical confidence interval (e.g., 90%) from repeated measurements of the same peptide (if available). Under the hypothesis that a peptide is not differentially expressed, the probability that the log ratio measurement z_i does not fall into this confidence interval is $q = 0.1$. Assuming a peptide is measured in n repeats, k times of which it falls outside of the confidence interval, its p-value for departure from the ratio of the majority would be:

$$p = \sum_{i \geq k}^{n} \binom{n}{i} q^i (1-q)^{n-i}.$$

3.9.2. Protein Level Analysis

In order to determine if a protein P exhibits a significantly larger mean SILAC ratio than a reference protein R, one can determine if the mean of all z_i^P that belong to protein P falls into a confidence interval constructed by bootstrapping from the observations z_i^R of the reference. Therefore, draw N sets of size n_P with replacement from the log ratio measurements $\{z_i^R\}$, where n_P is the number of measurements available for protein P. For each of these sets, calculate the mean and determine the empirical $(100p)\%$ confidence interval. If the mean of the observations $\{z_i^P\}$ falls into the confidence interval, the deviation is not significant at a $(1-p)$ level. Suitable parameters are, for example, $N = 1{,}000$, $p = 0.99$.

4. Notes

1. Stock solutions of Okadaic acid and Microcystine should be kept at –20°C. Okadaic acid should be protected from light. Both components are very toxic, so check Material Safety Data Sheets (MSDS) before working with these chemicals (see Subheading 2.2).

2. Suggested DTT stock solution is 1 M (in water), stored at −20°C. DTT should be added to the SDS buffer immediately prior to use (see Subheading 2.2).

3. If the myosin motor proteins dominate in the actin assay, adding 1 mM ATP to the lysis buffer and F-buffer would reduce the amount of myosin pelleting with actin (see Subheading 2.4.1).

4. Microtubule assay conditions can vary to favor binding of specific classes of proteins. For instance, adding 2–5 mM of AMPPNP to the lysis buffer will stabilize binding of motor proteins to microtubules (18) (see Subheading 2.4.2).

5. Store 1 M ammonium bicarbonate at 4°C and make this solution fresh every week (see Subheading 2.5).

6. Store iodoacetamide stock solution (500 mM), at −20°C in the dark (see Subheading 2.5).

7. For tryptic digestion, it is beneficial to label lysine and arginine since trypsin cleaves proteins after these amino acids. Labeling both residues increases the population of quantifiable peptides (see Subheading 3.1).

8. It is convenient to cryopreserve fully labeled heavy and light cells for future experiments. One can directly grow the cells from these stocks in heavy or light media without needing to passage the cells multiple times to incorporate the amino acids for each experiment. However, cells may change their morphology or differentiate over time; therefore, this is only advisable to generate and use these stocks in the short term to prevent divergence of heavy and light labeled cell lines (see Subheading 3.2).

9. As cells are semisynchronized at this stage, they can be grown at a higher density $2-5 \times 10^6$ cells/mL, to control the cost of SILAC media (see Subheading 3.3).

10. Perform a FACS analysis to confirm the synchrony and the cell stage of the collected cells (see Subheading 3.3).

11. Swapping the labels is crucial for reliable results and eliminates systematic errors (see Subheading 3.4).

12. All sample preparation should be performed on ice to minimize any enzyme activity. Buffers should always include a mixture of phosphatase inhibitors to prevent dephosphorylation. Alternatively, perform all lysis steps in a cold room at 4°C (see Subheading 3.5.1).

13. Separate dark- and light-stained regions to prevent masking of less abundant proteins (see Subheading 3.5.2).

14. Although trypsin is the most commonly used protease for LC–MS/MS experiments, using different proteolytic

enzymes will allow an increase in the analytical depth (the proteome coverage and the number of phosphopeptides (see Subheading 3.5.2).

15. We found it more convenient to mix the cell lysates before the sonication to minimize discrepancy during cell lysis (see Subheading 3.5.3).

16. It is important that all experiments are performed in the shortest time possible after the mixing of the heavy and light isotope labeled lysates as equilibration of the proteins can take place. For example, in the case of the cytoskeleton, it was observed if the lysates were incubated for extended periods in time the differences in the mitotic versus interphase samples were less pronounced (see Subheadings 3.6.1 and 3.6.2).

17. Acidification is necessary because phospho-groups on the proteins are chemically stable at the acidic or physiological pH values (see Subheading 3.7).

18. In our experience, this step significantly increases the specificity for phosphopeptides (see Subheading 3.7).

19. Phosphopeptides have a significantly higher number of missed cleavage events compared to other peptides due to hindering of proteases by phosphorylated residues that are in close proximity to sites of proteolytic cleavage. Therefore, it is recommended to allow a higher number of missed cleavage events for searching phosphopeptide-enriched samples (19) (see Subheading 3.8).

References

1. Taylor, S., and Peters, J. M. (2008) Polo and Aurora kinases: lessons derived from chemical biology. *Curr. Opin. Cell. Biol.* **20**, 77–84.
2. Zhang, J., Yang, P. L., and Gray, N. S. (2009) Targeting cancer with small molecule kinase inhibitors. *Nat. Rev. Cancer* **9**, 28–39.
3. Lapenna, S., and Giordano, A. (2009) Cell cycle kinases as therapeutic targets for cancer. *Nat. Rev. Drug Discov.* **8**, 547–566.
4. Lemeer, S., and Heck, A. J. (2009) The phosphoproteomics data explosion. *Curr. Opin. Chem. Biol.* **13**, 414–420.
5. Feng, Y., Mitchison, T. J., Bender, A., Young, D. W., and Tallarico, J. A. (2009) Multiparameter phenotypic profiling: using cellular effects to characterize small-molecule compounds. *Nat. Rev. Drug Discov.* **8**, 567–578.
6. Bantscheff, M., Eberhard, D., Abraham, Y., Bastuck, S., Boesche, M., Hobson, S., Mathieson, T., Perrin, J., Raida, M., Rau, C., Reader, V., Sweetman, G., Bauer, A., Bouwmeester, T., Hopf, C., Kruse, U., Neubauer, G., Ramsden, N., Rick, J., Kuster, B., and Drewes, G. (2007) Quantitative chemical proteomics reveals mechanisms of action of clinical ABL kinase inhibitors. *Nat. Biotechnol.* **25**, 1035–1044.
7. Kelly, A. E., and Funabiki, H. (2009) Correcting aberrant kinetochore microtubule attachments: an Aurora B-centric view. *Curr. Opin. Cell Biol.* **21**, 51–58.
8. Keen, N., and Taylor, S. (2004) Aurora-kinase inhibitors as anticancer agents, *Nat. Rev. Cancer* **4**, 927–936.
9. Harrington, E. A., Bebbington, D., Moore, J., Rasmussen, R. K., Ajose-Adeogun, A. O., Nakayama, T., Graham, J. A., Demur, C., Hercend, T., Diu-Hercend, A., Su, M., Golec, J. M., and Miller, K. M. (2004) VX-680, a potent and selective small-molecule inhibitor of the Aurora kinases, suppresses tumor growth in vivo. *Nat. Med.* **10**, 262–267.
10. Fang, G., Yu, H., and Kirschner, M. W. (1998) Direct binding of CDC20 protein family members activates the anaphase-promoting complex in mitosis and G1. *Mol. Cell* **2**, 163–171.

11. Ozlu, N., Monigatti, F., Renard, B. Y., Field, C. M., Steen, H., Mitchison, T. J., and Steen, J. J. Binding partner switching on microtubules and aurora-B in the mitosis to cytokinesis transition. *Mol. Cell Proteomics* **9**, 336–350.
12. Steen, J. A., Steen, H., Georgi, A., Parker, K., Springer, M., Kirchner, M., Hamprecht, F., and Kirschner, M. W. (2008) Different phosphorylation states of the anaphase promoting complex in response to antimitotic drugs: a quantitative proteomic analysis. *Proc. Natl. Acad. Sci. USA* **105**, 6069–6074.
13. Shevchenko, A., Wilm, M., Vorm, O., and Mann, M. (1996) Mass spectrometric sequencing of proteins silver-stained polyacrylamide gels. *Anal. Chem.* **68**, 850–858.
14. Budde, P. P., Desai, A., and Heald, R. (2006) Analysis of microtubule polymerization in vitro and during the cell cycle in Xenopus egg extracts. *Methods* **38**, 29–34.
15. Cox, J., and Mann, M. (2008) MaxQuant enables high peptide identification rates, individualized p.p.b.-range mass accuracies and proteome-wide protein quantification. *Nat. Biotechnol.* **26**, 1367–1372.
16. Cox, J., Matic, I., Hilger, M., Nagaraj, N., Selbach, M., Olsen, J. V., and Mann, M. (2009) A practical guide to the MaxQuant computational platform for SILAC-based quantitative proteomics. *Nat. Protoc.* **4**, 698–705.
17. Graumann, J., Hubner, N. C., Kim, J. B., Ko, K., Moser, M., Kumar, C., Cox, J., Scholer, H., and Mann, M. (2008) Stable isotope labeling by amino acids in cell culture (SILAC) and proteome quantitation of mouse embryonic stem cells to a depth of 5,111 proteins. *Mol. Cell Proteomics* **7**, 672–683.
18. Sawin, K. E., and Mitchison, T. J. (1991) Poleward microtubule flux mitotic spindles assembled in vitro. *J. Cell Biol.* **112**, 941–954.
19. Molina, H., Horn, D. M., Tang, N., Mathivanan, S., and Pandey, A. (2007) Global proteomic profiling of phosphopeptides using electron transfer dissociation tandem mass spectrometry. *Proc. Natl. Acad. Sci. USA* **104**, 2199–2204.

Chapter 16

Investigation of Acquired Resistance to EGFR-Targeted Therapies in Lung Cancer Using cDNA Microarrays

Kian Kani, Rafaella Sordella, and Parag Mallick

Abstract

Clinical tools to accurately describe, evaluate, and predict an individual's response to cancer therapy are a field-wide priority; in many advanced cancers, only 10–20% of individuals will have a clinical benefit from therapy, yet we treat the entire population. Furthermore, many therapies are initially effective, but lose effectiveness over time. Here we describe methods to derive in vitro models of resistance to EGFR tyrosine kinase inhibitors. We additionally describe approaches to characterize possible mechanisms of resistance by genomic and transcriptomic approaches.

Key words: Gefitinib, Erlotinib, Non-small-cell lung cancer, Therapeutic response, Proteomics, Resistance

1. Introduction

Mechanistically, changes in cancer cell growth patterns and rates may originate with alterations in growth signaling networks. The concept of "oncogene addiction" has been demonstrated in a variety of mouse tumorigenesis models in which continued expression of the transforming oncogene is required for tumor maintenance. Numerous targeted therapeutics attempt to halt the growth of a tumor via specific disruptions in these networks. For example, the efficacy of drugs such as imatinib illustrate the importance of BCR-ABL in chronic myelogenous leukemia and the dramatic responses of epidermal growth factor receptor (EGFR)-mutant lung tumors to EGFR tyrosine kinase inhibitors (TKIs), such as erlotinib and gefitinib, suggest that even complex epithelial cancers may exhibit dependency on a single activated kinase for survival. Specifically in the case of lung cancer, much excitement has recently been generated by the finding that a group of non-small-cell lung cancer (NSCLC) patients benefit highly from treatment with selective EGFR inhibitors (1). The clinical success of tyrosine kinase inhibitors (TKIs) has dramatically influenced research and medical oncology over the past decade. Unfortunately, these therapies are often only effective in a small percentage of patients. Furthermore, even when initially effective, therapies can lose effectiveness over time, presumably through the tumor's molecular evolution of resistance to the therapeutic. Despite extensive study, de novo and acquired resistance to targeted therapeutic agents remains a major obstacle to improving remission rates and achieving prolonged disease-free survival.

Through the use of derived models of resistance numerous mechanisms of response and resistance have been uncovered. NSCLC patients with activation mutations in the EGFR gene exhibit dramatic sensitivity to targeted TKIs (2). These mutations remove some or all of the negative allosteric regulatory mechanisms in the EGFR kinase domain (3). The most frequent activating mutations are the in-frame deletions of leucine-747 to glutamic acid-749 (DLRE) and the leucine to arginine substitution at codon 858 (L858R), which account for 44% and 41% of all the mutations in EGFR cases in NSLC, respectively (4, 5). Subsequent studies also identified a mutation of threonine to methionine at 790 that confers resistance. In addition to mutations in the EGFR, amplification of c-MET has recently been identified as another potential acquired resistance mechanism. In a preliminary study, 22% (4/18) of cases of NSCLC with acquired resistance to gefitnib/erlotinib have been shown to harbor c-MET amplification (6). Interestingly, some of these tumors contained both the T790M mutation and c-MET amplification. Although the role of c-MET amplification in EGFR TKI-acquired resistance has yet to be definitively proven, current studies suggest that the presence of T790M and c-MET amplification could account for approximately 50% of all cases (6). Thus, despite considerable progress in identifying acquired resistance mechanisms, new determinants of EGFR TKI have yet to be uncovered in the majority of tumors that have relapsed.

The accumulation of genetic/epigenetic aberrations that ultimately lead to the acquisition of resistance to a particular TKI treatment in fact usually results in dramatic changes in the expression pattern of multiple genes. In this regard, a strong correlation between gene expression and copy number variations has been observed. As such, gene expression profiling or microarray analysis, by enabling the measurement of thousands of genes in a single RNA sample, provides a powerful research tool for elucidating genetic interactions and response to drug treatments.

Simplistically, while DNA sequence analysis instructs us on what a cell could possibly do as a consequence of the accumulations of genetic aberrations, the expression profile data conveys us what it is actually happening in a given cell in a particular cell state. The basic idea behind all the different variety of microarray platforms that have been developed is simple: a glass slide or membrane is spotted or "arrayed" with DNA fragments or oligonucleotides that represent specific gene coding regions. Purified RNA is then fluorescently or radioactively labeled and hybridized to the slide/membrane. After thorough washing, the raw data is obtained by laser scanning or autoradiographic imaging. At this point, the data may then be entered into a database and analyzed by a number of statistical methods. The up-front design of a study is critical to a research study's ability to draw sound conclusions in the particular case of identifying signaling pathways or genes whose disregulation could contribute to the acquisition of resistance to a given drug treatment. Here, we introduce several techniques for deriving models of resistance. We also describe genomic and transcriptomic techniques for characterizing the mechanism of resistance of those models.

2. Materials

2.1. In Vitro Selection of Resistant Populations

1. NSCLC cell lines: e.g., HCC827 cells.
2. Type II classification biological hood and safety cabinet.
3. Cell growth media compatible for cells under investigation: e.g., Dulbecco's Modified Eagle's Medium (DMEM) containing 1% of dialyzed fetal bovine serum.
4. Gefitinib: 99% purità, prepare 10 mM stock solution in DMSO.
5. Cell counter, microscope.
6. 96-well plates: flat bottom for cell culture.
7. Cell viability assay kit: e.g., the MTS or MTT assays are commercially available from many sources.
8. Ethyl methane sulfonate (EMS): 600 µg/ml in cell culture medium.

2.2. DNA Sequencing

DNA can be prepared for sequencing by use of several commercially available kits.

1. DNeasy Blood and Tissue Kit.
2. Pipettes and pipette tips.
3. Vortexer.
4. Microcentrifuge tubes (1.5 ml or 2 ml).
5. Microcentrifuge with rotor for 1.5 ml and 2 ml tubes.
6. Ethanol: 96–100% purity.

7. Phosphate-based saline (PBS).
8. Lysis buffer: Autoclaved PBS supplemented with 1 mM EDTA, 0.5% NP40, 25 mM DTT, 5 mM $MgCl_2$, and 1× RNase Inhibitor.

2.3. RNA Isolation

1. Trizol reagent.
2. Chloroform.
3. Ethanol: 200 proof quality.
4. Dulbecco's phosphate-buffered saline (DPBS).
5. Sodium acetate: 3 M, pH 5.2.
6. RNAse-free water: 1 ml of 0.1% (v/v) diethylpyrocarbonate (DEPC) in 999 ml of water. Let stand overnight. Autoclave prior to use.
7. Cell scraper.
8. Centrifuge tubes: 15 ml, round bottom, polypropylene.
9. Centrifuge tubes: 50 ml, conical, polypropylene.
10. Plastic tubes: 1.5 ml.
11. PCR tubes: 0.2 ml, thin wall.
12. Centrifugal filter: MicroCon 100.
13. High-speed centrifuge.

2.4. Quantitative PCR

1. PCR tubes: 0.2 ml, thin wall (or plate).
2. Plastic tubes: 1.5 ml, RNAse free.
3. Primers for genes of interest.
4. DNA polymerase: JumpStart Taq kit.
5. Reverse transcription: ImProm-II Rt system.

2.5. Transcriptomic Profiling

1. Ethanol: 200 proof quality.
2. Dulbecco's phosphate-buffered saline (DPBS).
3. Sodium acetate: 3 M, pH 5.2.
4. Nucleotides: dATP, dCTP, dGTP, dTTP, 100 mM each, store frozen at –20°C.
5. Primers: 1 mg/ml pd(T)12–18 in water, store frozen at –20°C.
6. Oligo primer: anchored, 5′-TTT TTT TTT TTT TTT TTT TTV N-3′, resuspend at 2 mg/ml, store frozen at –20°C.
7. Fluorescent dyes: 1 mM CyTM3-dUTP and 1 mM CyTM5-dUTP, store at –20°C, protect from light.
8. Rnase inhibitor: RNasina, store at –20°C.
9. SUPERSCRIPTTM II Rnase H` Reverse Transcriptase Kit: store at –20°C.
10. Human C0t-1 DNA: 10 mg/ml, store frozen at –20°C.

11. Ethylenediaminetetraacetic acid (EDTA): 0.5 M, pH 8.0.
12. NaOH: 1 N.
13. Tris(hydroxymethyl)aminomethane (Tris)–HCL: 1 M, pH 7.5.
14. TE buffer (1×): 10 mM Tris, 1 mM EDTA pH 7.4.
15. Diethylpyrocarbonate (DEPC)-treated water: 0.1% v/v diethylpyrocarbonate in water.
16. Tris-Acetate electrophoresis buffer (TAE, 50×): 2 M Tris acetate pH 8.0, 55 mM EDTA in DEPC-treated water.
17. Centrifuge tubes: 15 ml, round bottom, polypropylene.
18. Centrifuge tubes: 50 ml, conical bottom, polypropylene.
19. Plastic tubes: 1.5 ml.
20. PCR tubes: 0.2 ml, thin wall.
21. Centrifugal filter: MicroCon 100.
22. High-speed centrifuge for 15-ml tubes.
23. Nucleotides: 100 mM dGTP, dATP, dCTP, and dTTP.
24. First-Strand Buffer: 5×, provided with Superscript II kit.
25. Poly d(A): 8 mg/ml in water.
26. Yeast tRNA: 4 mg/ml in water.
27. SSC buffer (20×): 3 M sodium chloride, 300 mM sodium citrate, pH 7.0.
28. Denhardt's blocking solution (50×): 1% Ficoll type 400, 1% polyvinylpyrrolidone, and 1% bovine serum albumin.
29. For our studies, we used the Affimetrix platform including the Affimetrix U95Av2 array that contains approximately 12,600 human genes and the Affymetrix GeneChip Scanner 3000. Other alternative systems may also be used.

3. Methods

3.1. Generation of Gefitinib Resistant Cell Populations in Cell Culture

3.1.1. Titration Method

1. Maintain cells for several passages to ensure normal growth (see Note 1).
2. Plate the cells at 3,500 cells per well in quadruplicate in 96-well plates (flat bottom, cell culture plated).
3. 18 h after cell plating, wash the cells with fresh medium and then add medium supplemented with different concentrations (e.g., threefold dilution series) of gefitinib (see Note 2). Incubate the cells for 2–3 days (see Note 3).

4. Measure cell viability, for example, using the MTS assay with UV detection at 490 nM in a plate reader. Determine the drug concentration at which 50% of all cells are viable (IC50 value). This drug concentration is used as a starting point for subsequent cell dosing.

5. Start dosing the cells at one order of magnitude below the determined IC50 value (e.g., 100 nM).

6. Plate the cells in a 10-cm cell-culture plate.

7. Incubate the cells with 10 nM gefitinib (see Note 4) and replenish drug containing media every 24 h.

8. Monitor cell viability and increase gefitinib concentration as the cells regain normal growth kinetics (see Note 5).

9. Expand the cells to desired quantities for subsequent experiments (see Notes 6 and 7).

3.1.2. Rapid Selection Method

In addition to the above described titration method, a rapid selection protocol with or without exposure to mutagen can be employed. A mutagen such as EMS can be used to increase genetic aberrations. In this case, cells are treated prior to selection with EMS at a concentration of 600 µg/ml and allowed to recover for 72 h.

1. Maintain the cells for several passages to ensure normal growth.

2. Measure IC50 by performing a MTS viability assay with different concentrations of gefitinib as described in Subheading 3.1.1.

3. Plate the cells in a 10 cm cell culture plate at a 30% confluency (i.e., 6×10^4 cells per 10 cm^2).

4. Incubate the cells with three times the IC50 in the presence of 5% serum (selection media). In the case of the HCC827 cells, this corresponds to 1 µM gefitinib.

5. Replenish every 24 h with new selection media (RPMI, 5% FBS, Strep/pen Invitrogen).

6. Expand the cells to the desired quantities for subsequent experiments.

3.2. Characterization of Resistant Cell Populations by DNA Sequencing

1. Grow cells to 65% confluence in 10-cm plates and wash three times with PBS.

2. Scrape the cells off the plate with 400 µl of lysis buffer.

3. Add 40 µl proteinase K. Check pH. If required, adjust pH using hydrochloric acid or glacial acetic acid.

4. Add 400 µl Buffer AL provided in the DNeasy kit (without added ethanol) to the sample and mix thoroughly by vortexing.

5. Add 400 µl ethanol (96–100%) and mix again thoroughly by vortexing. It is important that the sample and the ethanol are mixed thoroughly to yield a homogeneous solution.

6. Pipette the mixture from step 5 (including any precipitate) into the DNeasy Mini spin column placed in a 2-ml collection tube (provided). Centrifuge at ≥6,000×*g* for 1 min. Discard the flow-through and collection tube.

7. Place the DNeasy Mini spin column in a new 2-ml collection tube (provided), add 500 μl Buffer AW1 (provided in the DNeasy kit), and centrifuge for 1 min at ≥6,000×*g*. Discard the flow-through and collection tube.

8. Place the DNeasy Mini spin column in a new 2-ml collection tube (provided), add 500 μl Buffer AW2 (provided in the DNeasy kit), and centrifuge for 3 min at 20,000×*g* to dry the DNeasy membrane.

9. Place the DNeasy Mini spin column in a clean 1.5 ml or 2 ml microcentrifuge tube (not provided) and pipette 400 μl Buffer AE (provided in the DNeasy kit) directly onto the DNeasy membrane. Incubate at room temperature for 1 min and then centrifuge for 1 min at ≥6,000×*g* to elute the sample.

10. Measure the DNA quality and purity by use of OD 260/280 and send out for commercial sequencing (see Note 8).

3.3. Interrogation of Markers of Epithelial to Mesenchymal Transition by Quantitative PCR

Here, we provide a reliable protocol to assess the expression of most commonly used epithelial to mesenchymal transition (EMT) markers by using QPCR-based techniques (see Note 9).

3.3.1. RNA Isolation

Many protocols and commercially available kits are currently available for the generation of RNA. We routinely employ the following method based on a combination of phase extraction and chromatography.

1. Wash subconfluent cells (i.e., approximately 5×10^6 cells) twice with cold PBS on ice. Scrape the cells with 1 ml of cold PBS and transfer them into sterile RNase-free 1.5-ml microcentrifuge tubes. Pellet by centrifugation at 13,000×*g* for 10 s and remove the supernatant by gently aspiration.

2. Lyse cells by repetitive pipetting in 1 ml of Trizol.

3. Add two-tenth volume of chloroform (i.e., 200 μl) and shake vigorously for 15 s.

4. Let mixture stand for 3 min at room temperature. Centrifuge at 13,000×*g* for 15 min at 4°C.

5. Take off the aqueous phase (i.e., upper phase) and transfer it to a polypropylene tube.

6. Add 0.53 volumes of ethanol (i.e., 500 µl) slowly while vortexing (see Note 10).
7. Let mixture stand for 10 min at room temperature and centrifuge at 13,000×g for 10 min at 4°C.
8. The RNA forms a pellet on the side or bottom of the tube. Discard the supernatant.
9. Wash the pellet two times by adding 1 ml of 75% ethanol and centrifuging at 10,000×g for 5 min at 4°C.
10. Dry the pellet for 5–10 min and resuspend RNA in 80 µl of DEPC-treated water at 65°C.
11. Resuspend RNA at approximately 1 mg/ml in DEPC-treated water.
12. Concentrate the sample by centrifugation (500×g) in a MicroCon 100 filter unit (see Note 11).
13. Determine the concentration of RNA by spectrophotometry. Store at −80°C (see Note 12). To measure the RNA concentration, take 2–5 µl RNA sample and dilute with RNase-free water to a final volume of 1 ml in a 1.5-ml microcentrifuge tube (i.e., 200–500 dilution of the RNA sample). Transfer 1 ml of RNase-free water to a clean cuvette and read absorbance as blank. Pipette the diluted RNA sample in to a clean cuvette and read absorbance at 260 nm and 280 nm. To determine RNA concentration of the original sample, use the following formula: [RNA µg/µl] = A_{260} × 33 × dilution factor/1,000.

3.3.2. Reverse Transcriptase Reaction

Many commercial kits are available for the reverse transcriptase reaction. The following protocol has been optimized for the ImProm-II Rt system.

1. Preparation of a reaction master mix is highly recommended to give best reproducibility. Mix all reagents but template in a common mix, using ~10% more than needed. A 20 µl reaction contains 4 µl reaction buffer, 3 mM $MgCl_2$, 0.5 mM of each dNTP, 1 µ/µl ribonuclease inhibitor (we suggest recombinant RNAasin), and 1 µl of reverse transcriptase (we suggest the Improm-II system, see Note 13).
2. Anneal RNA and oligos for 5 min at 25°C.
3. For each reaction, combine 15 µl of reverse transcriptase mix with RNA and oligos for a final volume of 20 µl.
4. The first-strand cDNA is synthesized by incubating the reaction for 60 min at 42°C (i.e., the extension reaction) and terminated by incubating at 70°C for 15 min.

3.3.3. Quantitative PCR

Quantitative PCR uses the linearity of DNA amplification to determine relative amounts of a known sequence in a sample by using a fluorescent reporter in the reaction. When the DNA is in

Table 1
Pipetting scheme for QPCR

Volume*	Reagent	Final concentration
25 µl	2× JumpStart Taq ReadyMix	1.5 units Taq DNA polymerase, 10 mM Tris–HCl, 50 mM KCl, 1.5 mM MgCl$_2$, 0.001% gelatin, 0.2 mM dNTP, stabilizers
– µl	Forward primer	50–1,000 nM (see Notes 15 and 16)
– µl	Reverse primer	50–1,000 nM
– µl	Template DNA	10–100 ng
– to 50 µl	Water	
50 µl	Total volume	

Table 2
PCR cycle conditions

	Temperature	Time
Initial denaturation	94°C	2 min*
Denaturation	94 °C	15 s
Annealing/extension	60°C or 5°C below lowest primer T_M	1 min**
Cycle	40	
(Optional) Hold	4°C – only if products will be run out on a gel	

the log linear phase of amplification, the amount of fluorescence increases above the background. The point at which the fluorescence becomes measurable is called the Threshold Cycle (C_T) or crossing point.

1. A reaction master mix (see Note 14) of all reagents but template is assembled as a common mix according to Table 1.
2. Aliquot the master mix into a 200 µl PCR tube or plate.
3. Add 1 µl of RT reaction.
4. Mix gently by vortexing and briefly centrifuge to collect all components at the bottom of the tube.
5. Perform thermal cycling according to Table 2 (see Note 17).

3.4. Gene Expression Profiling

The first step in gene expression profiling analysis is the RNA isolation. We refer to Subheading 3.3.1 for a detailed protocol.

3.4.1. RNA Labeling

1. Anneal the oligo dT(12–18) primer to the RNA in the reaction mixture defined in Table 3 using a 0.2-ml thin-wall PCR

Table 3
Pipetting scheme for RNA annealing

Component	Addition for Cy5 labeling	Addition for Cy3 labeling
Total RNA (>7 mg/ml)	150–200 µg	50–80 µg
dT(12–18) primer (1 µg/µl)	1 µl	1 µl
DEPC H$_2$O	to 17 µl	to 17 µl

Table 4
Pipetting scheme for RNA labeling

Component	Volume [µl]
5× first-strand buffer	8
10× low T dNTPs mix	4
Cy5 or Cy3 dUTP (1 mM)	4
0.1 M DTT	4
Rnasin (30 µ/µl)	1
Superscript II (200 µ/µl)	2
Total volume	23

tube so that incubations can be carried out in a PCR cycler (see Note 18).

2. Heat to 65°C for 10 min and transfer on ice for 2 min.
3. Add 23 µl of the reaction mixture defined in Table 4 containing either Cy5-dUTP or Cy3-dUTP nucleotides, mix well by pipetting, and use a brief centrifuge spin to concentrate the liquid in the bottom of the tube.
4. Incubate at 42°C for 30 min. Then add 2 µl Superscript II. Make sure that the enzyme is well mixed in the reaction volume and incubate at 42°C for 30–60 min (see Note 19).
5. Stop the reaction by adding 5 µl of 0.5 M EDTA (see Note 20).
6. Add 10 µl of 1 N NaOH and incubate at 65°C for 30 min to hydrolyze residual RNA. Cool to room temperature (see Note 21).
7. Neutralize the reaction by adding 25 µl of 1 M Tris–HCl, pH 7.5.
8. Desalt the labeled cDNA by adding the following neutralized reaction: 400 µl of TE pH 7.5 and 20 µg of human C0t-1 DNA. Transfer the solution to a MicroCon 100 cartridge. Pipette to mix and spin for 10 min at 500×g.

9. Wash again by adding 200 μl TE pH 7.5 and concentrating to about 20–30 μl by centrifuging at 500×*g* for 8–10 min.

10. Recover the sample by inverting the concentrator over a clean collection tube and spinning for 3 min at 500×*g*.

11. Take a 2–3 μl aliquot of the Cy5-labeled cDNA for analysis, leaving the remaining 18–28 μl for hybridization.

12. Run this probe on a 2% agarose gel (6 cm wide×8.5 cm long, 2 mm wide teeth) in Tris Acetate Electrophoresis Buffer (TAE, see Note 22).

13. Scan the gel on a fluorescence scanner (setting: red fluorescence, 200 μm resolution, see Note 23).

3.4.2. Hybridization

1. As an initial step, it is necessary to determine the volume of the hybridization solution required (see Note 24). Usually, 0.033 μl of hybridization solution is used for each mm^2 of slide surface area covered by the coverslip for each array is used (i.e., an array covered by a 24 mm by 50 mm coverslip will require 40 μl of hybridization solution).

2. For a 40 μl hybridization, pool the Cy3- and Cy5-labeled cDNAs into a single 0.2-ml thin-wall PCR tube and adjust the volume to 30 μl by either adding DEPC-treated water, or by removing water in a vacuum concentrator. If using a vacuum device to remove water, do not use high heat or heat lamps to accelerate evaporation as the fluorescent dyes might be degraded.

3. For a 40-μl hybridization, combine the components specified in Table 5.

4. Mix the components well by pipetting, heat at 98°C for 2 min in a PCR cycler, cool quickly to 25°C, and add 0.6 μl of 10% SDS.

5. Centrifuge for 5 min at 14,000×*g*. The labeled cDNAs have a tendency to form small, very fluorescent, aggregates

Table 5
Pipetting scheme for array hybridization

Component	High sample blocking	High array blocking
Cy5 + Cy3 probe	30 μl	28 μl
Poly d(A) (8 mg/ml)	1 μl	2 μl
Yeast tRNA (4 mg/ml)	1 μl	2 μl
Human C0t-1 DNA (10 mg/ml)	1 μl	0 μl
20× SSC	6 μl	6 μl
50× Denhardt's blocking solution	1 μl (optional)	2 μl
Total volume	40 μl	40 μl

which result in bright, punctate background on the array slide. Hard centrifugation will pellet these aggregates, avoiding their introduction to the array.

6. Apply the labeled cDNA to a 24 mm × 50 mm glass coverslip and then touch with the inverted microarray (see Note 25).

7. Place the slide in a microarray hybridization chamber. Add 5 μl of 3× SSC to the reservoir and seal the chamber. Submerge the chamber in a 65°C water bath and allow the slide to hybridize for 16–20 h (see Note 26).

8. Wash off unbound fluorescent cDNA by incubating in prewarmed 2× SSC, 0.2% SDS washing solution at 65°C for 5 min. Then, wash the array three times in 2× SSC, 0.2% SDS washing solution at RT for 2 min. Subsequently, air-dry the array.

9. Remove the hybridization chamber from the water bath, cool and carefully dry off. Unseal the chamber and remove the slide (see Note 27).

10. Place the slide, with the coverslip still affixed, into a Coplin jar filled with 0.5× SSC/0.01% SDS wash buffer. Allow the coverslip to fall from the slide and then remove the coverslip from the jar with a forceps. Allow the slide to wash for 2–5 min.

11. Transfer the slide to a fresh Coplin jar filled with 0.06× SSC. Allow the slide to wash for 2–5 min (see Note 28).

12. Transfer the slide to a slide rack and centrifuge at low speed for 3 min in a clinical centrifuge equipped with a horizontal rotor for microtiter plates (see Note 29).

13. Obtain image of array. Images are typically obtained using microarray scanners. A large variety of microarrays scanners are available with different features such as sensitivity, resolution, scan area, rapidity of scan, excitation and emission filters, and autofocus capability. For our studies, we used the Affymetrix GeneChip Scanner 3000.

3.5. Data Analysis

3.5.1. Array Segmentation, Background Intensity Extraction, and Target Detection

1. The first step in any analysis of microarray data is the extraction of quantitative information from the images resulting from the readout of hybridizations. As a preliminary analysis, the data from each experiment is assessed for overall quality and to determine the extent of difference between the experimental sample and the reference sample. A segmentation of the array is initially performed to decode the array information. Since each element of an array is printed automatically to a predefined location and because specific orientation markers are given, the initial positioning of the grid can be automatically aligned.

2. The background of the microarray image is usually not uniform over the entire array. Therefore, it is necessary to extract local background intensities. Owing to many technical reasons,

the changes of fluorescent background across an array are usually gradual and smooth. In case more abrupt changes are observed, we recommend caution in the interpretations of the data. Conventionally, pixels near the bonding box edge are taken to be the background pixels, and the average gray level of these pixels are used for the estimation of the local background intensity.

3. A fixed thresholding method is used in image analysis to determine the signal corresponding to a specific target over the background. A threshold value (T) corresponding to changes of over three times the value of standard deviation (s) over the local background mean (m) is usually used (e.g., $T = m + 3s$). However, this method based on a simple fixed thresholding fails quite often due to variability of the background and the signal, particularly when the signal is weak (a frequent finding in cDNA array experiments). To avoid these problems, a more sophisticated thresholding method such as the Mann–Whitney method may be implemented (7).

4. The local background value is subtracted from the reported sample intensities from the red channel (R) and the green channel (G), and then the ratio (R/G) is calculated. Clearly, the ratio measurement is the ratio of two average intensity measurements. We usually use Affymetrix Expression Console QC metrics to pass the image data, although other software packages are available and can be used.

3.5.2. Data Visualization

A second general step in the analysis of gene expression profile data is the collection of experimental data into a database that supports both further mathematical analysis and connection to the available knowledge about the structure and function of the individual genes (Database Design & Development). Usually, this step is automatically generated by current software packages.

3.5.3. Gene Annotation

1. Gene annotation provides functional information on a given gene. In addition, depending on the tool utilized this analysis can also provide other useful information such as for example the location of each gene within a particular chromosome. Having identified some set of regulated genes, the next step in expression profiling analysis involves looking for patterns within the regulated set. The way in which particular genes' expression patterns vary across the samples can be analyzed in a variety of ways. In expression clustering analysis, a query asks whether the similarities of patterns between genes suggest involvement in common processes, or whether differences in the individual gene expression patterns can be aligned with differences in the sample types. In Discriminative Gene List analysis, genes having the most differential behavior between

samples can be used to try to identify the particular cellular activities that differ between classes of samples. By using these two types of analysis, one can start to make biological sense of expression profiling data. Many analytical tools are currently available for data mining and to determine whether, for example, proteins made from genes with similar patterns of expression perform related functions, whether they are chemically alike or have similar subcellular localization.

2. As part of available tools, Gene ontology analysis provides a standard way to define these relationships. Gene ontologies start with very broad categories, e.g., "metabolic process," and break them down into smaller categories, e.g., "carbohydrate metabolic process," and finally into quite restrictive categories such as "inositol and derivative phosphorylation." The Molecular Signatures Database, the Comparative Toxicogenomics Database and the Ingenuity Gene Network Diagram are examples of resources to further categorize genes.

3.5.4. Validation by Statistical Analysis

1. Data analysis of microarrays has become an area of intense research. Simply stating that a group of genes are regulated by at least twofold lacks a solid statistical footing. The usual typical three replicates in each group are in fact not sufficient from a statistical perspective and can easily create a deceptive difference greater than twofold. Rather than identifying differentially expressed genes using a fold change cutoff, one can use a variety of statistical tests such as ANOVA, all of which estimate how often we would observe the data by chance alone. This type of analysis also allows the identification of genes that, despite subtle variation in expression, could have important biological functions.

2. In addition to treatment (i.e., drug) or comparison of multiple cell lines, it is also helpful to include information such as hybridization, operator, scanner, etc. as variable control items.

3. The output of an ANOVA test includes two values: a p-value and a mean square for each factor tested. The mean of the mean square for each factor is used to quantify the contribution of each factor to the experimental variation. The p-values indicate instead the significance of an observed difference in the expression. The lower the p-value, the more confidence one has that the difference detected are not due to random chance. A p-value of 0.05 is typically defined to indicate significance, since it estimates a 5% probability of observing the data by chance. A p value alone of course is not sufficient since for example analysis of 10,000 genes on a microarray would result in the identification of 500 genes at $p < 0.05$ even if there were no difference between the experimental groups. A variety of analysis packages from bioinformatics

companies are available to account for this so-called multiple hypothesis testing. Among these tools, we use the Significance Analysis of Microarrays (SAM) system. In addition, we suggest following the MAQC Project recommendations for microarray analysis.

3.5.5. Validation by QPCR and Western Blot Analysis

Ultimately, changes in the expression of certain genes of interest should be further validated by more direct methods such as quantitative PCR and western blot analysis. While high throughput DNA microarrays lack the quantitative accuracy of QPCR, it takes about the same time to measure the gene expression of a few dozen genes via QPCR as it would to measure an entire genome using DNA microarrays. Thus, we suggest performing semiquantitative DNA microarray analysis experiments to identify candidate genes and then perform QPCR on some of the most interesting candidate genes to validate the microarray results. Western blot analysis of some of the protein products of differentially expressed genes is also recommended, since the mRNA levels do not necessarily correlate to the amount of expressed protein. We refer to the previous section for a detailed protocol for QPCR analysis.

4. Notes

1. Cell growth should be carefully monitored, as some cells take longer to obtain a resistant phenotype (see Subheading 3.1.1).

2. Drug resistance can be obtained by incremental titration of a particular drug over a several month time course. For example, the IC50 of the HCC827 cell line treated with gefitinib is in the nanomolar range (10–100 nM). Once the IC50 has been determined for a particular cell line and drug, the initial dosage can be set. For example, if the IC50 for the HCC827 cell line with gefitinib is ~100 nM, then one could begin dosing with 10 nM of gefitinib for 1 month. The exact concentration of gefitinib has to be established by a case-by-case basis, but initial dosing at concentrations above the IC50 can result in apoptosis and the release of cell debris that can prevent proper cell attachment and growth (see Subheading 3.1.1).

3. The rate of the development of an acquired resistance cell line also depends on the frequency of drug replenishment. Gefitinib is an anilinoquinazoline and thus will undergo latent hydrolysis in aqueous and is insoluble in alkaline pH. Therefore, the replenishment of the gefitinib containing media will determine the effective inhibition time of EGFR. The half-life of the therapeutic in vitro will determine the rate and possibly influence the mechanism of resistance. This parameter should

be addressed prior to dosing and documented in any manuscript (see Subheading 3.1.1).

4. Acquired resistance can develop over a course of several months. For the HCC827 example, if the initial dosing started at 10 nM, then one can incrementally increase gefitinib threefold until a particular stopping point is achieved. Cell viability should be monitored regularly and drug concentration increased as cells regain their normal growth kinetics at each dosing level. In our hands, HCC827 gefitinib-resistant cells demonstrated normal growth kinetics after 4 months and ultimately handled gefitinib up to 10 µM. However, as with any therapeutic in high concentration, the number of off-target hits increases leading to overlapping inhibition of multiple kinases. It would be reasonable to generate a line that is resistant to gefitinib at concentrations above 10 µM as long as the final resistant pool was maintained in 1 µM to avoid overlapping inhibition (see Subheading 3.1.1).

5. After approximately 2 weeks, resistant clones start to be visible at a frequency of 0.01% (i.e., 100 clones for 1×10^6 selected cells). Each clone can then be expanded from a 96-well plate to a 10 cm dish in the presence of selecting medium (see Subheading 3.1.1).

6. At this point, usually the resistant derived cell lines have become stably resistant to the drug treatment and can be grown in normal media without drug (see Subheading 3.1.1).

7. The in vitro development of acquired resistance starts with a homogenous cell type, which has been a priori deemed sensitive to a particular therapy. In the case of NSCLC tissue, several cell lines with activation mutations in the EGFR kinase domain have been isolated and cataloged at various bioresource centers (ATCC in the USA, JCRB in Japan). Once the appropriate cell line has been obtained, one should confirm the sensitivity to EGFR targeted tyrosine kinase inhibitors (TKIs) by performing a cell viability assay to demonstrate the half maximal inhibitory concentration (IC50) of the particular TKI (see Subheading 3.1.1).

Limitations: The described protocols make use of in vitro-based cell culture systems. Although these systems are easy to implement and are based on a limited number of variables, they do not represent the high complexity of actual tumors. New experimental evidence is now indicating that also the tumor microenvironment could play an important role in modifying the response of cells to drug treatment. As such new protocols based on in vivo selections are currently under development. In addition, one should also be aware that the cell lines currently in used are usually highly genetic unstable and therefore genomic abnormalities observed in this culture system could not reflect actual mechanism of resistance. The possibility of utilizing early passages tumors cells could overcome these limitations.

8. In order to characterize modes of acquired TKI resistance, it is imperative to sequence exon 18–20 of EGFR. This is particularly important because a low percentage of T790M is sufficient to confer resistance (8, 9) even when introduced in cis (10). As a result, traditional sequencing might not be sufficiently stringent enough to identify a small proportion of T790M mutant bearing EGFR genes. One such method relies on an exonuclease derived from celery (CEL I) (11). This enzyme demonstrates preference for cutting at 3′ to the mismatched nucleotides on both strands of DNA. CEL I recognizes deletions and insertion mutations irrespective of context within the DNA. This has been adapted to fully automated and commercially available sequencing such as the SURVEYOR (12). DNA should be prepared from any tissue using aseptic technique and purified highly. Polymerase chain amplification of the region of interest is then performed on heterozygote alleles followed by heat denaturation and slow reannealing generates a population of dsDNA heteroduplexes. Enzymatic digestion of the PCR product by SURVEYOR yields cleaved fragments. These fragments can be separated by HPLC column to further increase signal-to-noise prior to sequencing. This technique has been applied to EGFR mutation screens with success in the past (13) (see Subheading 3.2).

9. Resistant populations obtained either by rapid selection protocol or by progressive titration of drug usually display a high degree of heterogeneity in their morphological features. While the majority display characteristic of epithelial cells (i.e., cobble stone morphology, growth in patches) other are characterized by more mesenchymal like appearance (i.e., spindle shape). These morphological differences are usually associated with changes in their growth properties, motility, and invasive capabilities. At the molecular level the switch to a more mesenchymal phenotype (i.e., EMT) has been associated with the activation of complex network of signaling molecules and transcription factors (e.g., TGFβ, WNT, Notch, NF-KB, STAT3 signaling axis and transcriptional regulators such as Snail, Slug, ZEB1, ZEB2, TWIST, and FOXM1). Interestingly, the cell rewiring that lead to the acquisition of mesenchymal features has also been shown to lead to resistance to certain drug treatment. Decreased sensitivity to erlotinib in NSCLC derived cell lines has for example been recently associated with EMT-like properties (see Subheading 3.3).

10. The ethanol should be added drop by drop and allowed to mix completely with the supernatant before more ethanol is added.

If a high local concentration of ethanol is produced, the RNA will precipitate (see Subheading 3.3.1).

11. This step removes many residual, small to medium-sized molecules that inhibit the reverse transcription reaction in the presence of fluorescently derivatized nucleotides (see Subheading 3.3.1).
12. A ratio between 1.7 and 2 of absorbance at 260 over 280 represent good RNA (see Subheading 3.3.1).
13. The reverse transcriptase reaction is usually set up in 20 µl reaction and utilize up to 1 µg of RNA allowing the detection of all the target here described. We recommend using a mixture of random priers and oligo (dT) with a final concentration of 0.5 µg. It is important to use sterile, nuclease-free reaction tubes and to perform all the reactions on ice (see Subheading 3.3.2).
14. We usually use a volume for 50 µl reaction; however, volumes may be scaled to give the desired reaction volumes (see Subheading 3.3.3).
15. Primers are usually kept as a 100 µM stock (see Table 1).
16. Table 6 lists the primers that we successfully used to detect the expression of selective EMT markers. The following Web site provide a useful source of validated QPCR primers: http://web.ncifcrf.gov/rtp/gel/primerdb/default.asp (see Table 1)
17. Optimal cycling parameters vary with probe design and thermal cycler. We found that an initial denaturation step of greater than 2 min is unnecessary and it is actually not recommended (see Subheading 3.3.3).
18. Because the incorporation rate for Cy5-dUTP is less than that of Cy3-dUTP, more RNA is labeled in the former case to achieve equivalent signal (see Subheading 3.4.1).

Table 6
Validated primers for detecting the expression of EMT markers

Gene	Forward primer	Reverse primer
TGFB1	CAACAATTCCTGGCGATACCT	GCTAAGGCGAAAGCCCTCAAT
TGFB2	CCCCGGAGGTGATTTCCATC	CAGACAGTTTCGGAGGGGA
Ecad	CGAGAGCTACACGTTCACGG	GGCCTTTTGACTGTAATCACACC
Vim	AGAACTTTGCCGTTGAAGCTG	CCAGAGGGAGTGAATCCAGATTA
SNAIL	AATCGGAAGCCTAACTACAGCG	GTCCCAGATGAGCATTGGCA
ZEB2	GCTCCGAAGCTGGCAAGAA	GGGACTTGTCACTATGCAGGTT

19. The superscript polymerase is very sensitive to denaturation at air–liquid interfaces, so be very careful to suppress foaming in all handling of this reaction (see Subheading 3.4.1).

20. It is important to stop the reaction first with EDTA before adding NaOH, since nucleic acids precipitate in alkaline magnesium solutions (see Subheading 3.4.1).

21. The purity of the sodium hydroxide solution used in this step is crucial. Slight contamination or long storage in a glass vessel can produce a solution that will degrade the Cy5 dye molecule (see Subheading 3.4.1).

22. For maximal sensitivity, do not add ethidium bromide to the gel or running buffer (see Subheading 3.4.1).

23. Platforms: With the continue advances in microarray technologies multiple platforms are currently available both form commercial and for in-house generation. While in principle cDNA and oligos platforms can be easily generated, depending on the number of planned experiments, it can be more prudent to seek the service of an academic microarray core facility or a commercial service. The estimated cost for purchasing a clone set and/or an oligos library, robot, printing pins, and the reagents could vary significantly, but one can expect to need at least $100,000 to establish such a platform. Using commercial platforms it also eliminates the manufacturing expertise required and ensures more robust and reproducible results. In order to decide which commercial system to use one should consider the total content of the array, the availability of gene annotation, standardize protocol and reagents as well as platform performance, cost, and general acceptance. For our studies, we use an Affimetrix U95Av2 (Sata Clara,CA) that contains approximately 12,600 human genes (see Subheading 3.4.1).

24. The volume of the hybridization solution is critical. If not enough solution is used, the coverslip will bow toward the slide in the center and the hybridization will be nonuniform and likely air bubbles over some portion of the arrayed ESTs will be also introduced. On the contrary, if too much solution is added the coverslip will move too easily compromising the accuracy of the experiment (see Subheading 3.4.2).

25. The hybridization solution is added to the coverslip first, since some aggregates of fluor remain in the solution and will bind to the first surface they touch (see Subheading 3.4.2).

26. There are a wide variety of commercial hybridization chambers. It is worthwhile to prepare a mock hybridization with a blank slide, load it in the chamber, and incubate it to test for leaks, or drying of the hybridization fluid, either of which cause severe fluorescent noise on the array (see Subheading 3.4.2).

27. As there may be negative pressure in the chamber after cooling, it is necessary to remove water from around the seals so that it is not pulled into the chamber and onto the slide when the seals are loosened (see Subheading 3.4.2).

28. The sequence of washes may need to be adjusted to allow for more aggressive noise removal, depending on the source of the sample RNA. Useful variations are to add a first wash which is 0.5× SSC/0.1% SDS or to repeat the normal first wash twice (see Subheading 3.4.2).

29. If the slide is simply air dried, it frequently acquires a fluorescent haze. Centrifuging off the liquids results in a lower fluorescent background. As the rate of drying can be quite rapid, it is suggested that the slide be placed in the centrifuge immediately upon removal from the Coplin jar (see Subheading 3.4.2).

Limitations: Numerous gene expression profiling studies genes have identified statistically significant changes in expression that occur upon acquisition of resistance. Although informative, this type of analysis bears several limitations. First, because of financial constraints, usually expression profiling experiments are limited to a small number of observations (i.e., three biological replicas) reducing the statistical power of the experiment, making it impossible for the experiment and as such preventing the identification of subtle yet biologically important changes. In addition, cells in fact use many other mechanisms to regulate proteins in addition to altering the amount of mRNA, so these genes may stay consistently expressed even when protein concentrations are rising and falling.

References

1. Scaltriti, M., and Baselga, J. (2006) The epidermal growth factor receptor pathway: a model for targeted therapy. *Clin. Cancer Res.* 12, 5268–5272.
2. Lynch, T. J., Bell, D. W., Sordella, R., Gurubhagavatula, S., Okimoto, R. A., Brannigan, B. W., Harris, P. L., Haserlat, S. M., Supko, J. G., Haluska, F. G., Louis, D. N., Christiani, D. C., Settleman, J., and Haber, D. A. (2004) Activating mutations in the epidermal growth factor receptor underlying responsiveness of non-small-cell lung cancer to gefitinib. *N. Engl. J. Med.* 350, 2129–2139.
3. Choi, S. H., Mendrola, J. M., and Lemmon, M. A. (2007) EGF-independent activation of cell-surface EGF receptors harboring mutations found in gefitinib-sensitive lung cancer. *Oncogene* 26, 1567–1576.
4. Kumar, A., Petri, E. T., Halmos, B., and Boggon, T. J. (2008) Structure and clinical relevance of the epidermal growth factor receptor in human cancer. *J. Clin. Oncol.* 26, 1742–1751.
5. Shigematsu, H., and Gazdar, A. F. (2006) Somatic mutations of epidermal growth factor receptor signaling pathway in lung cancers. *Int. J. Cancer* 118, 257–262.
6. Engelman, J. A., Zejnullahu, K., Mitsudomi, T., Song, Y., Hyland, C., Park, J. O., Lindeman, N., Gale, C. M., Zhao, X., Christensen, J., Kosaka, T., Holmes, A. J., Rogers, A. M., Cappuzzo, F., Mok, T., Lee, C., Johnson, B. E., Cantley, L. C., and Janne, P. A. (2007) MET amplification leads to gefitinib resistance in lung cancer by activating ERBB3 signaling. *Science* 316, 1039–1043.
7. Jiang, N., Leach, L. J., Hu, X., Potokina, E., Jia, T., Druka, A., Waugh, R., Kearsey, M. J., and Luo, Z. W. (2008) Methods for evaluating gene expression from Affymetrix microarray datasets. *BMC Bioinformatics* 9, 284.

8. Kwak, E. L., Sordella, R., Bell, D. W., Godin-Heymann, N., Okimoto, R. A., Brannigan, B. W., Harris, P. L., Driscoll, D. R., Fidias, P., Lynch, T. J., Rabindran, S. K., McGinnis, J. P., Wissner, A., Sharma, S. V., Isselbacher, K. J., Settleman, J., and Haber, D. A. (2005) Irreversible inhibitors of the EGF receptor may circumvent acquired resistance to gefitinib. *Proc. Natl. Acad. Sci. USA* **102**, 7665–7670.

9. Pao, W., Miller, V. A., Politi, K. A., Riely, G. J., Somwar, R., Zakowski, M. F., Kris, M. G., and Varmus, H. (2005) Acquired resistance of lung adenocarcinomas to gefitinib or erlotinib is associated with a second mutation in the EGFR kinase domain. *PLoS Med.* **2**, e73.

10. Engelman, J. A., Mukohara, T., Zejnullahu, K., Lifshits, E., Borras, A. M., Gale, C. M., Naumov, G. N., Yeap, B. Y., Jarrell, E., Sun, J., Tracy, S., Zhao, X., Heymach, J. V., Johnson, B. E., Cantley, L. C., and Janne, P. A. (2006) Allelic dilution obscures detection of a biologically significant resistance mutation in EGFR-amplified lung cancer. *J. Clin. Invest.* **116**, 2695–2706.

11. Oleykowski, C. A., Bronson Mullins, C. R., Godwin, A. K., and Yeung, A. T. (1998) Mutation detection using a novel plant endonuclease. *Nucleic Acids Res.* **26**, 4597–4602.

12. Qiu, P., Shandilya, H., D'Alessio, J. M., O'Connor, K., Durocher, J., and Gerard, G. F. (2004) Mutation detection using Surveyor nuclease. *Biotechniques* **36**, 702–707.

13. Janne, P. A., Borras, A. M., Kuang, Y., Rogers, A. M., Joshi, V. A., Liyanage, H., Lindeman, N., Lee, J. C., Halmos, B., Maher, E. A., Distel, R. J., Meyerson, M., and Johnson, B. E. (2006) A rapid and sensitive enzymatic method for epidermal growth factor receptor mutation screening. *Clin. Cancer Res.* **12**, 751–758.

INDEX

A

Animal models 37, 40, 41, 42
Antibody-array 191
ATP-sepharose 120–122, 125–128, 131–133
Aurora kinase 218, 219, 224, 225

B

Binding assay 36, 71–76, 110, 111
Binding mode 5, 7–17, 23, 159

C

Cancer 1–26, 42, 56, 70, 84, 133, 149, 162,
     192, 201, 203, 207, 208, 213, 218, 219, 233–252
Capture compound mass spectrometry
     (CCMS) 135–147
Cellular imaging 84, 85
Chemical proteomics 136, 149
Chemoproteomics 161–176
Chronic myeloid leukemia (CML) 3, 5, 18–20,
     22, 56, 218
CML. *See* Chronic myeloid leukemia (CML)
Compound screening 25, 80, 113
Covalent crosslink 137, 145, 179–189
Crohn's disease 40–41

D

2D gel electrophoresis 121, 123–125, 129–131, 139
Differential scanning fluorimetry (DSF) 109–117
Discovery toxicology 83
Drug safety evaluation 86

E

Erlotinib 3, 4, 6, 14, 20, 22, 23, 112,
     203, 207, 213, 233, 234, 249

F

Fluorescence polarization 69–80

G

Gefitinib 3, 4, 6, 14, 19, 20, 22, 23, 112, 233,
     235, 237–238, 247, 248

H

Hepathocyte 22, 83–106, 136
Hepatocellular damage 92
HepG2 cells 138, 139–141
High content screening and analysis 83
High-throughput screening 65, 70, 78

I

Inhibitor selectivity 109–117, 223
In vitro kinase assay 46–47, 50
Isobaric mass tags 162, 166, 171

K

Kinase
     inhibitor 1–26, 35–42, 83–106, 109–117,
          119–133, 136, 149–159, 161–176, 180, 191–201,
          203–214, 217–230, 233
     profiling 163
     substrate 36, 42, 48, 53, 179, 180, 182, 184, 188, 225

L

Leucine-rich repeat kinase 2 (LRRK2) 45–53
Lipid kinase activity 55–66
LRRK2. *See* Leucine-rich repeat kinase 2 (LRRK2)
Lupus erythematosis 41

M

Mass spectrometry 116, 120, 121, 124–125,
     131–133, 135–147, 150, 151, 162, 218, 227
Mechanism based drug profiling 83
MEK inhibitor 24, 40,
     205, 207
Microtubulome 219
Multiplex bead-based sandwich immunoassay 191–201

N

Non-small cell lung cancer (NSCLC) 3, 5, 6, 8,
     19, 20, 234, 235, 248, 249

O

Oncogene 4, 17, 18, 233

Bernhard Kuster (ed.), *Kinase Inhibitors: Methods and Protocols*, Methods in Molecular Biology, vol. 795,
DOI 10.1007/978-1-61779-337-0, © Springer Science+Business Media, LLC 2012

P

Parkinson's disease (PD) 45–53
PBD. *See* Polo-box domain (PBD)
Pharmacodynamic biomarker 203
Phosphatidylinositol (PI) 55, 57–59, 61, 63–65
Phosphatidylinositol 3,4,5-trisphosphate 55, 59
Phosphoinositide 3-kinase (PI3K) 3, 6, 7, 11, 12, 18, 23, 36, 38, 40, 55–66, 204, 205, 207
    inhibitors 56, 62, 207
Phosphoproteome 179, 218, 219
PI3K. *See* Phosphoinositide 3-kinase (PI3K)
Polo-box domain (PBD) 69–80
Polo-like kinase 1 (PLK1) 11, 69–80
Primary cell culture 90, 105
Protein kinase CK2 .... 120, 122, 125, 132
Protein kinase inhibitors 4–7, 10–17, 20–23, 25, 26, 36, 119–133
Protein stability 79
Proteomics 86, 125, 133, 136, 149, 161

Q

Quantitative mass spectrometry 162
Quantitative proteomics 217–230

R

Receptor tyrosine kinases (RTK) 2, 18, 36, 55, 56, 58, 60, 174, 191–201
Resistance 22–23, 233–252
Reverse phase protein array 205
Rheumatoid and collagen-induced arthritis 39

S

Self assembling monolayers 149–159
Sepsis 37, 39
Small molecular weight compounds 24, 25
Staurosporine 14, 112, 135–147, 162

T

Target identification 127–128
Therapeutic response 233
Thiophene–2,3-dialdehyde 181
Tissue profiling 135
Toxicity test 89
Translational toxicology 83

U

Ulcerative colitis 40–41

```
QP              Kinase inhibitors.
606
.P76
K56
2012

                           35010000572824
$119.00
```

DATE			

BAKER & TAYLOR